THE LUNG IN RHEUMATIC
DISEASES

LUNG BIOLOGY IN HEALTH AND DISEASE

Executive Editor: **Claude Lenfant**

Director, National Heart, Lung, and Blood Institute
National Institutes of Health
Bethesda, Maryland

THE LUNG IN RHEUMATIC DISEASES

Edited by

Grant W. Cannon

Division of Rheumatology
Department of Medicine
University of Utah

VA Medical Center
Salt Lake City, Utah

Guy A. Zimmerman

Nora Eccles Harrison Cardiovascular Research
and Training Institute

Division of Respiratory Diseases
Department of Medicine
University of Utah
Salt Lake City, Utah

MARCEL DEKKER, INC.   New York • Basel

Library of Congress Cataloging-in-Publication Data

The Lung and rheumatic diseases / edited by Grant W. Cannon, Guy A.
Zimmerman.
      p.   cm. -- (Lung biology in health and disease ; v. 45)
    Includes bibliographical references.
    ISBN 0-8247-8211-9 (alk paper)
    1. Pulmonary manifestations of general diseases. 2. Rheumatism-
-Complications and sequelae. 3. Lungs--Diseases. I. Cannon, Grant
W., II. Zimmerman, Guy A. III. Series.
    [DNLM: 1. Lung--physiopathology. 2. Rheumatic Diseases-
-physiopathology. W1 LU62 v. 45 / WF 600 L9625]
RC732.L85 1990
616.7'23--dc20
DNLM/DLC
for Library of Congress   90-2909
                                          CIP

This book is printed on acid-free paper

MARCEL DEKKER, INC.
270 Madison Avenue, New York, New York 10016

Current printing (last digit):
10 9 8 7 6 5 4 3 2 1

PRINTED IN THE UNITED STATES OF AMERICA

To my parents, George I. and Isabel H. Cannon; my wife, Sandra W. Cannon; and my children, Christine, Lisa, Janae, Karen, and Suzanne

GWC

To my parents, who encouraged me

GAZ

INTRODUCTION

It is maintained that never has knowledge been so complex . . .

Harold Himsworth, 1953

Undoubtedly, the interaction between diseases and their mechanisms constitutes one of the most potent examples of the complexity of medical knowledge.

From the very inception of the series of monographs Lung Biology in Health and Disease, it was recognized that a comprehensive review of what we know about the lung should extend much beyond the organ itself. In 1616, at the dawn of our understanding of the human body, William Harvey asked the following question, "Do the lungs have any special function at all?" Much later, in 1953, Julius Comroe asked "Do the lungs have any other function?" (that is, other than respiration). Comroe's question started a long series of research pursuits which have established that the lung is far more than a bellows, that it performs complex nonrespiratory functions as well.

The lung's extraordinary complexity is exemplified by its interaction with other organs. Over the years, it has been clearly shown that the lung is an immunologic organ. As a consequence, any immune disorder may choose the lung as one of its targets and, conversely, a disruption of the lung immunologic function is likely to affect distant parts of the body. We now know that humoral and cellular factors are the links between pulmonary and other manifestations of immunologic disorders.

This volume, edited by Drs. Grant W. Cannon and Guy A. Zimmerman, discusses the interplay between lung and connective tissue disorders, with a special focus on rheumatic disease.

The editors first discuss structural and functional pulmonary alterations in the presence of rheumatic disease, and then focus attention upon specific connective tissue disorders with lung involvement. Such a topic and such an approach are new for the series Lung Biology in Health and Disease. The editors have assembled a roster of authors whose expertise in their field is well known, and there is no doubt that the product is an asset to this series of monographs. As the Executive Editor of the series, I am indebted to the editors and authors for their participation in this effort.

Claude Lenfant, M.D.

PREFACE

The rheumatic patient with lung disease presents diagnostic challenges, requires specific management skills, and poses perplexing questions on the interrelationship of these organ systems. Although musculoskeletal manifestations are the most noted clinical features of rheumatic diseases, pulmonary involvement is common.

Our understanding of pulmonary involvement in rheumatic diseases is still evolving. During the first part of this century, the coexistence of lung and musculoskeletal disorders was firmly recognized. As methods of testing pulmonary function matured, the prevalence and severity of the pulmonary processes were further defined. Presently, clinical and pathologic classifications have been developed to categorize the different types of lung disease seen with musculoskeletal disorders.

The future challenge in this arena will involve the investigation of the underlying pathologic processes through the development of new animal models and the assays of molecular biology. Inflammatory processes are certainly an important component of these disorders, but attention must also be given to understanding the immunologic pathways, alterations of host defense systems, and other mechanisms involved in these disorders.

This book is designed for the basic scientist and clinician. For the investigator, it should give a review of our present understanding of the pathophysiologic processes involved in the development of concomitant joint and lung disease. For the clinician, a description of the different clinical manifestations of these disorders and a rational approach to the rheumatic patient with lung disease are provided. As in all aspects of medicine, differences of opinion exist which serve to challenge our ingenuity in approaching patients with these problems. Presenting these contrasting approaches with the data used to reach these conclusions should help the clinician to apply these guidelines to the management of a specific patient.

This book is divided into four sections. The first section discusses our understanding of the pathophysiology of parenchymal and pleural lesions in rheumatic diseases. The second reviews our present methods of evaluation pulmonary disease in rheumatic patients. The third portion describes the pathophysiology, clinical features, and management of pulmonary complications of specific rheumatic disorders. The final section discusses multisystem diseases with concomitant lung and joint involvement.

It is our hope that this work will serve to expand our understanding of the fascinating relationships between joint and lung disease and improve our management of patients suffering from these conditions.

Grant W. Cannon

Guy A. Zimmerman

CONTENTS

CONTRIBUTORS

Irvin Broder, M.D., F.R.C.P.C. Professor, Department of Medicine, University of Toronto; Director, Gage Research Institute, Toronto Western Hospital, Toronto, Ontario, Canada

Grant W. Cannon, M.D. Assistant Professor of Medicine, Rheumatology Division, Department of Medicine, University of Utah; Associate Chief of Staff for Education, VA Medical Center, Salt Lake City, Utah

Thomas V. Colby, M.D. Department of Pathology and Laboratory Medicine, Division of Surgical Pathology, Mayo Clinic, Rochester, Minnesota

Thomas R. Cupps, M.D. Assistant Professor of Medicine, Division of Rheumatology, Immunology, Allergy, Georgetown University Medical Center, Washington, D.C.

C. Gregory Elliott, M.D. Medical Director, Respiratory Care, LDS Hospital; Associate Professor of Medicine, Pulmonary Disease Division, Department of Medicine, University of Utah, Salt Lake City, Utah

Mark R. Elstad, M.D. Assistant Professor, Respiratory Disease Division, Department of Internal Medicine, University of Utah, Salt Lake City, Utah

Duncan A. Gordon, M.D., F.A.C.P., F.R.C.P. (C) Professor of Medicine and Director, Rheumatic Disease Unit, University of Toronto; Toronto Western Hospital, Toronto, Ontario, Canada

Robert H. Hyland, M.D., F.A.C.P., F.R.C.P. (C) Associate Professor, University of Toronto; Chief, Division of Respirology, Wellesley Hospital, Toronto, Ontario, Canada

Takateru Izumi, M.D. Professor of Medicine, Chest Research Institute, Kyoto University, Kyoto, Japan

Lynell Klassen, M.D. Chief, Rheumatology/Immunology Section, University of Nebraska Medical Center, Omaha, Nebraska

Max S. Lundberg, M.D. Instructor of Medicine, Rheumatology Division, Department of Medicine, University of Utah, Salt Lake City, Utah

Joseph P. Lynch III, M.D. Associate Professor of Internal Medicine, Division of Pulmonary and Critical Care Medicine, University of Michigan Medical Center, Ann Arbor, Michigan

Steven Mathews, M.D. Jacksonville, Florida

Edward V. Reardon, D.O. Special Fellow, Department of Rheumatic and Immunologic Disease, Cleveland Clinic Foundation, Cleveland, Ohio

Stephen I. Rennard, M.D. Professor of Medicine, and Stokes-Shackelford Associate Chief, Pulmonary Section, Department of Internal Medicine, University of Nebraska Medical Center, Omaha, Nebraska

Perry J. Rush, M.D., F.R.C.P. (C) Assistant Professor of Medicine, Department of Physical Medicine and Rehabilitation, University of Toronto and Mount Sinai Hospital, Toronto, Ontario, Canada

Steven A. Sahn, M.D. Professor of Medicine, Director, Division of Pulmonary/Critical Care Medicine, Department of Medicine, Medical University of South Carolina, Charleston, South Carolina

Allen M. Segal, D.O. Head, Section of Clinical Pharmacology, Department of Rheumatic and Immunologic Disease, Cleveland Clinic Foundation, Cleveland, Ohio

Om P. Sharma, M.D. Professor of Medicine, Department of Medicine, University of Southern California, Los Angeles, California

Abraham Shore, M.D., F.R.C.P. (C) Assistant Professor of Pediatrics and Medicine, Division of Immunology and Rheumatology, Hospital for Sick Children, University of Toronto, Toronto, Ontario, Canada

Virginia D. Steen, M.D.   Associate Professor of Medicine, Division of Rheumatology and Clinical Immunology, University of Pittsburgh, Pittsburgh, Pennsylvania

Ira N. Targoff, M.D.   Assistant Professor of Medicine, University of Oklahoma Health Science Center; Arthritis and Immunology Program, Oklahoma Medical Research Foundation; Research Associate, Veterans Administration Medical Center, Oklahoma City, Oklahoma

Irena M. Tocino, M.D.   Associate Clinical Professor of Medicine, Department of Radiology, University of Utah; Department of Diagnostic Roentgenology and Nuclear Medicine, LDS Hospital, Salt Lake City, Utah

Galen B. Toews, M.D.   Associate Professor of Medicine and Chief, Division Pulmonary and Critical Care Medicine, University of Michigan Medical Center, Ann Arbor, Michigan

John R. Ward, M.D.   Professor of Medicine, Rheumatology Division, Department of Medicine, University of Utah, Salt Lake City, Utah

Guy A. Zimmerman, M.D.   Associate Professor of Medicine, Nora Eccles Harrison Cardiovascular Research and Training Institute, Department of Medicine, University of Utah, Salt Lake City, Utah

THE LUNG IN RHEUMATIC DISEASES

Part I

**PATHOGENESIS OF CONCURRENT LUNG
AND JOINT DISEASE**

1

Pathogenesis of Airway, Alveolar, and Interstitial Lesions

STEPHEN I. RENNARD and LYNELL KLASSEN

University of Nebraska Medical Center
Omaha, Nebraska

I. Introduction

The connective tissue diseases are a heterogeneous group of disorders that share many features including chronic inflammation. As a result of the inflammatory processes associated with these diseases, a variety of organs may be affected. Inflammation of the lung is frequent in these disorders, and clinically significant lung disease is widely recognized. This review will provide an overview of the pathogenetic mechanisms that can lead to impairment of lung function in the connective tissue diseases.

The function of the lung, to provide adequate gas exchange, can be conceptually divided into three parts: (a) a gas exchange surface, the alveoli; (b) a means to conduct gas between the alveoli and the environment, the airways; and (c) a means to conduct the cardiac output to the alveoli, the pulmonary vascular system (1). Connective tissue diseases can affect the alveoli, the airways, or the vascular system of the lung and can do so in varying combinations. The physiologic impact on lung function will depend on the extent and severity as well as the site of disease activity (Table 1).

3

Table 1 Physiologic Impairment of the Lung in the Connective Tissue Diseases

Site	Lung volumes	Air flow	Compliance	Diffusion capacity	Pulmonary hypertension	Dead space
Alveolitis (fibrosis)[a]	↓	Normal	↓	↓	No[b]	Normal
Bronchitis	[c]	↓	Normal	±[d]	No[b]	Normal
Vasculitis	Normal	Normal	Normal	↓	Yes	↑

[a]It is not possible, in general, to distinguish between alveolitis and fibrosis by physiology alone.
[b]Pulmonary hypertension does develop with severe loss of alveolar capillary bed in alveolitis and may develop as a secondary feature of ventilation-perfusion mismatching in bronchiolitis.
[c]Bronchiolitis may be associated with loss of lung volumes and other features of alveolitis perhaps because of associated alveolitis; air trapping may result in increased total lung capacity.
[d]Bronchiolitis may be associated with reduced diffusion capacity, perhaps due to involvement of respiratory bronchioles.

II. Pulmonary Structures Affected by Connective Tissue Diseases

A. Alveoli

Disease of the alveoli due to inflammation, i.e., fibrosis secondary to alveolitis, is the most commonly recognized parenchymal lung disorder associated with connective tissue disease (2-10). Alveolitis can lead to altered lung function by several mechanisms including the formation of edema, the accumulation of masses of inflammatory cells, and the disruption of the structure of the alveolar parenchyma (11). All these can disrupt the exchange of gas between the alveolar air space and the capillary bed. As a result, the most common physiological consequence of alveolitis is a reduced diffusion capacity (2,3,11-14). If the loss of diffusion capacity is due to edema or the accumulation of inflammatory cells, it may be reversible. If disruption of the alveolar structural framework has occurred, however, dysfunction may be permanent.

Alveolitis is often associated with the development of pulmonary fibrosis (11,15,16). This is the equivalent of "scar" formation within the alveolar structures. The normal pulmonary parenchyma becomes replaced by dense fibrous connective tissue that impedes pulmonary function in several ways. Because it cannot expand well to admit air during inspiration, fibrosis of the lung is associated with decreased pulmonary compliance.* Moreover, lung volumes in the fibrotic lung are decreased, perhaps as a result of "retraction"

---

*Compliance is defined as the increase in volume of the lung that results from an increase in inspiratory pressure. A fibrotic lung is stiff; i.e., an increase in pressure results in a lower than normal increase in volume.

of the fibrous parenchymal scar. The combination of decreased volumes, decreased diffusion capacity, and reduced compliance are the classic features of pulmonary restriction associated with inflammatory interstitial lung disease. A restrictive ventilatory defect is often the result of connective tissue disease affecting the lung.

B. Airways

Abnormalities of the airways are also frequent in the connective tissue diseases (17-23). Both small airways and glands may be affected. Loss of airway glands, as seen in Sjogren's syndrome, can lead to xerotrachea, chronic cough, difficulty with lower respiratory tract clearance, and recurrent infections (24). Disease of the airways, i.e., bronchitis, may lead to airflow obstruction and may be difficult to distinguish from airways obstruction from other causes. The smallest airways, the respiratory bronchioles, have a dual function: providing airflow to the more distal alveoli, and directly permitting gas exchange. In this latter capacity, the respiratory bronchioles resemble alveoli, and disease of these structures, bronchiolitis, can share features with alveolitis—e.g., reduction of diffusion capacity and development of restriction. The respiratory bronchioles are frequently involved in connective tissue disease syndromes (20-23,25). While inflammation of these airways may be reversible, this bronchiolitis is also associated with the development of fibrosis and permanent obliteration of the small airways.

C. Vessels

Vascular disease associated with connective tissue disease may also affect the pulmonary vascular bed (26-31). Endothelial cell damage is frequently observed in alveolar capillaries in connective tissue diseases (31), and disease of capillaries can lead to diffuse hemorrhage (30). Disease of larger vessels may lead to pulmonary hypertension (27,29). Pulmonary hypertension can also develop secondary to hypoxia, perhaps because of tissue remodeling mediated by vascular smooth muscle cells (32). Because vascular disease of the lung can lead to nonperfused but ventilated alveoli, wasted ventilation (i.e., increased "dead space") may result. Necrobiotic nodules similar to those at other tissue sites may also develop in the lung in rheumatoid arthritis (2,20,33). Isolated small nodules of this type probably do not contribute significantly to lung dysfunction. They may develop, however, in the face of massive pulmonary fibrosis. Necrobiotic nodules often must be distinguished from infections and neoplastic processes.

D. Secondary Effects Due to Drugs

Not only can connective tissue diseases have multiple effects on the lung, the drugs used to treat these systemic chronic inflammatory conditions have been associated with lung disease (34-40) (see Chap. 14). Separating the effects of drugs from the effects of the underlying connective tissue disease is often difficult. Nevertheless, it is likely that a variety of mechanisms of drug-induced disease will be involved including hypersensitivity and toxic and idiosyncratic pharmacologic reactions. Both penicillamine and gold have been implicated in the development of interstitial lung disease and bronchiolitis (35-39). A hypersensitivity mechanism has been suggested. Cytotoxic drugs such as methotrexate (34), cyclophosphamide, and azathioprine have also been associated with alveolitis (40). While hypersensitivity has been a suggested mechanism, direct toxic effects to the lung parenchyma are likely. The injury that results from these drugs is thought to lead to inflammation and subsequently to clinically recognized lung disease. Nonsteroidal, anti-inflammatory drugs, perhaps by altering the balance between leukotrienes and prostaglandins at local levels in the lung, can precipitate acute asthma (41).

Thus, the physiological consequences of connective tissue disease in the lung are complex. Several pathophysiological mechanisms can lead to lung dysfunction, and, in addition, the treatments patients receive can also adversely affect the lung. Nevertheless, while the "etiopathophysiology" of each connective tissue disease is not completely understood, certain generalizations about disease mechanisms can be made. For example, immune complex formation is a common feature of most of these disease syndromes (2, 26). Immune complexes may lead to varying forms of vasculitis or tissue inflammation, depending on the site of deposition. The alveolitis and bronchiolitis frequently lead to irreversible fibrosis and permanent lung dysfunction. While the specific disease etiologies may be quite different, it is likely that the mechanisms that affect the lung are similar in the various connective tissue diseases. The remainder of this overview will be a brief discussion of one of these mechanisms: the fibrotic process as it is thought to occur in the lung following inflammation of the alveolar structures—i.e., alveolitis.

III. Alveolitis and Pulmonary Fibrosis in Connective Tissue Diseases

The initial event in the development of parenchymal lung disease is thought to be the initiation of alveolitis, or inflammation of the lower respiratory tract (11,42-44).

A. Alveolitis

This inflammatory process can both damage the lung and initiate the complex process of repair. Fibrosis is thought to result from an incompletely effective repair process. Rather than complete restoration of lung function, which is often the case following lung injury, in fibrosis abnormal accumulations of fibroblasts and fibrous connective tissue replace the normal tissue structures. Under normal circumstances, the alveolar structures contain several types of inflammatory cells (11,42-44). Alveolar macrophages present in the alveolar space and within the alveolar interstitium are by far the most numerous. Lymphocytes are also present in a similar distribution. The cells present in the alveolar space can be sampled by bronchoalveolar lavage (43, 44). With this technique, approximately 85-90% of recovered cells are macrophages and 10-15% are lymphocytes. Of the lymphocytes, 10% are usually B cells and 70% T cells with a ratio of helper cells to suppressor cells of 1.8:1 (45). Basophils are probably present within the normal pulmonary interstitium but are not ordinarily sampled by bronchoalveolar lavage. The normal lung contains very few neutrophils or eosinophils.

Under "normal conditions," the cells present in the lung are not "activated." The alveolar macrophages, for example, do not release proinflammatory mediators. Rather, they release mediators such as PGE_2 that are thought to inhibit inflammatory responses (46,47). Lymphocytes are "resting" and do not express interleukin 2 (IL-2) production, IL-2 receptors, spontaneous replication, or other markers of lymphocyte activation (11). In contrast, alveolitis is characterized by active inflammation (48,49). Several overlapping types may occur. Thus, the various cell types normally present in the lower respiratory tract can increase in numbers and become activated (11,43,44). Eosinophilic granuloma, for example, is characterized by increased numbers and activation of alveolar macrophages. Sarcoidosis characteristically involves macrophage activation together with marked expansion and activation of T-helper cells. In hypersensitivity pneumonitis, in contrast, the T-cell population expands due to increased numbers of T-suppressor cells, and basophils are increased. Finally, cells not normally present within the lower respiratory tract can be recruited in various diseases. Neutrophils, for example, are frequently observed in cases of active idiopathic pneumonitis.

Alveolitis has been consistently observed in the connective tissue diseases. The patterns of inflammation, however, have been varied. Increased numbers and activation of macrophages, lymphocytes, and neutrophils have all been reported. It is likely that, even in a single disease such as rheumatoid arthritis, the pattern of inflammation of the pulmonary parenchyma will vary with disease activity, both among patients and in a single patient at various times. The detailed characterization of the alveolitis of these individual diseases promises to be a particularly exciting area of investigation and will be discussed in subsequent chapters. As a consequence of alveolitis, damage of the alveolar structures can occur with the development of fibrosis.

B. Alveolar Damage

Fibrosis is the replacement of normal tissue structures with fibrous connective tissue. It requires both the disruption of normal tissue and the deposition of new connective tissue, both thought to be consequences of tissue inflammation (15,16,42). Inflammatory cells are capable of damaging the normal cellular and matrix structures of the lung by releasing both reactive oxidant species (6,50,51) and potent proteolytic enzymes (11,42,52). Inflammatory cells also activate the coagulation system (53,54), which can provide an abnormal matrix on which repair is based (55). Activated inflammatory cells release a variety of mediators that can lead to the recruitment and accumulation of fibroblasts (16), a major source of connective tissue macromolecules. Finally, inflammatory cells can modulate the number and types of connective tissue macromolecules produced by fibroblasts (55-57). Taken together, inflammatory cells can both disrupt tissue architecture and activate all of the mechanisms that appear to be required to replace parenchymal structures with morphologically abnormal fibrous connective tissue.

The alveoli and small airways of the lung are delicate structures composed of a single layer of epithelium resting on a basement membrane with a small amount of subjacent connective tissue. Proper tissue function requires preservation of this delicate anatomic architecture: fusion of the alveolar and capillary basement membranes is required for gas exchange, and the continuity of the alveolar interstitial connective tissue with that of the respiratory and terminal bronchioles is required to maintain airflow in small airways (1). It is likely that the preservation of normal tissue architecture depends on the relationship between the epithelial cells and the subjacent basement membrane and connective tissue (58). The basement membrane appears to "direct" the morphologic aspects of "repair" during normal epithelial cell replacement in the adult lung. Conversely, the epithelial cells are probably the major source of basement membrane synthesis in the lung (59-62). Lung fibroblasts, however, have also been reported to produce basement membrane components (63), and it is likely that maintenance of normal lung architecture depends on complex interactions between epithelial cells and fibroblasts.

Activated inflammatory cells present in the lower respiratory tract can directly injure both epithelial cells and fibroblasts. Cells recovered from the lower respiratory tract of patients with connective tissue disease have been demonstrated to release active oxidant species (6). Moreover, both epithelial cells and fibroblasts are susceptible to oxidant-induced injury (51,64). Tissue damage in the lung due to release of oxidants is likely similar to that thought to occur at other tissue sites (50). It is likely, however, that if cellular injury were the only consequence of inflammation, the replication of epithelial cells would lead to restoration of normal tissue structures. While such repair processes are incompletely understood, it is likely that their failure to occur results, at least in part, from damage to the basement membranes and subsequent connective tissues (58).

Basement membranes are complex structures containing a major specialized collagen, type IV collagen; a major glycoprotein, laminin; a major species of proteoglycan; and other macromolecules (61). On one side, basement membranes are associated with interstitial connective tissue. In the lung, this interstitial connective tissue is composed of collagen, predominantly types I and III; elastic fibers; and proteoglycans (62). While these structural components are relatively stable, they are subject to degradation. Importantly, inflammatory cells are potent sources of proteases that have varying capacities to degrade connective tissue macromolecules, thus leading to disruption of tissue supporting structures. Neutrophils, macrophages, mast cells, and eosinophils have all been described to release proteases that can degrade connective tissue components. In combination, these proteases can degrade all components of lung connective tissue (62). Moreover, oxidation of connective tissue components may increase their subsequent degradation (65). Thus, the structural components of the lung can be disrupted as a consequence of active inflammation.

The lung is thought to be protected from proteolytic attack, in part, by soluble antiproteases. Alpha-1 antiprotease, for example, is a major inhibitor of neutrophil elastase, a broad-spectrum protease that can degrade elastin and most components of basement membrane (61,62,66). Antiproteases, however, have a limited capacity, and it is likely that within a tissue, at a site of intense local inflammation, there will be protease excess and destruction of basement membrane and other matrix components. Consistent with this, ultrastructural studies have noted disruptions of the basement membrane in inflammatory lesions leading to fibrosis (67). These observations led to Vrako's suggestion that basement membrane disruption precludes, or at least impairs, normal tissue restoration during the deposition of fibrous connective tissue (58).

Inflammatory processes not only injure normal tissue cells and matrix, they can lead to the rapid deposition of an abnormal extracellular matrix through activation of the coagulation system (53,54). During inflammation, leakage of plasma proteins, including fibrinogen, occurs. Activation of the coagulation system, by inflammatory proteases or by release of procoagulant activity from alveolar macrophages, can then lead to deposition of fibrin within alveoli and small airways. The formation of these fibrin-containing membranes is a frequent feature of inflammatory processes within the lung. Fibronectin, a serum glycoprotein that is also produced by alveolar macrophages and other cells within the lung, can bind to this fibrin and provide a matrix for fibroblasts to accumulate at abnormal tissue locations (see below) (68). Thus, the "temporary" matrix that is deposited by activation of the coagulation system following inflammation in the lung can provide a basis for the replacement of normal lung tissue with morphologically abnormal fibrous connective tissue.

C. Fibrosis

The major cell type that accumulates in fibrosis of the lung is the mesenchymal fibroblast. While fibroblasts normally comprise up to one third of pulmonary parenchymal cells, their population is significantly increased in fibrosis (69). Moreover, several "types" of fibroblasts are found within the lung, and the cells that accumulate in fibrosis may not reflect the "normal" mesenchymal cell distribution (70,71). Thus, factors that alter the accumulation of fibroblasts within the lung play a major role in the development of fibrosis. This accumulation of cells can be thought to take place in three interconnected phases: recruitment, attachment, and proliferation.

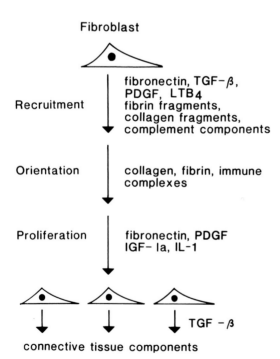

Figure 1 Potential mediators for fibroblast accumulation and connective tissue synthesis in fibrosis in the lung. Shown are the potential mediators of the various stages of fibroblast accumulation and connective tissue biosynthesis in the lung. (See text for details.) Note that the various stages of fibroblast recruitment are also subject to inhibition. This is discussed in the text.

Recruitment

Fibroblasts are capable of directed migration in response to a number of mediators (Fig. 1). These include species derived from components present in the extracellular milieu: degraded and denatured connective tissue components (72-74), fibronectin (75,76), fibrin fragments (77), and activated complement components (78), as well as several factors released from a variety of cell types, including macrophages (79-81), platelets (82), lymphocytes (83), and epithelial cells (84). These factors are not completely characterized but include leukotriene B4 (85), fibronectin (79,80), and the growth factors PDGF (81,82) and TGF-β (86). Thus, there are a number of mechanisms by which fibroblasts can be recruited to sites of inflammation in the lung. It is likely that the importance of specific factors and specific sources of factors will vary with different disease states.

While the identities and sources of chemotactic factors for fibroblasts in the lung in connective tissue disease have not been defined, observations from other interstitial lung diseases are useful. Alveolar macrophages recovered by bronchoalveolar lavage are activated in several interstitial lung diseases, including idiopathic pulmonary fibrosis, sarcoidosis, and others, to release increased amounts of fibronectin (80). The fibronectins are a group of large multifunctional proteins that possess binding sites for both cell surface receptors and components present in the extracellular milieu (87,88). They are thought to mediate a variety of interactions between the components of the extracellular space and cells. A single gene gives rise to several different forms of fibronectin through differential splicing of the mRNA (89). The liver is the major source of plasma fibronectin, which also comprises the major form present in the lung (87,88). Alveolar macrophages, however, produce a "cellular form" of fibronectin that has been reported to be a potent chemotactic stimulus for fibroblasts (79,80,90). The increased chemotactic potency of macrophage fibronectin compared to plasma fibronectin is thought to derive from the structural differences between the molecular species. Because of its increased chemotactic potency, macrophage fibronectin has been suggested to be capable of recruiting fibroblasts to sites of macrophage activation even in the presence of large amounts of plasma fibronectin.

Normal alveolar macrophages produce fibronectin, but in interstitial lung disease, the amounts produced are increased 10- to 20-fold. Total fibronectin in lung epithelial fluid estimated by studies of bronchoalveolar lavage is also increased. The majority of the fibronectin in lavage fluid, however, appears to be derived from plasma, either through leakage or through active transport (91). Nevertheless, since alveolar macrophages cluster at sites of disease activity and since the macrophage fibronectin appears to be a much more potent chemotactic factor for fibroblasts, it is likely that macrophage fibronectin is one mediator that can recruit fibroblasts on a local level within the lung. Finally, fibronectin can be cleaved by various proteases present at sites of inflammation (92,93), and the proteolytic fragments can retain biologic activity (76,94). Thus, macrophage fibronectin may be not only a direct chemotactic factor, but a substrate for other mediators of inflammation. Undoubtedly, other chemotactic factors will also have a role, and it is very likely that recruitment of fibroblasts will result from an interaction of several distinct factors.

Attachment

Once recruited to sites of inflammation, fibroblasts must attach to the extracellular matrix as a necessary requirement prior to proliferation. The attachment of fibroblasts to matrix components is a complex process mediated by a number of molecular interactions. At least two components of normal plasma, fibronectin (87,88,95) and vitronectin (95,96), are capable of mediating fibroblast attachment, as are a number of components of extracellular matrix, including collagen, with which fibroblasts can interact directly (95). The attachment of cells to matrix proteins is mediated through a family of cell surface receptors termed integrins. These are heterodimeric molecules that share a common 95,000-dalton beta subunit and have unique 150,000-180,000-dalton alpha subunits. These receptors span the cell membrane and, by virtue of being able to bind to extracellular matrix components, can both attach cells to extracellular matrix and interact with intracellular components—e.g., the cytoskeletal actin network.

While cell attachment under normal circumstances is likely a complex process involving several components, fibronectin may play a unique role in inflammatory states owing to its multifunctionality. Thus, fibronectin could lead to fibroblast attachment at abnormal tissue locations by at least three mechanisms: (a) Although it binds poorly to fibrinogen, fibronectin binds and can be cross-linked to fibrin (97). Since fibrin deposition is a frequent feature of inflammatory lesions, this interaction may serve as a nidus for fibroblast adhesion following inflammation (68). While such a mechanism may be an important aspect of wound healing, it may have serious adverse consequences in the lung. (b) Hyaline membranes, of which fibronectin and fibrin are major components (98), are deposited in alveoli in a variety of syndromes of lung injury. Fibronectin does not bind the soluble C1 components of complement, but can bind the C1q component after release of C1r and C1s which takes place after C1 binds to immune complexes. The C1rs is released in soluble form, and the C1q remains bound to the immune complex where fibronectin can subsequently bind (99). One consequence of the interaction of fibronectin with C1q may be a means to augment the phagocytic clearance of immune complexes through fibronectin opsonin function.

Alternatively, fibronectin bound to C1q is also able to mediate fibroblast cell attachment (100). In lung diseases where immune complexes are deposited within tissues, this could be an important means by which fibroblasts accumulate at abnormal tissue locations. (c) Fibronectin binds to denatured collagens more readily than to native collagen fibers (87,88). While the major tissue collagenases that degrade interstitial collagens destroy the site with which fibronectin interacts (101), this may not be the case in inflammatory conditions. Reactive oxidant species, for example, can also lead to collagen degradation and may leave an intact fibronectin binding site that could then serve as a nidus for cell attachment (65).

In connective tissue diseases, any of these three mechanisms may be important. Acute pneumonitis could lead to fibrin and fibronectin (hyaline membrane) deposition; immune complex deposition within tissues is a frequent feature of several diseases; and release of reactive oxidant species is thought to be a frequent mechanism of tissue injury. Any of these, through subsequent binding of fibronectin to components of the extracellular milieu, could lead to the attachment of fibroblasts at abnormal sites within tissues. As these cells accumulate at abnormal sites within tissues, normal tissue architectural relationships are disrupted. As the fibroblasts accumulate and produce new matrix, normal tissue morphology may be lost.

Proliferation

Once fibroblasts have been recruited and oriented at a tissue site, their subsequent replication and accumulation are regulated by the interaction of several growth factors (102-104). In general, maximal fibroblast proliferation involves the interaction of at least one member from each of two classes of growth factors. While the precise cellular mechanisms are complex competence factors, the first class can be thought of as acting early in the G1 phase of the cell cycle. These factors transiently make the cell "competent" to respond to members of the second class of growth, termed "progression factors." Examples of competence factors include PDGF and fibronectin, both of which can be produced by activated macrophages in the lung (80,81, 105). The second class of growth factors acts later in the G1 phase of the cell cycle and causes an appropriately primed cell to proceed with subsequent DNA synthesis and cell division. Examples of these progression factors include insulin and insulinlike growth factors (IGFs) (103,104). Activated alveolar macrophages produce AMDGF (alveolar macrophage-derived growth factor) (106), which is the same as IGF1a, a form of IGF-1 that differs from the plasma form because of differential splicing of the mRNA (107). Thus, alveolar macrophages are capable of producing both competence and progression factors and can therefore stimulate fibroblast proliferation.

In addition to factors that stimulate replication, fibroblast replication can be inhibited by factors present in the extracellular milieu (108-110). The prostaglandin PGE_2, for example, can inhibit fibroblast replication, including that stimulated by AMDGF and fibronectin (47). PGE_2 can be produced by a variety of lung cells including macrophages and fibroblasts. Moreover, the production of PGE_2 by fibroblasts can be markedly stimulated by a partially characterized macrophage-derived peptide that can thus inhibit fibroblast replication (109,110). Thus, fibroblast replication can be inhibited by both paracrine and autocrine mechanisms. While the role of these inhibitory factors in lung diseases is not fully known, the concentration of PGE_2 present in the epithelial lining fluid of the lower respiratory tract is sufficient to inhibit fibroblast growth under normal conditions (111). Decreases have been observed in interstitial diseases (112).

D. Evidence for Macrophage-Derived Factors

A role for macrophage-produced growth factors in human lung disease is supported by several lines of circumstantial evidence:

1. Alveolar macrophages recovered from the lower respiratory tract produce increased amounts of both fibronectin (80) and AMDGF (113).

2. In one study, patients with interstitial lung disease whose macrophages were producing increased amounts of both factors showed progressive worsening of their restrictive ventilatory defects (114). In contrast, patients whose macrophages were releasing increased amounts of neither, or only one, mediator did not deteriorate and tended to improve slightly during follow-up.

3. Studies of subjects in a family with a form of hereditary pulmonary fibrosis revealed increased production of both fibronectin and AMDGF in individuals without detectable lung abnormalities (115). Longer follow-up will be required to determine if these biochemical abnormalities will predict disease.

4. Prolonged exposure to high concentrations of oxygen causes pulmonary fibrosis. Studies in normal human volunteers indicate that brief exposure to high concentrations of oxygen, which causes no permanent pulmonary abnormalities, results in transient activation of macrophages to produce increased amounts of fibronectin and AMDGF (116).

5. Animal models of pulmonary fibrosis yield similar results. A study in monkeys given paraquat, for example, demonstrated the activation of alveolar macrophages to release fibronectin and alveolar

macrophage-derived fibroblast growth factor, preceding the development of fibrosis (117).

Taken together, these observations suggest that macrophages can be activated to release increased amounts of fibronectin and AMDGF by stimuli or circumstances that lead to progressive pulmonary fibrosis and that the prolonged release of these mediators is associated with progressive disease. This suggests a pathogenetic role for these mediators.

The role of other mediators is less clear, largely because investigations to define their roles are incomplete. Macrophages can produce an array of mediators in addition to fibronectin and AMDGF. Undoubtedly, the roles of these factors in specific diseases will be the topic of future studies.

E. Phenotypes of Fibroblasts in Pulmonary Fibrosis

The fibroblasts that accumulate in lung fibrosis differ from normal fibroblasts in several important ways. They have features that resemble smooth muscle cells and have been called "myofibroblasts" (70,71). The retraction of these cells may be in part responsible for the tissue collapse with loss of lung volume that characterizes restrictive ventilating defects (118). Fibroblasts in the lungs of patients with fibrosis also appear to produce increased amounts of collagen (119).

While it is unclear how the phenotype of lung fibroblasts changes in fibrosis, several mechanisms are possible. First, the recruitment and subsequent proliferation of fibroblasts could lead to selection of cells with a characteristic phenotype. Second, interactions of cells with extracellular matrix can have dramatic effects on differentiated cell function. While this has not been demonstrated for lung fibroblasts, it may be that fibroblast function is altered as a consequence of altered matrix composition. Third, growth factors can alter fibroblast function. For example, transforming growth factor beta (TGF-β) can interact with lung fibroblasts and lead to both increased expression of collagen and fibronectin mRNA and increased production of both macromolecules (58,120,121). Since TGF-β can be released by macrophages or platelets at sites of inflammation, fibroblast behavior could be altered by this mediator. Fourth, fibroblasts can modulate the amount of collagen released by degrading a portion inside the cell prior to secretion, and this process can be regulated by several agents that alter cellular cAMP levels (122). Thus, fibroblast function within the lung could be altered in interstitial lung diseases by any combination of (a) changes in the type and number of cells present, (b) changes in the interaction of cells with matrix, (c) changes in the genetic expression of fibroblasts induced by specific mediators, and (d) changes in the "metabolic behavior" of fibroblasts induced by specific mediators.

F. Biological Basis for Therapy

It is premature to make therapeutic recommendations based on the current understanding of the fibrotic process. Inasmuch as specific mediators appear to lead to organ dysfunction, attempts to alter the release or action of these mediators are reasonable therapeutic goals. While specific inhibitors are not available, several lines of evidence suggest that such approaches may be possible. Colchicine can block alveolar macrophage release of both fibronectin and AMDGF, a response not achieved by glucocorticoids (123). Suramin can block the action of certain growth factors (124). Inhibitors of fibroblast chemotaxis have been described (125-127). Thus, it may be possible to design clinical trials where the target of therapeutic agents will be the interference with mechanisms of fibrosis.

IV. Summary

Finally, studies of the lung in the connective tissue diseases may offer fundamental insights in at least two ways. First, it is likely that the activation of the inflammatory processes in the lung are similar to those at other sites in the body. However, because the lung is relatively accessible (by bronchoalveolar lavage), the inflammatory process within the lung can be characterized. Insights derived from such studies may well have important implications for connective tissue disease in general. Second, patients with connective tissue diseases are often treated with potent antiinflammatory drugs. By monitoring the effects of these therapies on lung inflammation, it may be possible to develop new therapeutic strategies for other chronic inflammatory lung diseases.

The connective tissue diseases can affect the lung in a number of ways. Application of currently available methods has begun to shed light on the mechanisms by which inflammation and alveolitis proceed to fibrosis. Studies of these mechanisms promise both improved understanding of the connective tissue diseases at the cellular and biochemical level and the development of novel therapeutic strategies. Moreover, similar investigational approaches may provide insight into mechanisms of injury and fibrosis at other sites and in other organ systems.

References

1. Comroe, J. H. (1974). *Physiology of Respiration*. Year Book Medical Publishers. Chicago.
2. Hunninghake, G. W., and Fauci, A. S. (1979). Pulmonary involvement in the collagen vascular diseases. *Am. Rev. Respir. Dis.* **119**:471-503.

3. Turner-Warwick, M. (1981). Interstitial pulmonary fibrosis with and without associated collagen vascular disease. *Am. Rev. Respir. Dis.* **123**:73.

4. Turner-Warwick, M. (1986). Connective tissue disorders and the lung. *Aust. N.Z. J. Med.* **16**:257-262.

5. Wallaert, B., Hatron, P. Y., Grosbois, J. M., et al. (1986). Subclinical pulmonary involvement in collagen-vascular diseases assessed by bronchoalveolar lavage. *Am. Rev. Respir. Dis.* **133**:574-579.

6. Garcia, J. G. N., James, H. L., Zinkgraf, S., Perlman, M. B., and Keogh, B. A. (1987). Lower respiratory tract abnormalities in rheumatoid interstitial lung disease. *Am. Rev. Respir. Dis.* **136**:811-817.

7. Lovell, D., Lindsley, C., and Langston, C. (1984). Lymphoid interstitial pneumonia in juvenile rheumatoid arthritis. *J. Pediatr.* **105**:947-950.

8. Schwarz, M. I., Mattas, R. A., Sahn, S. A., Standford, R. E., Marmorstein, P. L., and Scheinhorn, D. J. (1976). Interstitial lung disease in polymyositis and dermatomyositis: Analysis of six cases and review of the literature. *Medicine* **55**:89-104.

9. Salmeron, G., Greenberg, S. D., and Lidsky, M. D. (1981). Polymyositis and diffuse interstitial lung disease. *Arch. Intern. Med.* **141**:1005.

10. Wiener-Kronish, J. P., Solinger, A. M., Warnock, M. L., Chung, A., Ordonez, N., and Golden, J. A. (1981). Severe pulmonary involvement in mixed connective tissue disease. *Am. Rev. Respir. Dis.* **124**:499-503.

11. Crystal, R. G., Bitterman, P. B., Rennard, S. I., Hance, A., and Keogh, B. A. (1984). Interstitial lung disease of unknown etiology: Disorders characterized by chronic inflammation of the lower respiratory tract. *N. Engl. J. Med.* **310**:154-156, 235-244.

12. Vitali, C., Viegi, G., Tassoni, S., et al. (1986). Lung function abnormalities in different connective tissue diseases. *Clin. Rheum.* **5**:181-188.

13. Frank, S. T., Weg, J. G., Harkleroad, L. E., and Fitch, R. F. (1973). Pulmonary dysfunction and rheumatoid arthritis. *Chest* **63**:27-34.

14. Sharp, G. C., Irwin, W. S., May, C. M., et al. (1976). Association of antibodies to ribonucleoprotein and 5n antigens with mixed connective tissue disease, systemic lupus erythematosis and other rheumatic diseases. *N. Engl. J. Med.* **295**:1149-1154.

15. Keogh, B. A., and Crystal, R. G. (1982). Alveolitis: The key to the interstitial lung disorders. *Thorax* **37**:1-10.

16. Rennard, S. I., Bitterman, P. B., and Crystal, R. G. (1984). Current concepts of the pathogenesis of fibrosis: Lessons from pulmonary fibrosis. In: *Myelofibrosis and the Biology of Connective Tissue.* Edited by Berk, P. Alan R. Liss, New York, pp. 359-377.

17. Collins, R. L., Turner, R. A., Johnson, A. M., Whitley, N. O., and McLean, R. L. (1971). Obstructive pulmonary disease in rheumatoid arthritis. *Arth. Rheum.* **19**:623-628.

18. Geddes, D. M., Corrin, B., Brewerton, D. A., Davies, R. J., and Turner-Warwick, M. (1977). Progressive airway obstruction in adults and its association with rheumatoid disease. *Q. J. Med.* **46**:427-444.
19. Guttadauria, M., Ellman, H., and Kaplan, D. (1979). Progressive systemic sclerosis: Pulmonary involvement. *Clin. Rheum. Dis.* **5**:151.
20. McCann, B. G., Hart, G. J., Stokes, T. C., and Harrison, B. D. W. (1983). Obliterative bronchiolitis and upper-zone pulmonary consolidation in rheumatoid arthritis. *Thorax* **38**:73-74.
21. Lahdensuo, A., Mattila, J., and Vilppula, A. (1985). Bronchiolitis in rheumatoid arthritis. *Chest* **5**:705-708.
22. Fortoul, T. I., Cano-Valle, F., Oliva, E., and Barrios, R. (1985). Follicular bronchiolitis in association with connective tissue diseases. *Lung* **163**:305-314.
23. Hakala, M., Paakko, P., Sutinen, S., Huhti, E., Koivisto, O., and Tarkka, M. (1986). Association of bronchiolitis with connective tissue disorders. *Ann. Rheum. Dis.* **45**:656-662.
24. Constantopoulos, S. H., and Moutsopoulos, H. M. (1986). Respiratory involvement in patients with Sjogren's syndrome: Is it a problem? *Scand. J. Rheum.* **61**:146-150.
25. Yousem, S. A., Colby, T. V., and Carrington, C. B. (1985). Lung biopsy in rheumatoid arthritis. *Am. Rev. Respir. Dis.* **131**:770-777.
26. Leavitt, R. Y., and Fauci, A. S. (1986). Pulmonary vasculitis. *Am. Rev. Respir. Dis.* **134**:149-166.
27. Steckel, R. J., Bein, M. E., and Kelley, P. M. (1975). Pulmonary arterial hypertension in progressive systemic sclerosis. *A.J.R.* **124**:461.
28. Norton, W. L., and Nardo, J. M. (1970). Vascular disease in progressive systemic sclerosis (scleroderma). *Ann. Intern. Med.* **73**:317.
29. Kay, J. M., and Banik, S. (1977). Unexplained pulmonary hypertension with pulmonary arteritis in rheumatoid disease. *Br. J. Dis. Chest* **71**:53.
30. O'Brodovich, H. M., Way, R. C., Andrew, M., and Dent, P. B. (1983). Noninvasive diagnosis of pulmonary hemorrhage in rheumatoid arthritis. *Pediatrics* **72**:720-723.
31. Hammar, S. P., Winterbauer, R. H., Bockus, D., Remington, F., Sale, G. E., and Myers, J. D. (1983). Endothelial cell damage and tubuloreticular structures in interstitial lung disease associated with collagen vascular disease and viral pneumonia. *Am. Rev. Respir. Dis.* **127**:77-84.
32. Meacham, R. P., Whitehouse, L. A., Wrenn, D. S., et al. (1987). Smooth muscle mediated connective tissue remodeling in pulmonary hypertension. *Science* **237**:423-426.
33. Nusslein, H. G., Rodl, W., Giedel, J., Missmahl, M., and Kalden, J. R. (1987). Multiple peripheral pulmonary nodules preceding rheumatoid arthritis. *Rheumatology* **7**:89-91.

34. Miller, D. R., Letendre, P. W., DeJong, D. J., and Fiechtner, J. J. (1986). Methotrexate in rheumatoid arthritis: An update. *Pharmacotherapy* **6**:170-178.
35. Manthorpe, R., Horvob, S., Sylvest, J., and Vinterberg, H. (1986). Auranofin versus penicillamine in rheumatoid arthritis. *Scand. J. Rheum.* **15**:13-22.
36. Heyd, J., and Simmeran, A. (1983). Gold-induced lung disease. *Postgrad. Med. J.* **59**:368-370.
37. Cooke, N. T., and Bamji, A. N. (1983). Gold and pulmonary function in rheumatoid arthritis. *Br. J. Rheum.* **22**:18-21.
38. Morley, T. F., Komansky, H. J., Adelizzi, R. A., and Giudice, J. C. (1984). Pulmonary gold toxicity. *Eur. J. Respir. Dis.* **65**:627-632.
39. Shettar, S. P., Chattopadhyay, C., Wolstenholme, R. J., and Swinson, D. R. (1984). Diffuse alveolitis on a small dose of penicillamine. *Br. J. Rheum.* **23**:220-224.
40. Csuka, M., Carrera, G. F., and McCarty, D. J. (1986). Treatment of intractable rheumatoid arthritis with combined cyclophosphamide, azathioprine and hydroxychloroquine. *J.A.M.A.* **255**:2315-2319.
41. Samter, M., and Beers, R. F. (1968). Intolerance to aspirin. Clinical studies and consideration of its pathogenesis. *Ann. Intern. Med.* **68**: 975.
42. Crystal, R. G., Fulmer, J. D., Roberts, W. C., Moss, M. L., Line, B. R., and Reynolds, H. Y. (1976). Idiopathic pulmonary fibrosis: Clinical, histologic, radiographic, physiologic, scintigraphic, cytologic and biochemical aspects. *Ann. Intern. Med.* **85**:769-788.
43. Reynolds, H. Y. (1987). Bronchoalveolar lavage. *Am. Rev. Respir. Dis.* **135**:250-263.
44. Linder, J., and Rennard, S. I. (1988). *Bronchoalveolar Lavage.* American Society of Clinical Pathology Press, Chicago.
45. Hunninghake, G. W., Fulmer, J. D., Young, R. C. Jr., Gadek, J. E., and Crystal, R. G. (1979). Localization of the immune response in sarcoidosis. *Am. Rev. Respir. Dis.* **120**:49-57.
46. Morely, J., Bray, M. A., Jones, R. W., Nngtason, D. H., and Van Dorp, P. A. (1979). Prostaglandin and thromboxane production by human and guinea pig macrophages and leukocytes. *Prostaglandins* **17**:719-746.
47. Bitterman, P. B., Wewers, M. D., Rennard, S. I., Adelberg, S., and Crystal, R. G. (1986). Modulation of alveolar macrophage-driven fibroblast proliferation by alternative macrophage mediators. *J. Clin. Invest.* **77**:700-708.
48. Hunninghake, G. W., Bedell, G. N., Zavala, D. C., Monick, M., and Brady, M. (1983). Role of interleukin-2 release by T-cells in active sarcoidosis. *Am. Rev. Respir. Dis.* **128**:634-638.

49. Pinkston, P., Bitterman, P. B., and Crystal, R. G. (1983). Spontaneous release of IL-2 by lung T-lymphocytes in active sarcoidosis. *N. Engl. J. Med.* **308**:793-800.
50. Halliwell, B. (1987). Oxidants and human disease: Some new concepts. *FASEB J.* **1**:358-364.
51. Martin, W. J. II, Gadek, J. E., Hunninghake, G. W., and Crystal, R. G. (1981). Oxidant injury of lung parenchymal cells. *J. Clin. Invest.* **68**: 1277-1288.
52. Weiland, J. E., Garcia, J. G. N., Davis, W. B., and Gadek, J. E. (1987). Neutrophil collagenase in rheumatoid interstitial lung disease. *J. Appl. Physiol.* **62**:628-633.
53. Chapman, H. A. Jr., Allen, C. L., Stone, O. L., and Fair, D. S. (1985). Human alveolar macrophages synthesize factor VII in vitro. Possible role in interstitial lung disease. *J. Clin. Invest.* **75**:2030-2037.
54. Chapman, H. A. Jr., Bertozzi, P., and Reilly, J. J. Jr. (1988). Role of enzymes mediating thrombosis and thrombolysis in lung disease. *Chest* **93**:1256-1263.
55. Rennard, S. I., Stier, L. C., and Crystal, R. G. (1982). Intracellular degradation of newly synthesized collagen. *J. Invest. Dermatol.* **79**:77S-82S.
56. Varga, J., Rosenbloom, J., and Jimenez, S. A. (1987). Transforming growth factor β (TGF β) causes a persistent increase in steady-state amounts of type I and type III collagen and fibronectin mRNAs in normal human dermal fibroblasts. *Biochem. J.* **247**:597-604.
57. Rosenbloom, J., Feldman, G., Freundlich, B., and Jimenez, S. A. (1984). Transcriptional control of human diploid fibroblast collagen synthesis by α-interferon. *Biochem. Biophys. Res. Commun.* **123**:365-372.
58. Vrako, R. (1972). Significance of basal lamina for regeneration of injured lung. *Virchows Arch.* (*Pathol. Anat.*) **355**:264-274.
59. Stoner, G. D., Katoh, Y., Foidant, J. M., Trump, B. F., Steinert, P. M., and Harris, C. C. (1981). Cultured human bronchial epithelial cells: Blood group antigens, keratin, collagens and fibronectin. *In Vitro* **17**: 577-587.
60. Sage, H., Farin, F. M., Striker, G. E., and Fisher, A. B. (1983). Granular pneumocytes in primary culture secrete several major components of the extracellular matrix. *Biochemistry* **22**:2148-2155.
61. Martin, G. R., and Timpl, R. (1987). Laminin and other basement membrane components. *Ann. Rev. Cell. Biol.* **3**:57-85.
62. Rennard, S. I., Ferrans, V. J., Bradley, K. H., and Crystal, R. G. (1982). Lung connective tissue. In: *Mechanisms in Respiratory Toxicology*, Vol. 2. CRC Press, Boca Raton, FL, pp. 115-153.
63. Kuhl, U., Ocalan, M., Timpl, R., Mayne, R., Hay, E., and Von der Mark, K. (1984). Role of interstitial fibroblasts in the deposition of type IV collagen in the basal lamina of myotubes. *Differentiation* **28**:164-172.

64. Skillrud, D. M., and Martin, W. J. II. (1984). Paraquat-induced injury of type II alveolar cells. An in vitro model of oxidant injury. *Am. Rev. Respir. Dis.* **129**:995-999.
65. Curran, S. F., Amoruso, M. A., Goldstein, B. D., and Berg, R. A. (1984). Degradation of soluble collagen by ozone or hydroxyl radicals. *FEBS Lett.* **176**:155-160.
66. Gadek, J. E., and Crystal, R. G. (1983). 1-Antitrypsin deficiency. In: *Metabolic Basis of Inherited Disease.* Edited by Stanbury, J. B., et al. McGraw-Hill, New York, pp. 1450-1467.
67. Campbell, E. J., Senior, R. M., and Welgus, H. G. (1987). Extracellular matrix injury during lung inflammation. *Chest* **92**:161-167.
68. Grinnell, F., Feld, M., and Minter, D. (1980). Fibroblast adhesion to fibrinogen and fibrin substrata: Requirement for cold insoluble globulin. *Cell* **19**:517-525.
69. Crapo, J. D. (1986). Morphologic changes in pulmonary oxygen toxicity. *Ann. Rev. Physiol.* **48**:721-731.
70. Crystal, R. G., Bradley, K. H., Baum, B. J., Fulmer, J. D., Bernardo, J., Bruel, S. D., Elson, N. A., Fells, G. A., Ferrans, V. J., Gadek, J. E., Hunninghake, G. W., Kawanomi, O., Kelman, J. H., Line, B. R., McDonald, J. A., McLees, B. D., Roberts, W. C., Rosenberg, D. M., Tolstoshev, P., Von Gal, E., and Weinberger, S. E. (1978). Cells, collagen and idiopathic pulmonary fibrosis. *Lung* **155**:199-224.
71. Woodcock-Mitchell, J., Adler, K. B., and Low, R. B. (1984). Immunohistochemical identification of cell types in normal and in bleomycin-induced fibrotic rat lung. Cellular origins of interstitial cells. *Am. Rev. Respir. Dis.* **130**:910-916.
72. Postlethwaite, A. E., Seyer, J. M., and Kang, A. H. (1978). Chemotactic attraction of human fibroblasts to type I, II and III collagen and collagen-derived peptides. *Proc. Natl. Acad. Sci. USA* **75**:871-875.
73. Albini, A., and Adelmann-Grill, B. C. (1985). Collagenolytic cleavage products of collagen type I as chemoattractants for human dermal fibroblasts. *Eur. J. Cell Biol.* **36**:104-107.
74. Senior, R. M., Griffin, G. L., and Mechan, R. P. (1982). Chemotactic response of fibroblasts to tropoelastin and elastin-derived peptides. *J. Clin. Invest.* **70**:614-618.
75. Gauss-Muller, E., Kleinman, H. K., Martin, G. R., and Schiffmann, E. (1980). Role of attachment factors and attractants in fibroblast chemotaxis. *J. Lab. Clin. Med.* **96**:1071-1080.
76. Postlethwaite, A. E., Kesky-Oja, J., Balian, G., and Kang, A. H. (1980). Induction of fibroblast chemotaxis by fibronectin: Localization of the chemotactic region to a 140,000 molecular weight non-gelatin binding fragment. *J. Exp. Med.* **153**:494-499.

77. Senior, R. M., Skogen, W. F., Griffin, G. L., and Wilner, G. D. (1986). Effects of fibrinogen derivatives upon the inflammatory response. *J. Clin. Invest.* **77**:1014-1019.
78. Postlethwaite, A. E., Snyderman, R., and Kang, A. H. (1979). Generation of a fibroblast chemotactic factor in serum by activation of complement. *J. Clin. Invest.* **64**:1379-1385.
79. Tsukamoto, Y., Helsel, W. E., and Wahl, S. M. (1981). Macrophage production of fibronectin, a chemoattractant for fibroblasts. *J. Immunol.* **127**:673-678.
80. Rennard, S. I., Hunninghake, G. W., Bitterman, P. B., and Crystal, R. G. (1981). Production of fibronectin by the human alveolar macrophage: A mechanism for the recruitment of fibroblasts to sites of tissue injury in interstitial lung disease. *Proc. Natl. Acad. Sci. USA* **78**:7147-7151.
81. Martinet, Y., Rom, W. N., Grotendorst, G. R., Martin, G. R., and Crystal, R. G. (1987). Exaggerated spontaneous release of platelet-derived growth factor by alveolar macrophages from patients with idiopathic pulmonary fibrosis. *N. Engl. J. Med.* **317**:202-209.
82. Seppa, H., Grotendorst, G., Seppa, S., Schiffmann, E., and Martin, G. R. (1982). The platelet-derived growth factor is chemotactic for fibroblasts. *J. Cell Biol.* **92**:584-588.
83. Postlethwaite, A. E., Snyderman, R., and Kang, A. H. (1976). The chemotactic migration of human fibroblasts to a lymphocyte-derived factor. *J. Exp. Med.* **144**:1188-1203.
84. Shoji, S., Ertl, R. F., Rickard, K. A., and Rennard, S. I. (1987). Bronchial epithelial cells produce chemotactic activity for lung fibroblasts. *ATS* (submitted).
85. Mensing, H., and Czarnetzki, B. M. (1984). Leukotriene B₄ induces in vitro fibroblast chemotaxis. *J. Invest. Dermatol.* **82**:9-12.
86. Postlethwaite, A. E., Keski-Oju, J., Moses, H. L., and Kang, A. H. (1987). Stimulation of the chemotactic migration of human fibroblasts by transforming growth factor. *J. Exp. Med.* **165**:251-256.
87. Hynes, R. O. (1985-86). Fibronectins: A family of complete and versatile adhesive glycoproteins derived from a single gene. *Harvey Lect.* **81**:133-152.
88. Ruoshlahti, E., Engrall, E., and Hayman, E. G. (1981). Fibronectin. *Collagen Rel. Res.* **1**:95-128.
89. Paul, J. I., Schwarzbaner, J. E., Tamkun, J. W., and Hynes, R. O. (1986). Cell-type-specific fibronectin subunits generated by alternative splicing. *J. Biol. Chem.* **261**:12258-12265.
90. Alitalo, K., Hori, T., and Vaheri, A. (1980). Fibronectin is produced by human macrophages. *J. Exp. Med.* **151**:607-613.

91. Peters, J. H., Ginsberg, M. H., Bohl, B. P., Sklar, L. A., and Cochrane, C. G. (1986). Intravascular release of intact cellular fibronectin during oxidant-induced injury of the in vitro perfused rabbit lung. *J. Clin. Invest.* **78**:1596-1603.

92. McDonald, J. A., and Kelly, D. G. (1980). Degradation of fibronectin by human leukocyte elastase. Release of biologically active fragments. *J. Biol. Chem.* **255**:8848-8858.

93. Senior, R. M., and Campbell, E. J. (1983). Neutral proteinases from human inflammatory cells. A critical review of their role in extracellular matrix degradation. *Clin. Lab. Med.* **3**:345-366.

94. Seppa, H. E. J., Yamada, K. M., Seppa, S. T., Silver, M. H., Kleinman, H. K., and Schiffmann, E. (1981). The cell binding fragment of fibronectin is chemotactic for fibroblasts. *Cell. Biol. Int. Rep.* **5**:813-819.

95. Rouslahti, E., Hayman, E. G., and Pierschbacher, M. D. (1985). Extracellular matrices and cell adhesion. *Arteriosclerosis* **5**:581-594.

96. Barnes, D. W., and Silnutzer, J. (1983). Isolation of human serum spreading factor. *J. Biol. Chem.* **258**:12548-12552.

97. Mosher, D. F. (1975). Crosslinking of cold-insoluble globulin by fibrin stabilizing factor. *J. Biol. Chem.* **250**:6614-6621.

98. Fukuda, Y., Ferrans, V. J., Schoenberger, C. I., Rennard, S. I., and Crystal, R. G. (1985). Patterns of pulmonary structural remodeling after experimental paraquat toxicity. *Am. J. Pathol.* **118**:452-475.

99. Menzel, E. J., Smolen, J. L., Liotta, L., and Reid, K. B. (1981). Interaction of fibronectin with C1q and its collagen-like fragment. *FEBS Lett.* **129**:188.

100. Rennard, S. I., Chen, Y. F., Robbins, R. A., Gadek, J. E., and Crystal, R. G. (1983). Fibronectin mediates cell attachment to C1q: A mechanism for the localization of fibrosis in inflammatory disease. *Clin. Exp. Immunol.* **97**:1925-1932.

101. Kleinman, H. K., McGoodwin, E. B., Martin, G. R., Klebe, R. J., Fletzek, P. P., and Woolley, D. E. (1978). Localization of the binding site for cell attachment in the alpha-1-(1) chain of collagen. *J. Biol. Chem.* **253**:5642-5646.

102. Goldstein, R. H., and Fine, A. (1986). Fibrotic reactions in the lung: The activation of the lung fibroblast. *Exp. Lung Res.* **11**:245-261.

103. Ross, R. (1986). The biology of platelet derived growth factor. *Cell* **46**:155-169.

104. Harrington, M. A., and Pledger, W. J. (1987). Characterization of growth factor modulated events regulating cellular proliferation. *Methods Enzymol.* **147**:400-407.

105. Bitterman, P. B., Rennard, S. I., Adelberg, S., and Crystal, R. G. (1983). Role of fibronectin as a growth factor for fibroblasts. *J. Cell Biol.* **97**:1925-1932.

106. Bitterman, P. B., Rennard, S. I., Hunninghake, G. W., and Crystal, R. G. (1982). Human alveolar macrophage growth factor for fibroblasts: Regulation and partial characterization. *J. Clin. Invest.* **70**:806-822.
107. Rom, W. N., Nukima, T., and Crystal, R. G. (1988). Alveolar macrophages express the IGF-Ia gene and spontaneously release exaggerated amounts of IGF-1 in interstitial lung disease. *Clin. Res.* **36**:624A.
108. Duncan, M. R., and Berman, B. (1985). α-Interferon is the lymphokine and β-interferon the monokine responsible for inhibition of fibroblast collagen production and late but not early fibroblast proliferation. *J. Exp. Med.* **162**:516-527.
109. Clark, J. G., Kostal, K. M., and Marino, B. A. (1983). Bleomycin induced pulmonary fibrosis in hamsters. *J. Clin. Invest.* **72**:2082-2091.
110. Elias, J. A., Rossman, M. D., Zurier, R. B., and Daniele, R. P. (1985). Human alveolar macrophage inhibition of fibroblast growth. A prostaglandin dependent process. *Am. Rev. Respir. Dis.* **131**:94-99.
111. Ozaki, T., Rennard, S. I., and Crystal, R. G. (1987). Cyclooxygenase metabolites are compartmentalized in the human lower respiratory tract. *J. Appl. Physiol.* **62**:219-222.
112. Ozaki, T., Rennard, S. I., and Crystal, R. G. (1983). Arachindonic acid cyclooxygenase metabolites in lung epithelial lining fluid. *Clin. Res.* **31**:165A.
113. Bitterman, P. B., Adelberg, S., and Crystal, R. G. (1983). Mechanisms of pulmonary fibrosis. Spontaneous release of the alveolar macrophage-derived growth factor in the interstitial lung disorders. *J. Clin. Invest.* **72**:1801-1813.
114. Bitterman, P. B., Rennard, S. I., Keogh, B., Adelberg, S., and Crystal, R. G. (1983). Chronic alveolar macrophage release of fibronectin and alveolar macrophage derived growth factor correlates with functional deterioration in fibrotic lung diseases. *Clin. Res.* **31**:414A.
115. Bitterman, P. B., Rennard, S. I., Keogh, B. A., et al. (1986). Familial pulmonary fibrosis: Evidence of lung inflammation in unaffected family members. *N. Engl. J. Med.* **314**:1343-1347.
116. Davis, W. B., Rennard, S. I., Bitterman, P. B., and Crystal, R. G. (1983). Pulmonary oxygen toxicity: Early reversible biologic changes in human alveolar structures induced by hyperoxia. *N. Engl. J. Med.* **309**:879-883.
117. Schoenberger, C. I., Rennard, S. I., Bitterman, P. B., Fukuda, Y. F., Ferrans, V. J., and Crystal, R. G. (1984). Paraquat induced pulmonary fibrosis: Role of the alveolitis in modulating the development of fibrosis. *Am. Rev. Respir. Dis.* **1129**:168-173.
118. Evans, J. N., Kelley, J., Low, R. B., and Adler, K. B. (1982). Increased contractility of isolated lung parenchyma in an animal model of pulmonary fibrosis induced by bleomycin. *Am. Rev. Respir. Dis.* **125**:89-94.

119. McDonald, J. A., Broekelman, T. J., Matheke, M. L., Crouch, E., Koo, M., and Kuhn, C. (1986). A monoclonal antibody to the carboxy terminal domain of procollagen type I visualizes collagen synthesizing fibroblasts. Detection of an altered fibroblast phenotype in lungs of patients with pulmonary fibrosis. *J. Clin. Invest.* **78**:1237-1244.

120. Ignotz, R. A., and Massagae, J. (1986). Transforming growth factor-beta stimulates the expression of fibronectin and collagen and their incorporation into the extracellular matrix. *J. Biol. Chem.* **261**:4337-4345.

121. Fine, A., and Goldstein, R. H. (1987). The effect of transforming growth factor-beta on cell proliferation and collagen formation by lung fibroblasts. *J. Biol. Chem.* **262**:3897-3902.

122. Rennard, S. I., Stier, L. C., and Crystal, R. G. (1982). Intracellular degradation of newly synthesized collagen. *J. Invest. Dermatol.* **79**: 77S-82S.

123. Rennard, S. I., Bitterman, P. B., Ozaki, T., Rom, W. N., and Crystal, R. G. (1988). Colchicine suppresses the release of fibroblast growth factors from alveolar macrophages in vitro: The basis of a possible therapeutic approach to the fibrotic disorders. *Am. Rev. Respir. Dis.* **137**:181-185.

124. Betsholtz, C., Johnsson, A., Heldin, C. H., and Westermark, B. (1986). Efficient reversion of simian sarcoma virus-transformation and inhibition of growth factor induced mitogenesis of suramin. *Proc. Natl. Acad. Sci. USA* **83**:6440-6444.

125. Ochs, M. E., Postlethwaite, A. E., and Kang, A. H. (1987). Identification of a protein in sera of normal humans that inhibits fibroblast chemotactic and random migration in vitro. *J. Invest. Dermatol.* **88**:183-190.

126. Adelmann-Grill, B. C., Hein, R., Wach, F., and Krieg, T. (1987). Inhibition of fibroblast chemotaxis by recombinant human interferon gamma and interferon alpha. *J. Cell. Physiol.* **130**:270-275.

127. Peoschl, A., Rehn, D., Dumant, J. M., Mueller, P. K., and Hennings, G. (1987). Malotilate reduces collagen synthesis and cell migration activity of fibroblasts in vitro. *Biopharm. Drug Dispos.* **22**:3957-3963.

2

Pathogenesis of Pleural Effusions and Pleural Lesions

STEVEN A. SAHN

Medical University of South Carolina
Charleston, South Carolina

I. Introduction

At postmortem examination, thoracotomy, and thoracoscopy, pleural lesions are frequently observed in the collagen vascular diseases. However, pleural thickening or pleural effusions are uncommon and rarely problematic clinically, except in systemic lupus erythematosus and rheumatoid arthritis. It is logical that these systemic diseases can affect the pleura, as the lung is commonly involved and pleural pathology is often a reflection of underlying pulmonary disease. With a localized subpleural inflammatory process, such as pneumonia or pulmonary infarction, or with diffuse lung injury as in the adult respiratory distress syndrome, pleural effusions are a common accompaniment as extravascular fluid moves along a pressure gradient from the interstitium to the pleural space across the relatively permeable mesothelium. Inflammatory injury to the pleural or subpleural tissues causes effusions in other diseases as well, including rheumatic syndromes. Thus, pleural effusions in collagen vascular diseases result from increased

Table 1 Pleural Lesions in the Collagen Vascular Diseases

Disease	Incidence	Probable pathogenesis	Pleural lesion	Pleural fluid	Clinical course
Rheumatoid arthritis	Hx of pleurisy (20%) effusions (5%) postmortem (38-73%)	Local immune pleuritis Trapped lung Cholesterol effusion	Effusions Fibrosis Trapped lung	Small-moderate unilateral; serous, turbid, yellow-green, milky, necrotic; protein > 3.5; PMN or mono predominant; pH 7.00, glucose 30, LDH > 1,000; complement low, IC present, RF $\geq$ 1:320	Variable; effusion resolves over months; some require decortication
Systemic lupus erythematosus	Effusion or pleuritic pain (50-75%) Postmortem acute fibrinous pleuritis (40%) fibrosis (30%)	Local immune pleuritis	Effusion Fibrosis	Small-moderate bilateral; serous, turbid, or bloody; PMN or mono predominant; pH and glucose low (20%), LE cells diagnostic, complement low, IC present, ANA $\geq$ 1:160 or PF/S $\geq$ 1.0 suggestive	Dramatic response to corticosteroids; minimal sequelae
Mixed connective tissue disease	Pleuritic pain (40%) Effusion (0-6%)	Unknown	Effusion Fibrosis	Small unilateral or bilateral serous; normal glucose; normal complement	No clinical importance
Sjögren's syndrome	Effusion <1% in primary SS	Lymphocytic infiltration of pleura; local immune pleuritis	Effusion	Analysis not reported	No clinical importance
Polymyositis/ dermatomyositis	Only in association with ILD Postmortem effusion rare fibrosis rare	Lymphocytic or plasma cell infiltration of pleura	Pleuritis Fibrosis	Small volume noted at postmortem; analysis not reported	No clinical importance

Disease	Features	Pathogenesis	Pleural manifestation	Fluid analysis	Clinical importance
Wegener's granulomatosis	Chest pain (20-56%) Effusion (5-55%)	Subpleural vascular lesions; hemorrhagic infarcts	Effusion Fibrosis	Small unilateral; analysis not reported	No clinical importance; effusion resolves simultaneously or with R_x of vasculitis
Progressive systemic sclerosis	Postmortem pleural adhesions (67%) pleural fibrosis (86%) effusion rare	Direct pleural involvement by systemic disease; infectious complication	Adhesions Fibrosis	Analysis not reported	No clinical importance
Ankylosing spondylitis	Effusion (rare) Fibrosis (common) Pneumothorax (8%)	Subpleural infection; noninfectious inflammation; *Aspergillus* colonization; rupture of subpleural bulla	Effusion Pleural fibrosis Pneumothorax	Small-moderate effusion; serous exudate; normal glucose	No clinical importance
Churg-Strauss syndrome	Effusion (29%)	Eosinophilic and other inflammatory cell infiltration of pleura; pulmonary infarction	Pleural vasculitis Effusion Fibrosis	Serous, bloody; exudate high % eosinophils	Response to corticosteroids
Behçet's disease	Effusion (<5%)	SVC obstruction thoracic duct rupture	Effusion	Transudate; chylothorax	As with chylothorax

Abbreviations: IC, immune complexes; ILD, interstitial lung disease.

capillary permeability from immune and nonimmune inflammation, either subpleurally or directly involving the pleura. The severity and persistence of the injury will determine whether resolution or pleural fibrosis results.

Increased capillary permeability is the cardinal feature of pleural involvement in the collagen vascular diseases. The capillary leak may be due to pleural infiltrative processes that may occur with Sjögren's syndrome, polymyositis/dermatomyositis, and progressive systemic sclerosis; however, these diseases are rarely accompanied by pleural effusions. Immune mechanisms appear to be a more important cause of pleural lesions and are responsible for pleural disease seen in the rheumatoid arthritis, systemic lupus erythematosus, Churg-Strauss syndrome, and possibly Sjögren's syndrome. Circulating immune complexes have been demonstrated in both blood and pleural fluid in patients with both rheumatoid arthritis and systemic lupus erythematosus (1). Circulating immune complexes can localize either subpleurally or in pleural capillaries per se. This can result in the generation of activated complement components (C3a and C5a) that can lead to increased vascular permeability, allowing proteinaceous fluid to escape into the lung interstitium or directly into the pleural space. Immune complexes and complement precursors can accumulate in the pleural space as they are locally generated, or arrive indirectly from the leaky vascular bed and potentiate the pleural injury, possibly by their interaction. This concept is supported by the finding of immune complexes and reduced levels of complement components in pleural fluid in both lupus and rheumatoid arthritis (1,2).

The release of polymorphonuclear (PMN) leukocyte chemotaxins, including activated complement components, and the activation of phagocytic cells may further potentiate the pleural injury by the release of oxygen radicals and lysosomal enzymes. Even though many long-standing rheumatoid and lupus effusions have a predominance of mononuclear leukocytes, for several days following the acute injury the polymorphonuclear leukocyte is the predominant cell. The mechanisms responsible for the transition from pleural fluid neutrophilia to lymphocytosis has not been clearly elucidated and may be due to release of lymphocyte chemotaxins (3), removal of immune complexes and activated complement components, or inhibitory factors for neutrophil chemotaxis. Once the T lymphocyte enters the pleural space, it is capable of releasing lymphokines that may contribute to the inflammatory process (4,5). Furthermore, extracellular release of proteolytic enzymes from neutrophils and macrophages not only affects capillary permeability but also may modulate fibroblast migration and growth and collagen metabolism and determine the extent and degree of pleural injury (see Chap. 1).

In the remainder of this chapter I will address the pathologic findings in the pleural space, the current concepts of pathogenesis of pleural lesions and pleural fluid, and the salient clinical features of pleural involvement in the collagen vascular diseases. Table 1 summarizes the characteristic features and probable pathogenesis of pleural effusions in these conditions.

II. Rheumatoid Pleurisy

Involvement of the pleura is probably the most common thoracic manifestation of rheumatoid arthritis. Approximately 20% of patients with rheumatoid arthritis will relate a history of pleurisy (6), but in only 5% of patients will pleural effusions be documented (6,7). Rheumatoid pleural effusions are more commonly found in males with rheumatoid nodules who have had articular disease for several years; it is unusual for patients less than 35 years of age to present with rheumatoid pleurisy (6-8).

Over a century ago, several reports considered pleurisy and empyema complications of rheumatoid arthritis (9,10); however, it was not generally accepted that these common entities were specific for rheumatoid arthritis. In 1943, Baggenstoss and Rosenberg (11) reported that 22 of 30 patients with rheumatoid arthritis had evidence of pleurisy at postmortem examination. Fingerman and Andrus (12) found evidence of severe fibrous pleurisy in 23 of 61 patients. The clinical-pathologic discrepancy suggests that many patients have inconsequential symptoms, or minimal symptoms masked by anti-inflammatory drugs.

Patients with a rheumatoid pleural effusion may present with symptoms mimicking an acute bacterial pneumonia; chronic, intermittent chest discomfort; or a finding on a routine chest film (6,13). The typical radiograph shows a small to moderate unilateral pleural effusion, although effusions may be bilateral and large in volume (6, 13). Other manifestations of rheumatoid lung disease such as necrobiotic nodules or interstitial disease may be concomitant in approximately 30% of patients (6).

Pleural fluid analysis will usually support the diagnosis of rheumatoid pleurisy. The fluid may be serous, turbid, yellow-green, or milky. It may appear to contain necrotic or caseous material (13,14); it also may be described as having a sheen (15). The effusion generally has a total protein concentration of greater than 3.5 g/dl and may be dominated by either PMN or mononuclear leukocytes depending on the acuteness of the inflammatory process in relation to thoracentesis (6,16). The characteristic biochemical features include a pH of approximately 7.00, a glucose less than 30 mg/dl, and a lactate dehydrogenase (LDH) level greater than 1,000 U/L (13,17,18). Total hemolytic complement and complement components have been reported to be low, and immune complexes have been found to be increased in rheumatoid pleural fluid (1,2). The rheumatoid factor in the fluid is usually greater than or equal to 1:320 and greater than the concomitant serum value (2).

In some chronic rheumatoid effusions, usually present for several years the pleura becomes thickened and calcific, and fluid persists because the lung is "trapped," resulting in increased negative intrapleural pressure. This fluid is likely to contain cholesterol crystals, which can be identified under polarized light and impart a sheen to the fluid when visualized at the bedside under proper lighting (15,19). However, if the cholesterol is present in the esterified form, crystals will not be seen, and the characteristic sheen is absent. Coe and Aikawa (20) reported that cholesterol exited from the pleural space at a slow rate, suggesting that the increased cholesterol in the pleural space originated from cell destruction; however, Newcombe and Cohen (21), in studies with labeled acetate, suggested that local biosynthesis contributed to cholesterol accumulation.

Nosanchuk and Naylor (14) have described unique cytologic findings in patients with rheumatoid pleural effusions that suggested a mechanism for pleural fluid formation. The characteristic findings were a background of granular material; large, elongated cells; and giant, round, or oval multi-nucleated cells. These authors postulated that the characteristic histopatho-logic lesion of rheumatoid arthritis, the rheumatoid nodule, can occur not only subcutaneously but in a multitude of organs. The palisade of cells in the rheumatoid lesion may occur as distinct pleural nodules or in a linear pattern over the entire pleural surface (see Chap. 6). The isolated nodules may leak slowly or rupture their necrotic contents into the pleural space; with diffuse pleural involvement, inflammatory cells may desquamate into preexistent pleural fluid. This may result in both viable and degenerative cells in the pleural fluid; the cells and granules found in pleural fluid closely resemble the components of the rheumatoid nodule. Aru and colleagues (22) have commented on the absence of mesothelial cells during thoracoscopic biopsies in patients with rheumatoid pleurisy. Thus, the final barrier to in-terstitial fluid leak into the pleural space may not exist owing to the rheuma-toid inflammatory process in the pleura.

Halla and associates (23) demonstrated that pleura and pleural fluid mononuclear cells from patients with rheumatoid pleuritis synthesized IgM and IgM rheumatoid factor; this was not observed with peripheral blood monocytes. Their findings support the local production of IgM and IgM rheumatoid factor in patients with rheumatoid pleuritis and suggest that these events contribute to the pathogenesis of rheumatoid effusions.

A low pleural fluid glucose, with a pleural fluid to serum (PF/S) ratio (< 0.5) and low pleural fluid pH (< 7.30) are found concomitantly in 80% of rheumatoid pleural effusions (8,24,25). These biochemical findings are characteristic of chronic rheumatoid effusions, while those with normal glucose and pH (15-20%) tend to be found with acute rheumatoid pleurisy (18). Thickening of the pleural membrane and metabolic activity of cells in the pleura and pleural fluid appear to be the most important factors in the development of low-pH and low-glucose effusions, as in vitro incubation of rheumatoid pleural fluid results in minimal utilization of glucose, genera-tion of CO_2 and lactate, and fall in pH (26). The thickened and inflamed pleura is thought to inhibit glucose movement from blood to pleural space; furthermore, the glucose that does enter is utilized at a normal or slightly increased rate by either pleural fluid cells or inflamed pleural tissue with the production of its end products, CO_2 and lactic acid. Because of the abnormally thick membrane, these end products cannot escape from the pleural space at a normal rate and accumulate until a new steady state is reached, resulting in a glucose of less than 30 mg/dl and pH about 7.00 (24,25).

III. Lupus Pleuritis

Postmortem studies had found that approximately two thirds of patients with systemic lupus erythematosus (SLE) have evidence of pleural involvement, in the form of adhesions, thickening, or effusions (27,28). Approximately 50% of patients with SLE will report pleuritic chest pain at some time during the course of their illness, and about a third will have chest radiographic evidence of pleural effusions (29). Pleuritis may be the presenting manifestation of SLE in approximately 5% of cases (30).

Patients with lupus pleuritis and pleural effusions universally have pleuritic pain and commonly associated dyspnea, cough, and fever (31). In contrast to patients with rheumatoid pleurisy, patients with lupus pleural effusions almost always have pleural symptoms at the time the effusion is discovered (31). Pleural effusions in SLE are most commonly bilateral and small to moderate in volume, but may be unilateral and massive (31-33). Alveolar infiltrates, atelectasis, and a large cardiac silhouette are common accompaniments on the chest radiograph (31).

Pleural effusions in SLE are exudates with protein concentrations generally greater than 3.5 g/dl and LDH concentrations rarely exceeding 500 U/L (31). Cell counts vary from a few hundred up to 15,000 cells/μl, and the differential counts vary from PMN to mononuclear predominant depending on the timing of thoracentesis and the acuteness of the pleural injury (31). Most commonly, the pleural fluid pH is greater than 7.30 and the glucose is greater than 60 mg/dl; however, effusions with low glucose and/or low pH have been reported with both native and drug-induced lupus (31). The finding of LE cells in pleural fluid appears diagnostic. A pleural fluid antinuclear antibody (ANA) titer greater than or equal to 1:160, or a pleural fluid/serum ANA ratio of greater than or equal to 1, is supportive of the diagnosis (31,34,35).

Kelley and colleagues (36) have noted atypical cells in pleural effusions from patients with SLE. These cells, when studied by light, electron, and fluorescent microscopy, resemble plasma cells and appear to be derived from the inflammatory pleural infiltrate. The atypical cells are generally intermixed

with other inflammatory cells, fibrinoid debris, red cells, and scarce mesothelial cells. The origin of these cells appears to be from mesenchyme, and
supports the concept that the cells are exfoliated into the pleural fluid at the
time of active inflammation (see also Chap. 6).

Low total hemolytic complement, C1q binding, C3, and C4 have been
found in patients with lupus pleural effusions (37). A diffusion block to
movement of complement components into the pleural space is an unlikely
explanation for the low concentrations, as high concentrations of protein
are generally found. It is likely that increased complement utilization in
pleural fluid may be triggered by anticomplementary factors. The high incidence and levels of pleural fluid immune complexes in rheumatoid pleurisy
have not been found in lupus pleuritis; furthermore, the levels of immune
complexes in pleural fluid from patients with SLE have not been found to
be different from levels in serum, in contrast to rheumatoid pleurisy, where
the pleural fluid/serum ratio is increased (1). Thus, the mechanisms responsible for the generation of pleural fluid immune complexes appear to be different in rheumatoid and lupus pleuritis lupus.

Riska and colleagues (38) demonstrated high antibody levels to double-
stranded DNA in pleural fluid from five patients with lupus pleuritis, four
with lung cancer, and one with tuberculous pleurisy; normal values were
found in the other 43 fluids (38). Following incubation with DNase, the DNA
antibody level rose only in patients with lupus pleuritis, and not in the others
with high DNA antibody levels. Since all five patients with lupus pleuritis
had serum values of double-stranded DNA that correlated with pleural fluid
values, the data suggest that pleural fluid DNA-anti-DNA complexes may
be involved in the pathogenesis of lupus pleuritis and pleural effusion. Wysenbeek et al. (39) reported a single case of a patient with pleural effusion and
SLE and moderately high pleural fluid levels of double-stranded DNA, which
were undetectable in the serum.

A specific immunofluorescent pattern characterized by nuclear staining of pleural lining cells with either anti-IgM, anti-IgG, or anti-C3 has been
reported in patients with both native and drug-induced lupus pleuritis (40,
41).

Patients with lupus pleuritis or rheumatoid pleurisy appear to develop
both pleuritis and pleural effusions due to localized immune responses, though
presumably through different mechanisms. Clinically, effusions in SLE patients also differ from effusions in rheumatoid arthritis patients. Pleuritis in
SLE patients tends to be symptomatic, to cause larger pleural effusions, not
to develop clinically important pleural fibrosis, and to respond dramatically
to corticosteroids. In contrast, patients with rheumatoid pleurisy have less
symptomatic pleuritis, smaller pleural effusions, a tendency toward clinically significant fibrosis, and no obvious response to corticosteroid.

IV. Mixed Connective Tissue Disease

Mixed connective tissue disease (MCTD) is a syndrome characterized by clinical features of scleroderma, SLE, polymyositis/dermatomyositis (PM/DM), and rheumatoid arthritis associated with high titer of antibody to ribonucleoprotein (RNPN). Pulmonary involvement in MCTD is common but may be clinically silent. In a study of 34 patients with MCTD, Sullivan and colleagues (42) found that 12 (35%) had evidence of pleuritis and 13 (40%) had pleuritic chest pain during the course of their disease; pleuritic pain was second only to dyspnea as the most common clinical symptom. However, on chest radiograph no pleural effusions were documented, and only one patient had pleural thickening.

Two of the five patients reported by Wiener-Kronish et al. (43) with severe pulmonary involvement in MCTD had pleuritic chest pain, and one of the two had a pleural friction rub. However, the authors did not report pleural effusion on chest radiograph and did not comment on the pleural space at autopsy.

In a review of 81 patients at the Mayo Clinic with MCTD, Prakash and associates (44) found that chest pain was the second most common symptom and was present in six (7%) patients; in one patient chest pain was pleuritic. Small pleural effusions were detected on chest radiograph in five (6%) patients. The effusion was unilateral in three and bilateral in two. Thoracentesis in one patient showed straw-colored fluid with a total protein concentration of 3.8 g/dl, a glucose of 80 mg/dl, and normal total hemolytic complement. Two (2%) patients had pleural thickening.

Hoogsteden et al. (45) reported a young woman with MCTD who presented with bilateral pleural effusions; the effusions were exudative with a total protein of 4.2 g/dl and an LDH concentration of 411 U/L. The cells were predominantly granulocytes, with only 5% mononuclear cells. No B lymphocytes and only 1% T lymphocytes were found. The pleural effusions resolved without corticosteroid therapy.

The pathogenesis of pleural lesions in MCTD has not been elucidated. The relative frequency of pleuritic pain and apparent low incidence of pleural effusions suggest pathogenetic mechanisms similar to those in rheumatoid pleurisy, as opposed to lupus pleuritis.

V. Sjögren's Syndrome

Sjögren's syndrome, the consequence of lymphocyte-mediated injury to exocrine glands, is characterized by keratoconjunctivitis sicca and xerostomia and is frequently associated with a collagen vascular disease, most commonly rheumatoid arthritis.

In a review of 343 patients with Sjögren's syndrome seen at the Mayo Clinic over a 7-year period, 31 (9%) had pulmonary involvement; three patients had pleuritic chest pain, one with associated SLE; and five additional patients had pleural effusions on chest radiograph (two bilateral, three unilateral) three of them having associated autoimmune diseases, either SLE or rheumatoid arthritis (46).

A more recent study did not find evidence of pleurisy in 40 patients with primary Sjögren's syndrome (no associated rheumatic disease), while only 2 of 26 (7.7%) patients with secondary Sjögren's syndrome had evidence of pleurisy (47).

Presumably, pleural involvement in Sjögren's syndrome is due to either lymphocytic infiltration of the pleura or immune complex deposition in the subpleural or pleural tissue, as suggested by the presence of cryoglobulins and low serum complement levels in patients with Sjögren's syndrome and interstitial lung disease.

VI. Polymyositis/Dermatomyositis

Pulmonary disease in PM/DM can result from interstitial pneumonitis, aspiration pneumonia, and diaphragmatic failure. Pleural disease in PM/DM has not been reported as an isolated finding but only in association with severe interstitial lung disease (48). Small amounts of pleural fluid have been noted at postmortem examination in patients dying with interstitial lung disease. Examination of the lungs of these patients has shown both pleural inflammation and fibrosis (49-51), a common finding in patients with idiopathic interstitial pneumonitis. However, clinically apparent or important pleural disease has not been reported in patients with PM/DM. In a single patient with PM and a pleural effusion, the effusion was most likely parapneumonic in etiology (52). Two children with DM have been reported with spontaneous pneumothoraces (53); in one patient pleural fibrosis was noted at surgery.

With the frequency of aspiration pneumonia and respiratory muscle weakness leading to atelectasis, it is difficult to be certain about the etiology of the pleural disease in PM/DM; however, lymphocytic and plasma cell infiltration of the pleura or subpleural connective tissue may be responsible for the small pleural effusions noted.

VII. Wegener's Granulomatosis

The lungs are universally involved in Wegener's granulomatosis. Radiologically, the lesions are solitary or multiple nodular densities or infiltrates that are variable in size, are often bilateral and transient, and have a tendency to cavitate (54) (see also Chap. 4). The pleura has received little attention, either clinically or pathologically, in this disease. Godman and Churg (55), however, commented that "when close to the pleura [referring to the pulmonary parenchymal lesions], they often induced deposition of fibrin on the surface." These authors also noted hemorrhagic infarcts with vessels occluded with thrombi, which may be one explanation for the pleural effusions in Wegener's granulomatosis.

Clinically, patients with Wegener's granulomatosis can present with pleurisy or nonpleuritic chest pain. Ten percent of the 56 patients reported by Walton (56) (10 personal and 46 from the literature) had chest pain as a presenting symptom. Twenty percent (2 of 10) of Walton's patients and 20% (9 of 46) of the cases in the literature had chest pain at some time during the course of their disease (56). Fauci and Wolff (57) reported that 56% (10 of 18) of patients experienced chest pain, whereas 38% (6 of 16) of Carrington and Liebow's (58) cases had pleurisy.

Pleural effusions have been reported in 5-55% of cases. In a series reported by Flye and colleagues (59), 4 of 47 (9%) patients had pleural effusions, and an additional 4 patients (9%) had pleural thickening only on chest radiograph; thus, 8 of 47 (17%) patients had evidence of pleural involvement. Pleural effusions have not been noted in the absence of parenchymal lesions, are small in size, and are usually unilateral (60).

To my knowledge, the characteristics of pleural fluid in Wegener's granulomatosis have not been reported. Presumably, the fluid is an inflammatory exudate without distinguishing features, except for the tendency to be hemorrhagic. Based on the observation that these lesions may occur close to the pleura, it is likely that the effusions are due to either subpleural necrotizing vascular lesions or hemorrhagic infarcts. As with pleural effusions from pulmonary embolism, the effusions in Wegener's granulomatosis are not large and generally resolve rapidly.

These speculations relating to the pathogenesis of the effusions are compatible with the clinical spectrum of pleural disease in Wegener's granulomatosis. With respect to clinical management, pleural effusion and thickening have not been major clinical problems, and the effusions have resolved spontaneously or with therapy directed at the vasculitis. Not only rheumatoid pleurisy, but also pleural involvement in Wegener's granulomatosis, should be considered in the differential diagnosis of bilateral nodular lesions and pleural effusions.

VIII. Progressive Systemic Sclerosis (PSS)

Interstitial fibrosis is found at autopsy in almost all cases of PSS (61), usually is evident radiographically (62), and may have important clinical implications.

In contrast, clinical pleural disease is uncommon, although pleural abnormalities are frequently found at postmortem examination. However, the direct relationship between PSS and pleural disease is uncertain.

In an autopsy series of 28 patients with PSS, pleural adhesions were found in two thirds (63). The adhesions frequently involved the complete surface of both lungs but were most likely to be found at the bases and apices. Pleural effusion and pulmonary edema occurred on occasion. Subpleural fibrotic nodules and cystic changes were frequently present.

Pleural thickening was demonstrated histologically in 24 of the 28 cases; it was moderate in 5 and focal or minimal in the remaining 19 cases. Pleural thickening predominated in the upper lobes in 7 cases, was greatest in the lower lobes in 4 cases, and had no predilection in the remaining 13 cases. Subpleural cystic involvement was a common finding and may be the etiology for some of the pneumothoraces that develop in PSS (64). Increased pleural vascularity, a finding infrequently reported in other diseases in the literature, was also noted.

With the predilection for aspiration and anaerobic pleuropulmonary infection, it is difficult to be certain whether the pleural disease is secondary to complications of PSS or there is direct pleural involvement by the primary pathologic process. It is surprising that with the degree of cystic changes that occur subpleurally, an extremely low incidence of secondary spontaneous pneumothorax is reported. Possibly, many of these patients have partial or complete pleural symphysis, due to either infectious complications of the disease or a primary pleural process.

IX. Ankylosing Spondylitis

The incidence of pleuropulmonary disease in cases of ankylosing spondylitis reported in the literature varies from nonexistent to up to 30%. Rosenow and colleagues (65) reviewed the records of 2,080 patients with ankylosing spondylitis and found 28 (1.3%) with pleuropulmonary manifestations that they thought were typical of those associated with the disease. In none of the 28 cases did pleuropulmonary disease precede the diagnosis of ankylosing spondylitis. Twenty-six of the 28 patients had upper lobe fibrobullous disease. There were three patients with pleural effusions, one with diffuse pleural thickening, and one with a spontaneous pneumothorax. All patients with fibrobullous disease had apical pleural thickening, and five with complicated aspergillomas had extensive localized pleural thickening. Nonapical pleural thickening occurred in two patients and was extensive in one, leading to respiratory failure.

Three of the patients reported by Rosenow et al. (65) had small to moderate pleural effusions of a few weeks' duration. One patient had bilateral effusions, and two had the effusion localized to the left hemithorax. In two of the three patients, pleuritic chest pain was reported. In one patient the fluid was recurrent after a 9-month interval. The effusions were characterized as exudates with negative cytology and a pleural fluid glucose similar to blood glucose. Pleural biopsy in two of the patients revealed pleural thickening and minimal inflammation. Kinnear and Shneerson (66) reported a patient with ankylosing spondylitis and quiescent joint disease who developed bilateral pleural effusions. The fluid was a straw-colored exudate with a protein concentration of 3.5 g/dl, PMNs, negative gram and AFB stains, and negative routine and AFB culture. No other cause for the effusion was documented, and it resolved in 1 month on steroid therapy. Dudley-Hart et al. (67) reported that 2 of 65 patients with ankylosing spondylitis had a history of pleurisy, and 1 had a pleural effusion; however, no details of the pleurisy or the effusion were provided. Zorab (68) reported that 1 of 53 patients with ankylosing spondylitis had a pleural effusion; no details were provided.

With the small number of cases of pleural effusions associated with ankylosing spondylitis and the frequency of effusions in the general population, it is unclear whether pleural effusion is an extraskeletal manifestation of ankylosing spondylitis. If it is, it has rarely been a clinical problem. Furthermore, the pathogenesis of pleural effusions in ankylosing spondylitis is also uncertain but may be related to underlying subpleural infectious or noninfectious inflammation.

The pleural thickening found almost universally in patients with fibrobullous disease may be related to the chronic inflammatory process or to *Aspergillus* colonization or microinvasion. It has been documented that progressive pleural thickening is an early radiographic clue to the presence of aspergilloma (69).

Spontaneous pneumothorax has been reported in 8 of 100 patients in the literature, suggesting an increased incidence (65). The subpleural bullous lesions would be a predisposing factor to the development of pneumothorax.

X. Churg-Strauss Syndrome

Churg-Strauss syndrome is characterized by hypereosinophilia and systemic vasculitis in association with asthma. Pulmonary infiltrates are a cardinal feature and occur in about 75% of patients, often predating the onset of systemic vasculitis (70). The pulmonary infiltrates are frequently transient, have no predilection for a particular area of the lung, and tend not to be lobar or segmental.

Pleural effusions have been noted in 18 of 61 (29%) patients reported in the literature (70-72). Some patients have presented with pleuritic chest pain or a pleural rub without manifesting pleural involvement radiographically (73).

The effusions have been described as serous or bloody, have been sterile, and have consistently had high percentages of eosinophils, in some cases with all the pleural fluid cells being eosinophils (71). Postmortem studies have revealed eosinophilic infiltration of the pleura with subpleural and pleural vasculitis characterized by vessel wall encroachment with eosinophils, neutrophils, lymphocytes, and plasma cells (71). Vascular involvement has ranged from eosinophilic perivascular cuffing to a panmural necrotizing arteritis. Fibrosed lesions have been noted as well as substantial pleural thickening and evidence of adhesive pleuritis. In some patients, pulmonary infarctions have been a prominent finding.

Pleural effusions in Churg-Strauss syndrome presumably result from eosinophilic and other inflammatory cell infiltration of the pleura with vasculitis, leading to increased capillary permeability of pleural or subpleural microvessels and movement of the interstitial fluid into the pleural space due to the interstitial-pleural pressure gradient. Major basic protein, constituting the core of the eosinophil granule, or other eosinophilic constituents may be responsible for the capillary leak (74). The progression of eosinophils from the lung to the pleural space may occur because of increased vascular permeability; however, a pleural space eosinophilic chemotactic factor has not been excluded. Pulmonary infarction secondary to the vasculitis may be an explanation for the hemorrhagic effusions that have been described. Pleural effusions have not been reported in the absence of parenchymal lesions.

XI. Behçet's Disease

Caval thrombosis appears to be an integral manifestation of Behçet's disease (oral and genital ulceration and ocular inflammation) and may be responsible for the pleural effusions that have been observed. Five of 32 patients seen by Hannun and Frayha (75) had superior vena cava (SVC) syndrome associated with Behçet's disease. Only one of the five patients had a pleural effusion; this was reported to be a pseudochylothorax, but the data suggest that it was a true chylothorax. Others have reported that none of four (76) and two of five (77) patients with SVC obstruction had an associated pleural effusion. In the latter series, one patient developed bilateral transudative pleural effusions, while the other had a moderate right pleural effusion without pleural fluid analysis. Thrombosis of the jugulosubclavian confluence, or the SVC syndrome, has been associated with chylothorax whether the obstruction is secondary to embolism, inflammation, or malignancy. Chylothorax due to Behçet's disease with SVC obstruction could result from interference with lymph flow and chylous reflux (78). The bilateral transudative effusions demonstrated in a single case may have been related to acute systemic venous hypertension (77).

References

1. Halla, J. T., Schrohenloher, R. E., and Volanakis, J. E. (1980). Immune complexes and other laboratory features of pleural effusions. *Ann. Intern. Med.* **92**:748-752.
2. Hunder, G. C., McDuffie, F. C., Hutson, K. A., Elveback, L. R., and Hepper, N. G. (1977). Pleural fluid complement, complement conversion, and immune complexes in immunologic and non-immunologic diseases. *J. Lab. Clin. Med.* **90**:971-980.
3. Dauber, J. H., and Daniele, R. P. (1980). Secretion of chemotaxins by guinea pig lung macrophages. I. The spectrum of inflammatory cell responses. *Exp. Lung Res.* **1**:23-32.
4. Koster, F. T., McGregor, D. D., and MacKaness, G. B. (1971). The mediator of cellular immunity. II. Migration of immunologically committed lymphocytes into inflammatory exudates. *J. Exp. Med.* **133**:400-409.
5. Asherson, G. L., and Allwood, G. G. (1972). Inflammatory lymphoid cells. Cells in immunized lymph nodes that move to sites of inflammation. *Immunology* **22**:493-502.
6. Walker, W. C., and Wright, V. (1968). Pulmonary lesions and rheumatoid arthritis. *Medicine* **47**:501-519.
7. Horler, A. R., and Thompson, M. (1959). The pleural and pulmonary complications of rheumatoid arthritis. *Ann. Intern. Med.* **51**:1179-1203.
8. Lillington, G. A., Carr, D. T., and Mayne, J. G. (1971). Rheumatoid pleurisy with effusion. *Arch. Intern. Med.* **128**:764-768.
9. Fuller, H. W. (1860). *On Rheumatism, Rheumatic Gout and Sciatica, Their Pathology, Symptoms and Treatment*, 3d ed. John Churchill, London.
10. Charcot, J. M. (1881). *Clinical Lectures on Senile and Chronic Diseases*, Vol. XCV. New Sydenham Society, London.
11. Baggenstoss, A. H., and Rosenberg, E. F. (1943). Visceral lesions associated with chronic infectious (rheumatoid) arthritis. *Arch. Pathol.* **35**:503-516.
12. Fingerman, D. L., and Andrus, F. C. (1943). Visceral lesions associated with rheumatoid arthritis. *Ann. Rheum. Dis.* **3**:168-181.
13. Carr, D. T., and Mayne, J. G. (1962). Pleurisy with effusion in rheumatoid arthritis, with reference to the low concentration of glucose in pleural fluid. *Am. Rev. Respir. Dis.* **85**:345-350.
14. Nosanchuk, J. S., and Naylor, B. (1968). A unique cytologic picture in pleural fluid from patients with rheumatoid arthritis. *Am. J. Clin. Pathol.* **50**:330-335.
15. Bower, G. C. (1968). Chyliform pleural effusion in rheumatoid arthritis. *Am. Rev. Respir. Dis.* **97**:455-459.

16. Pettersson, T., Klockars, M., and Hellstrom, P.-E. (1982). Chemical and immunologic features of pleural effusions: Comparison between rheumatoid arthritis and other diseases. *Thorax* **37**:354-361.
17. Berger, H. W., and Seckler, S. G. (1966). Pleural and pericardial effusions in rheumatoid disease. *Ann. Intern. Med.* **64**:1291-1297.
18. Sahn, S. A., Kaplan, R. L., Maulitz, R. M., and Good, J. T. Jr. (1980). Rheumatoid pleurisy: Observations on the development of low pleural fluid pH and glucose. *Arch. Intern. Med.* **140**:1237-1238.
19. Ferguson, G. C. (1966). Cholesterol pleural effusion in rheumatoid lung disease. *Thorax* **21**:577-582.
20. Coe, J., and Aikawa, J. K. (1961). Cholesterol pleural effusion. *Arch. Intern. Med.* **108**:763-774.
21. Newcombe, D. S., and Cohen, A. S. (1965). Chylous synovial effusion in rheumatoid arthritis: Chemical and pathogenetic significance. *Am. J. Med.* **38**:156-164.
22. Aru, A., Engel, U., and Francis, D. (1986). Characteristic and specific histological findings in rheumatoid pleurisy. *Acta Pathol. Microbiol. Immunol. Scand.* **94**:57-62.
23. Halla, J. T., Koopman, W. J., Schrohenloher, R. E., Darby, W. L., and Heck, L. W. (1983). Local synthesis of IgM and IgM rheumatoid factor in rheumatoid pleuritis. *J. Rheumatol.* **10**:204-209.
24. Sahn, S. A. (1985). Pathogenesis and clinical features of diseases associated with a low pleural fluid glucose. In *The Pleura in Health and Disease.* Edited by Chretien, J., et al. Marcel Dekker, New York, pp. 267-285.
25. Sahn, S. A. (1985). Pleural fluid pH in the normal state and in diseases affecting the pleural space. In *The Pleura in Health and Disease.* Edited by Chretien, J., et al. Marcel Dekker, New York, pp. 253-266.
26. Taryle, D. A., Good, J. T. Jr., and Sahn, S. A. (1979). Acid generation by pleural fluid: Possible role in determination of pleural fluid pH. *J. Lab. Clin. Med.* **93**:1041-1046.
27. Purnell, D. C., Baggenstoss, A. H., and Olsen, A. M. (1955). Pulmonary lesions in disseminated lupus erythematosus. *Ann. Intern. Med.* **42**:619-628.
28. Ropes, M. W. (1976). Characteristics, manifestations, and pathologic findings. In *Systemic Lupus Erythematosus.* Harvard University Press, Cambridge, MA, p. 54.
29. Rothfield, N. F. (1981). Clinical features of systemic lupus erythematosus. In *Textbook of Rheumatology.* Edited by Kelly, W. N., et al. Saunders, Philadelphia, p. 1124.
30. Winslow, W. A., Ploss, L. N., and Loitman, J. B. (1958). Pleuritis in systemic lupus erythematosus: Its importance as an early manifestation in diagnosis. *Ann. Intern. Med.* **49**:70-88.

31. Good, J. T. Jr., King, T. E., Antony, V. B., and Sahn, S. A. (1983). Lupus pleuritis. Clinical features and pleural fluid characteristics with special reference to pleural fluid antinuclear antibodies. *Chest* **84**:714-718.
32. Bulgrin, J. G., Dubois, E. L., and Jacobson, G. (1960). Chest roentgenographic changes in systemic lupus erythematosus. *Radiology* **74**: 42-49.
33. Taylor, T. L., and Ostrum, H. (1959). The roentgenographic evaluation of systemic lupus erythematosus. *A.J.R.* **82**:95-107.
34. Carel, R. S., Shapiro, M. S., Shoham, D., and Gutman, A. (1977). Lupus erythematosus cells in pleural fluid. *Chest* **72**:670-672.
35. Reda, M. G., and Baigelman, W. (1980). Pleural effusion in systemic lupus erythematosus. *Acta Cytol.* **24**:553-557.
36. Kelley, S., McGarry, P., and Hutson, Y. (1971). Atypical cells in pleural fluid characteristic of systemic lupus erythematosus. *Acta Cytol.* **15**: 357-362.
37. Hunder, G. G., McDuffie, F. C., and Hepper, N. G. G. (1972). Pleural fluid complement in systemic lupus erythematosus and rheumatoid arthritis. *Ann. Intern. Med.* **76**:357-363.
38. Riska, H., Fyhrquist, F., Selander, R.-K., and Hellstrom, P.-E. (1978). Systemic lupus erythematosus and DNA antibodies in pleural effusions. *Scand. J. Rheumatol.* **7**:159-160.
39. Wysenbeek, A. J., Pick, A. I., Sella, A., Beigel, Y., and Yeshurun, D. (1980). Eosinophilic pleural effusion with high anti-DNA activity as a manifestation of systemic lupus erythematosus. *Postgrad. Med.* **56**:57-58.
40. Chandrasekhar, A. J., Robinson, J., and Barr, L. (1978). Antibody deposition in the pleura: A finding in drug-induced lupus. *J. Allergy Clin. Immunol.* **61**:399-402.
41. Pertschuk, L. P., Moccia, L. F., Rosen, Y., Lyons, H., Marino, C. M., Rashforo, A. A., and Wollschlager, C. M. (1977). Acute pulmonary complication in systemic lupus erythematosus. Immunofluorescence and light microscopic study. *Am. J. Clin. Pathol.* **68**:553-557.
42. Sullivan, W. D., Hurst, D. J., Harmon, C. E., Esther, J. H., Agia, A. G., Maltby, J. D., Lillard, S. B., Held, C. N., Wolfe, J. F., Sunderrajan, E. V., Maricq, H. R., and Sharp, G. C. (1984). A prospective evaluation emphasizing pulmonary involvement in patients with mixed connective tissue disease. *Medicine* **63**:92-107.
43. Wiener-Kronish, J. P., Solinger, A. M., Warnock, M. L., Churg, A., Ordonez, N., and Golden, J. A. (1981). Severe pulmonary involvement in mixed connective tissue disease. *Am. Rev. Respir. Dis.* **124**:499-503.
44. Prakash, U. B. S., Luthra, H. S., and Divertie, M. B. (1985). Intrathoracic manifestations in mixed connective tissue disease. *Mayo Clin. Proc.* **60**:813-821.

45. Hoogsteden, H. C., van Dongen, J. J. M., Van der Kwast, T. H., Hooij-kaas, H., and Hilvering, C. (1985). Bilateral exudative pleuritis. An unusual pulmonary onset of mixed connective tissue disease. *Respiration* **48**:164-167.
46. Strimlan, C. V., Rosenow, E. C., Divertie, M. B., and Harrison, E. G. (1976). Pulmonary manifestations of Sjogren's syndrome. *Chest* **70**:354-361.
47. Constantopoulos, S. H., and Moutsopoulous, H. M. (1986). Respiratory involvement in patients with Sjogren's syndrome: Is it a problem? *Scand. J. Rheumatol.* (Suppl.) **61**:146-150.
48. Dickey, B. F., and Myers, A. R. (1984). Pulmonary disease in polymyositis/dermatomyositis. *Semin. Arthritis Rheum.* **14**:60-76.
49. Schwarz, M. I., Matthay, R. A., Sahn, S. A., Stanford, R. E., Marmorstein, B. L., and Scheinhorn, D. J. (1976). Interstitial lung disease in polymyositis and dermatomyositis: Analysis of six cases and review of the literature. *Medicine* **55**:89-104.
50. Goldfischer, J., and Rubin, E. H. (1959). Dermatomyositis with pulmonary lesions. *Ann. Intern. Med.* **50**:194-206.
51. Salmeron, G., Greenberg, S. D., and Lidsky, M. D. (1981). Polymyositis and diffuse interstitial lung disease: A review of the pulmonary histopathologic findings. *Arch. Intern. Med.* **141**:1005-1010.
52. Roach, D. G., and Salter, W. M. (1980). Polymyositis with pulmonary infiltrate and pleural effusion. *Minn. Med.* **63**:277-281.
53. Singsen, D. H., Tedford, J. C., Platzker, A. C. G., and Hanson, V. (1978). Spontaneous pneumothorax: A complication of juvenile dermatomyositis. *J. Pediatr.* **92**:771-774.
54. Felson, B. (1959). Less familiar Roentgen patterns of pulmonary granulomas. *Am. J. Roentgenol. Radium Ther. Nucl. Med.* **81**:211-223.
55. Godman, G. C., and Churg, J. (1954). Wegener's granulomatosis: Pathology and review of the literature. *Arch. Pathol.* **58**:533-553.
56. Walton, E. W. (1958). Giant-cell granuloma of the respiratory tract (Wegener's granulomatosis). *Lancet* **2**:265-270.
57. Fauci, A. S., and Wolff, S. M. (1973). Wegener's granulomatosis: Studies in eighteen patients and a review of the literature. *Medicine* **52**:535-561.
58. Carrington, C. B., and Liebow, A. A. (1966). Limited forms of angiitis and granulomatosis of the Wegener's type. *Am. J. Med.* **41**:497-527.
59. Flye, M. W., Mundinger, G. H., and Fauci, A. S. (1979). Diagnostic and therapeutic aspects of the surgical approach to Wegener's granulomatosis. *J. Thorac. Cardiovasc. Surg.* **77**:331-337.
60. Gonzalez, L., and Van Ordstrand, H. S. (1973). Wegener's granulomatosis. *Radiology* **107**:295-300.

61. D'Angelo, W. A., Fries, J. F., Masi, A. T., and Shulman, L. E. (1969). Pathologic observations in systemic sclerosis (scleroderma): A study of fifty-eight autopsy cases and fifty-eight matched controls. *Am. J. Med.* **46**:428-440.
62. Gondos, B. (1960). Roentgen manifestations in progressive systemic sclerosis (diffuse scleroderma). *A.J.R.* **84**:235-247.
63. Weaver, A. L., Divertie, M. B., and Titus, J. L. (1968). Pulmonary scleroderma. *Dis. Chest* **54**:4-12.
64. Edwards, W. G. Jr., and Dines, D. E. (1966). Recurrent spontaneous pneumothorax in diffuse scleroderma. *Dis. Chest* **49**:96-98.
65. Rosenow, E. C. III, Strimlan, C. V., Muhm, J. R., and Ferguson, R. H. (1977). Pleuropulmonary manifestations of ankylosing spondylitis. *Mayo Clin. Proc.* **52**:641-649.
66. Kinnear, W. J. M., and Shneerson, J. M. (1985). Acute pleural effusions in inactive ankylosing spondylitis. *Thorax* **40**:150-151.
67. Dudley-Hart, F., Bogdanovitch, A., and Nichol, W. D. (1950). The thorax in ankylosing spondylitis. *Ann. Rheum. Dis.* **9**:116-131.
68. Zorab, P. A. (1962). The lungs in ankylosing spondylitis. *Q. J. Med.* **31**:267-280.
69. Libschitz, H. I., Atkinson, G. W., and Israel, H. (1974). Pleural thickening as a manifestation of *Aspergillus* superinfection. *Am. J. Radiol. Radiother. Nucl.* **120**:883-886.
70. Lanham, J. G., Elkon, K. B., Pusey, C. D., and Hughes, G. R. (1984). Systemic vasculitis with asthma and eosinophilia: A clinical approach to the Churg-Strauss syndrome. *Medicine* **63**:65-81.
71. Harkavy, J. (1943). Vascular allergy. *J. Allergy* **14**:507-537.
72. Crofton, J. W., Livingstone, J. L., Oswald, N. C., and Roberts, A. T. M. (1952). Pulmonary eosinophilia. *Thorax* **7**:1-35.
73. Varriale, P., Minogue, W. F., and Alfenito, J. C. (1964). Allergic granulomatosis. *Arch. Intern. Med.* **113**:235-240.
74. Granthan, J. G., Meadows, J. A. III, and Gleich, G. J. (1986). Chronic eosinophilic pneumonia. Evidence for eosinophilic degranulation and release of major basic protein. *Am. J. Med.* **80**:89-94.
75. Hannun, Y., and Frayha, R. (1985). Behçet's disease with pseudochylothorax. *J. Rheum.* **12**:817-818.
76. Chajek, T., and Fainaru, M. (1975). Behçet's disease: Report of 41 cases and review of the literature. *Medicine* **54**:179-196.
77. Kansu, E., Ozer, F. L., Akalin, E., Guler, Y., Zileli, T., Tanman, E., Kaplaman, E., and Muftuoglu, E. (1972). Behçet's syndrome with obstruction of the venae cavae. *Q. J. Med.* **41**:151-168.
78. Maier, H. C. (1968). Chylous reflux in the lungs and pleurae. *Thorax* **23**:281-296.

Part II

**EVALUATION OF STRUCTURAL AND FUNCTIONAL
ALTERATIONS IN THE LUNGS OF
PATIENTS WITH LUNG DISEASES**

3

Functional Evaluation of the Airways, Lung Vessels, and Ventilatory Muscles

C. GREGORY ELLIOTT

LDS Hospital and University of Utah
Salt Lake City, Utah

This chapter outlines an approach to the assessment of respiratory function in patients who have collagen vascular disease. The text considers the reasons for functional evaluation of airways, lung vessels, and ventilatory muscles in patients with rheumatic diseases; selected techniques that are available to the clinician and investigator; the results of functional assessment for specific rheumatic disorders; and strategies for respiratory evaluation of patients with rheumatic diseases.

I. Rationale for Functional Assessment

The evaluation of lung function in the patient with known rheumatic disease serves several purposes. Pulmonary function studies can provide prognostic information, detect occult pulmonary disease, and screen for drug-induced lung disease. Serial measurements of lung function can quantitate the response to therapy or the progression of disease. Spirometric data and carbon monoxide diffusion studies help to determine impairment and disability for patients with rheumatic disease and respiratory involvement. Careful measurement of physiologic variables also helps to characterize clinical, roentgenographic, and biological observations in investigations of collagen vascular disease of the lung.

A. Prognosis

Pulmonary involvement associated with rheumatic diseases often limits life expectancy. Stupi et al. described 20 patients with CREST syndrome and pulmonary hypertension (1). These patients had a 2-year cumulative survival rate of 40%. They also had markedly decreased diffusion capacity for carbon monoxide (DL_{CO}) (mean 39% of predicted normal). The reduced DL_{CO} provided the earliest clue to the development of progressive pulmonary vascular injury. Similarly, Peters-Golden et al. reported that a DL_{CO} less than 40% of predicted was associated with a 9% 5-year survival for patients with systemic sclerosis (2). The data did not exclude the possibility that cigarette smoking in association with systemic sclerosis accounts for the increased mortality observed among men with severely reduced DL_{CO}.

The occurrence of pulmonary fibrosis in association with connective tissue disease also influences survival. Turner-Warwick et al. studied 220 patients with idiopathic pulmonary fibrosis including 22 who had rheumatoid arthritis (3). Pulmonary fibrosis was the cause of death for a number of patients with rheumatoid arthritis. The presence of right heart failure, the degree of dyspnea, and a low PaO_2 each predicted a poor outcome.

These studies suggest that pulmonary hypertension and right heart failure are unfavorable prognostic signs when pulmonary involvement complicates rheumatic diseases. Therefore, when assessing prognosis, the clinician should pay particular attention to the status of the pulmonary circulation. Moderate or severe dyspnea and marked DL_{CO} reductions provide clinical and laboratory clues to occult pulmonary vascular disease. Right heart catheterization should be performed if the clinician suspects significant pulmonary vascular disease.

B. Detection of Occult Pulmonary Disease

Pulmonary function tests detect and characterize clinically occult pulmonary disease. History and physical examination remain the most basic methods for detecting pulmonary parenchymal involvement associated with rheumatic diseases. A symptom or a sign suggesting pulmonary involvement, e.g., cough, exertional dyspnea, or late inspiratory rales, often leads the clinician to seek additional evidence of pulmonary disease. The chest roentgenogram provides visual documentation of lung disease in many instances. However, in some situations, the chest roentgenogram may remain normal. In these situations, pulmonary function tests may provide physiologic evidence of lung disease. For example, Epler et al. described 44 patients who had histologically confirmed

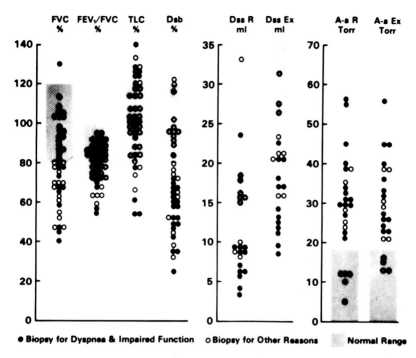

Figure 1   Physiologic observations in patients with biopsy-proven diffuse infiltrative lung disease and normal chest roentgenograms. FVC, forced vital capacity; FEV₁, forced expired volume in one second; TLC, total lung capacity; Dsb, single-breath CO diffusing capacity; A-aR and A-aEx, rest and exercise alveolar to arterial PO₂ difference. The stippled areas represent the normal range. (From ref. 4.)

diffuse infiltrative lung diseases and normal standard chest roentgenograms (4). Abnormalities of pulmonary function were commonly observed in these patients. Reductions of DL_{CO} and increased alveolar to arterial PO₂ gradient (P_AO_2-PaO₂) at rest and during exercise were usually present (Fig. 1). Patients with rheumatoid arthritis and systemic lupus erythematosus often have abnormally low DL_{CO} in the absence of symptoms, signs, and abnormal chest roentgenograms (5-9). Abnormal reductions of forced vital capacity (FVC), total lung capacity (TLC), and the ratio of forced expired volume in 1 s to forced vital capacity (FEV₁/FVC) were observed less frequently.

C. Screening for Drug-Induced Pulmonary Disease

A number of drugs that are prescribed for the treatment of rheumatic disorders may cause pulmonary injury (Chap. 14, Table 1). Although there are no studies that demonstrate the value of periodic monitoring for drug toxicity, noninvasive monitoring is difficult to fault. Since pulmonary toxicity from gold salts typically occurs within a few months of initiating this therapy (10), measurement of baseline spirometry, DL_{CO}, and TLC with a follow-up at 3 months appears reasonable. Similarly, periodic spirometric measures can be performed to monitor penicillamine therapy. At the very least, baseline spirometry and DL_{CO} measurements should be obtained and symptomatic patients can then be retested. This practice can contribute to earlier recognition of pulmonary dysfunction since the range of predicted normal values is larger than the reproducibility of spirometry and DL_{CO} for an individual patient.

D. Assessment of Response to Therapy or Progression of Disease

Routine pulmonary function tests provide objective measurements of the response to therapy or the progression of pulmonary disease. However, important questions remain unanswered for patients with rheumatic diseases. Which tests should be performed? How often should the patient be tested? What constitutes a significant change? For the present, only general clinical recommendations and extrapolation from studies of other patient groups are possible.

The patient with interstitial pneumonitis and pulmonary fibrosis can be followed every 3 months with measurements of vital capacity, TLC, and DL_{CO}. Greater than 10% reduction of vital capacity or TLC and greater than 15% reduction of DL_{CO} suggest progressive disease (11).

The patient with bronchiolitis obliterans may require spirometric monitoring. Timed variables (e.g., FEV_1, FEV_3) are best for comparison with baseline when airflow obstruction is present. Owens et al. reported that the FEV_1 of patients with stable chronic obstructive pulmonary disease ($\overline{X}$ FEV_1 = 1.15 L) who returned for monthly tests had a coefficient of variation of 16.4% (12). This suggests that changes in FEV_1 of less than 17% can be viewed as stable when moderate or severe airflow obstruction is present. Smaller changes may be used to guide therapeutic decisions when the patient's individual variability is known.

E. Impairment/Disability Evaluation

Impairment and disability are often important issues for patients with rheumatic diseases, whether or not they have pulmonary involvement. When lung dysfunction predominates, the assessment of impairment usually involves spirometry measurements and the single-breath DL_{CO}. These tests require patient cooperation, but it is unusual for systemic manifestations of

Table 1 Assessment of Impairment Directly Related to Reduced Lung Function[a]

Degree of impairment	FEV$_1$[b] % Predicted	FVC[b] % Predicted	[FEV$_1$/FVC] × 100 %	DL$_{CO}$[c] % of Predicted
Mild	60-70	60-99	60-94	60-79
Moderate	41-59	51-59	41-59	41-59
Severe	≤40	≤50	≤40	≤40

[a]Adapted from Reference 14.
[b]Evaluate subjects only after accurate diagnosis and optimal therapy.
[c]Corrections should be made for hemoglobin concentration and back pressure exerted by COHb.

rheumatic diseases to preclude testing. Exceptions may be patients with severe systemic sclerosis or for rheumatoid arthritis of the temporomandibular joint who cannot insert a mouthpiece. Exercise tests are also useful for the assessment of impairment and disability (13), but exercise tests are often difficult for patients with rheumatic diseases to perform. For this reason, the approach outlined by the American Thoracic Society is recommended (Table 1) (14). These recommendations also consider a number of modifying conditions—e.g., cor pulmonale, arterial hypoxemia, and upper airway obstruction—that may affect patients with rheumatic diseases.

II. Techniques for Functional Assessment of the Respiratory System*

Studies of respiratory function cover a spectrum from readily available and inexpensive methods, e.g., spirometry, to less widely available, expensive, and invasive studies, e.g., right heart catheterization. Because standardization of pulmonary function methodologies is so important and interlaboratory variability is so prevalent, the clinician should encourage the patient to attend the same laboratory if at all possible.

A. Spirometry and Flow Volume Curves

Spirometry represents one of the more basic measures of respiratory mechanics, providing important information about airflow and vital capacity. Spirometric measurements require patient cooperation. Potential problems exist with the accuracy of some commercially available instruments, and serious measurement errors are possible if the laboratory does not

*Reference 17 provides detailed descriptions of methodologies.

adhere to established standards. Recently, Nelson reported that one commercially available spirometer erred by 1.5 L (25%) in the measurement of forced vital capacity (15). Although such severe errors are uncommon, Nelson also noted that 26 of 53 spirometers did not meet the instrument standards proposed by the American Thoracic Society in 1987 (16). These findings should lead clinicians to carefully examine the instrumentation and laboratory methods where their patients are studied.

B. Clinical Abnormalities

Clinical abnormalities of spirometry can be divided into patterns of airflow obstruction and chest restriction. Definition of the lower limit of normal varies from laboratory to laboratory, creating problems in the overlap area between mild abnormality and low-normal values. A practical solution to this problem is to make clinical decisions based on both the spirometry result and other clinical data—e.g., physical examination.

Reductions in the ratio of FEV_1 to FVC define airflow obstruction (17). Bronchodilator response is usually assessed when airflow obstruction is present. The patient repeats the spirograms 15 min after a slow inhalation of bronchodilator aerosol. Some patients with airflow obstruction may not exhale long enough to deliver their entire vital capacity. Under these conditions, the FEV_1/FVC will change with changing total expiratory time. For this reason, pre- and postbronchodilator comparisons are best made with FEV_1 rather than FEV_1/FVC. Measurement of expiratory flow between 25% and 75% of forced vital capacity (FEF_{25-75}) allows examination of more peripheral airways than FEV_1. However, the range of normal values for FEF_{25-75} is quite large, making differentiation between normal and diseased peripheral airways difficult.

Obstruction of the large airways, e.g., trachea, can result from a number of rheumatic diseases (Table 2). Spirometry with a good forced inspiration or maximal inspiratory and expiratory flow-volume curves can detect upper airway obstruction whether it is fixed or varies as intratracheal pressure changes from positive (expiration) to negative (inspiration) (21).

Chest restriction can be suggested by spirometry but is best assessed by measurement of lung volume. When airflow obstruction is present, techniques that do not utilize gas dilution for lung volume measurement (plethysmography or radiographic TLC) avoid the error introduced by trapped air. Reduced lung volumes may result from diseases of the respiratory muscles or thoracic skeleton as well as from parenchymal lung diseases. Differentiation of these causes requires an integrated history, physical examination, and additional laboratory tests—e.g., measurements of maximal respiratory pressures or lung compliance.

Table 2 Rheumatic Diseases Associated with Upper Airway Obstruction

Disease	Clinical Observations
Wegener's granulomatosis	Usually accompanies widespread parenchymal pulmonary disease (18)
Relapsing polychondritis	Usually occurs without pulmonary or renal disease (19)
Rheumatoid arthritis	Occurs with involvement of cricoarytenoid cartilage (20)

C. Arterial Blood Gas Analysis

Because the prescription of oxygen relies heavily on the measurement of arterial PO_2, sampling arterial blood remains important for the assessment of patients with rheumatic pulmonary disease. Methodologic pitfalls are few, e.g., excessive heparin in the dead space of the syringe, but the clinician should be aware that PaO_2 can change dramatically during the exercise when interstitial lung disease is present.

The difference between alveolar PO_2 and arterial PO_2 (P_AO_2-P_aO_2) assesses the oxygen transfer function of the lung. Normal PaO_2 and P_AO_2-P_aO_2 change with increasing age so that the lower limit of normal PaO_2 at sea level is 84 at age 20 and 67 at age 80. The upper limit of normal P_AO_2-P_aO_2 is 17 at age 20 and 38 at age 80 (17). The arterial PCO_2 changes less with age. The upper limit of normal is approximately 39 mmHg at age 20 and 43 mmHg at age 80.

D. Diffusing Capacity of Carbon Monoxide

Carbon monoxide diffusing capacity (DL_{CO}) is a sensitive test for the detection of pulmonary dysfunction, but it lacks diagnostic specificity. The test measures the rate of CO uptake by the lungs (mL CO/min/mm Hg). Impaired matching of ventilation and perfusion, alterations in the alveolar-capillary membrane itself, and/or decreases in the pulmonary capillary blood volume cause an abnormal reduction of DL_{CO} (see Chap. 1) (22). The DL_{CO} is frequently abnormal in chest diseases when other clinical tests, e.g., chest roentgenograms, do not reveal abnormalities (4). However, abnormalities of the DL_{CO} do not point directly to interstitial pneumonitis or fibrosis associated with rheumatic diseases. Common diseases such as emphysema also lower DL_{CO} (23). Therefore, the test finds its widest application in the detection of lung dysfunction associated with rheumatic diseases and in serial evaluation of patients. Several methods exist for the measurement of DL_{CO}. These include the single-breath, steady-state, and rebreathing techniques. The single-breath technique represents the most widely used of these methods (17).

In order for the DL_{CO} to be clinically useful, care must be taken to avoid a number of technical pitfalls (Table 3). For example, a spuriously low DL_{CO} can result from the inadvertent collection of dead-space gas or from failure to correct the measurement for the subject's hemoglobin concentration. The latter point is particularly important because many patients with rheumatic diseases are anemic. Correction equations allow reasonable approximations of DL_{CO} for anemic patients (24) and for patients who have an elevated carboxyhemoglobin (25). The subject's lung volume represents yet another confounding variable. Pneumonectomy reduces the DL_{CO} dramatically, and yet the remaining lung may be normal. Therefore, indexing DL_{CO} to a simultaneously measured lung volume (DL/VA) can aid in the recognition of DL_{CO} reductions that result from decreased lung volume (17).

Standardization of methods for the measurement and calculation of DL_{CO} remains an important issue for the clinician. Mobile patients and additional consultations often lead to DL_{CO} measurements in more than one laboratory. Under such circumstances, changes in DL_{CO} may reflect inter-

Table 3 Common Technical Pitfalls in the Measurements of DL_{CO}

Problem	Solution
Collection of dead space gas	Discard the first 750 ml exhaled gas before collecting the expired sample
DL_{CO} reduced by anemia	Correct DL_{CO} for a simultaneously measured hemoglobin concentration. DL_{CO} corr = measured $DL_{CO} \times [(10.22 + Hb)/(1.7 \times Hb)]$ (24)
DL_{CO} reduced by the presence of COHb	Correct DL_{CO} for COHb measured in the patient's blood. COHb corrected DL_{CO} DL_{CO} = measured $DL_{CO} \times (1 + \%COHb/100\%)$ (25)
Effect of reduced lung volume (VA)	Index to a simultaneously measured lung volume (DL/VA) (17)

laboratory differences of methodology rather than changes in the patient's lung function. Investigators have described 50-90% interlaboratory variation in the DL_{CO} of the same subject (26). Other investigators have demonstrated that differences in calculation algorithms can cause the DL_{CO} to vary by more than 40% (27). These observations point out that serious errors in the interpretation of DL_{CO} may result from methodologic differences. For this reason, the clinician who is serially testing the DL_{CO} of a patient with rheumatic disease should use the same laboratory, preferably one that has matched predicted DL_{CO} values to studies of a representative group of healthy subjects (28).

The measurement of DL_{CO} at different altitudes contributes to interlaboratory variation of DL_{CO}. This occurs because of the decrease in alveolar PO_2 as ambient pressure decreases. It is possible to correct for altitude by altering the test gas oxygen concentration (29) or by the use of a correction equation (30).

Once the problems of technical error and standardization have been addressed, the reproducibility of DL_{CO} measurements becomes a critical issue. For example, the clinician needs to know whether a change in DL_{CO} from 16 ml CO/min/mmHg to 12 ml CO/min/mmHg represents deteriorating lung function or the variability of the DL_{CO} measurement in a stable patient. DL_{CO} variability is influenced by the presence and severity of lung disease. Therefore, proper interpretation of sequential DL_{CO} measurements requires knowledge of the patient's spirometry. Crapo has provided guidelines based upon five clinical categories: healthy, restrictive chest disease, mild, moderate, and severe airflow obstruction (Table 4) (31).

A decreased DL_{CO}, after correction for anemia and carboxyhemoglobin, generally reflects pulmonary disease. The underlying pulmonary diseases are not limited to interstitial lung diseases. Emphysema and pulmonary vascular diseases also reduce DL_{CO}. In one study, reductions in DL_{CO} ranging from 36% to 69% of predicted were observed in smokers who had a normal FEV_1/FVC ratio and who had emphysema demonstrated pathologically (23). The clinicians had not suspected emphysema prior to the lung biopsy. This observation that reduced DL_{CO} may be the evaluation of patients with rheumatic diseases who are cigarette smokers. In such a patient, a reduced DL_{CO} may reflect clinically occult emphysema rather than pulmonary disease associated with rheumatic disease. Conversely, rheumatic diseases often involve the lung, and an abnormally decreased DL_{CO} offers an important clue to presence of pulmonary disease (1,32).

Measurement of DL_{CO} following a cold stimulus (33-35) or in the upright and supine positions (36) may allow the detection of structural or functional abnormalities of the pulmonary vascular bed. In patients with progressive systemic sclerosis (PSS), failure of the DL_{CO} to increase when

Table 4 Estimated Variability of DL_{CO} Based on Patient Classification Prior to Testing

Patient Category	Upper Limit of Percent Change Expected Due to Test Variability (%)
Healthy	9
Restrictive chest disorder	9
Airflow obstruction	
Mild	7
Moderate	9
Severe	12

the patient is tested recumbent suggests an impairment of normal recruitment and distension of the pulmonary vascular bed (36). Similarly, failure of DL_{CO} to change when patients with rheumatic disease (e.g., PSS and Raynaud's phenomenon) are subjected to cold stress suggests abnormalities of the pulmonary vascular bed (33-35). The nature of the cold stimulus (digital vs. total body) and the time interval between the cold stimulus and the measurement of DL_{CO} represent important methodologic considerations for the clinician-investigator.

Abnormal increases of DL_{CO} accompany asthma and less commonly accompany left-to-right intracardiac shunts. Intrapulmonary hemorrhage, as may occur with pulmonary vasculitis, can cause markedly increased CO uptake. This occurs because intraalveolar red blood cells provide an additional reservoir for the uptake of CO. Serial DL_{CO} measurements can be used to monitor intrapulmonary hemorrhage (37).

E. Lung Volume Measurements

Total lung capacity (TLC) can be measured by gas dilution (multiple-breath nitrogen or single-breath helium), body plethysmography, or standard posteroanterior and lateral chest roentgenograms (38). Gas dilution techniques may substantially underestimate TLC in the presence of airflow obstruction because the indicator gas does not enter obstructed lung compartments. Body plethysmographic and roentgenographic measurements are not subject to this phenomenon. Therefore, simultaneous measurements of TLC by gas dilution and a nondilution technique allow an estimation of the volume of gas trapped in the chest (17).

Total lung capacity may be abnormally decreased (restriction) or abnormally increased (overinflation). Restriction commonly accompanies fibrotic lung diseases with or without neuromuscular or chest wall disease, whereas overinflation commonly results from obstructed airflow. Because pulmonary fibrosis and airflow obstruction may coexist, TLC can be within normal limits even though extensive pulmonary disease is present (39).

F. Exercise Testing and Blood Gas Analysis

Exercise tests and the analysis of arterial blood gases during exercise provide laboratory evidence of pulmonary dysfunction associated with rheumatic disorders. Decreases in arterial PO_2 and increases in P_AO_2-P_aO_2 are physiologic characteristics of interstitial fibrosis and pneumonitis (40,41). Fulmer et al. have demonstrated that the ratio of the change in P_AO_2-P_aO_2 to the change in oxygen consumption during exercise (ΔP_AO_2-$P_aO_2/\Delta \dot{V}O_2$) correlates best with quantitative histologic scoring of pulmonary fibrosis from lung biopsy specimens (42). Exercise testing can also detect pulmonary vascular disease earlier than resting measurements of pulmonary artery pressure, pulmonary arteriograms, or radionuclide perfusion scans (43). However, many patients with rheumatic diseases are unable to perform exercise tests because of synovial or muscle disease. Therefore, the clinician must assess the indications for exercise testing and the ability of the patient to exercise before ordering an exercise evaluation.

Exercise testing can be performed according to several protocols that make measurements during "steady state" (42) or during incrementally increasing work loads (44). Failure to sample arterial blood within 10 s of maximal exercise may result in failure to identify significant exercise-induced hypoxemia (45,46). Noninvasive oximetry represents an important potential alternative to sampling arterial blood during exercise. Watters et al. found that exercise-induced changes in O_2 saturation measured by ear oximetry parallel changes in exercise P_AO_2-P_aO_2 (47). However, Ries et al. reported that the 95% confidence limit (± 2 SEE) for an oximeter reading in estimating SaO_2 from the arterial blood of patients with lung disease was $\pm 3.8\%$; and the presence of COHb, jaundice, or darkly pigmented skin made estimations of arterial O_2 saturation more difficult (48). Patients with rheumatic disease may present additional problems because of vasculitis or skin disease.

Measurements of P_aO_2 and P_AO_2-P_aO_2 during exercise serve two purposes in the assessment of interstitial lung disease associated with rheumatic diseases. First, abnormal increases in P_AO_2-P_aO_2 provide physiologic evidence for pulmonary dysfunction when intracardiac shunts and severe cardiac disease are not present. Abnormal increases in P_AO_2-P_aO_2 during exercise characterize pulmonary fibrosis associated with rheumatic and nonrheumatic diseases (32,49), but abnormalities of gas exchange during exercise lack specificity for interstitial lung diseases. Pulmonary emphysema (50) and pulmonary vascular diseases (51) also cause abnormal P_aO_2 and P_AO_2-P_aO_2 during exercise.

Second, exercise-induced changes in P_aO_2 and P_AO_2-P_aO_2 per liter of oxygen consumed allow staging and monitoring of the severity of fibrotic lung diseases. Fulmer et al. reported that measurements of gas exchange during exercise correlate better than vital capacity, TLC, or DL_{CO} with the severity of fibrosis in lung biopsy specimens (42).

A number of studies have focused on the detection of physiologic abnormalities in patients with interstitial lung diseases. Because DL_{CO} measurement does not involve risk or discomfort, investigators have examined the predictive value of DL_{CO} for the detection of abnormal gas exchange during exercise. Sue et al. observed that a $DL_{CO} \geqslant 70\%$ of predicted did not identify men who had normal P_aO_2 and P_AO_2-P_aO_2 changes during exercise (44). These two tests of pulmonary gas exchange function, although correlated, do not mirror each other. For this reason, the clinician may use one or both to assess suspected rheumatic lung disease.

The normal ratio of dead space to tidal volume (Vd/Vt) is approximately 0.3. During exercise, this ratio decreases as tidal volume increases and increased cardiac output perfuses more of the pulmonary capillary bed (52). Chronic pulmonary vascular obstruction can cause an abnormal increase in Vd/Vt during exercise (43). For some patients, the increase in Vd/Vt during exercise may be present although pulmonary angiograms, radioisotope lung scans, and pulmonary artery pressures at rest and during exercise are normal (43). Conversely, measurements of Vd/Vt during exercise may fail to detect hemodynamically significant pulmonary vascular abnormalities accompanying collagen vascular disease (32).

G. Pulmonary Hypertension

Pulmonary hypertension accompanies a number of rheumatic diseases (Table 5). Measurement of pulmonary artery pressure and cardiac output with flow-

Table 5 Rheumatic Diseases Associated with
Pulmonary Hypertension

CREST variant of systemic sclerosis
Systemic lupus erythematosus
Rheumatoid arthritis
Mixed connective tissue disease
Dermatomyositis
Polymyositis

directed catheters may be necessary to diagnose mild pulmonary hypertension associated with rheumatic diseases. Mean pulmonary artery pressure greater than 20 mmHg at rest or greater than 24 mmHg during exercise that doubles cardiac output is abnormal. Combinations of DL_{CO} reductions with electrocardiographic and chest roentgenographic abnormalities may help to identify patients with pulmonary hypertension (44). Exercise measurements are particularly useful when resting pulmonary artery pressure is normal.

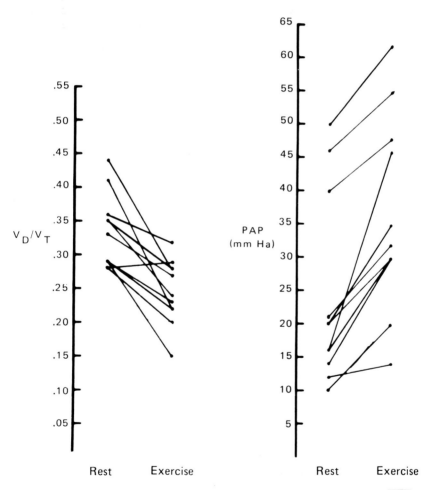

Figure 2 Measurements of Vd/Vt and mean pulmonary artery pressure ($\overline{PAP}$) at rest and during exercise in 11 patients with rheumatic diseases. $\overline{PAP}$ greater than 24 mm Hg during exercise is abnormal (from ref. 32).

Mohsenifar et al. found that mean pulmonary artery pressure increased abnormally with exercise in five of seven patients with collagen vascular disease who had normal pulmonary artery pressure at rest (Fig. 2) (32). The increase in pulmonary artery pressure during exercise was a more sensitive test for the detection of pulmonary vascular disease than increasing Vd/Vt.

H. Maximal Inspiratory and Expiratory Pressures

Measurement of maximal inspiratory pressure (MIP) requires that the patient exhale to residual volume and then make a maximal effort to inhale into a mouthpiece connected to a pressure gauge or transducer. The system requires a 1 mm diameter $\times$ 15 mm length leak, which prevents the cheek muscles from contributing to the pressure measurement. Measurement of maximal expiratory pressure (MEP) requires that the patient make a maximal effort to exhale from total lung capacity into the same system.

Maximal inspiratory and expiratory pressures are abnormally decreased when a variety of neuromuscular disorders impair the function of respiratory muscles. Black and Hyatt have provided normal values for men and women (ages 20-86) (53). Before attributing an abnormally low measurement to neuromuscular dysfunction, the clinician must exclude poor patient effort, pain, or a poorly fit mouthpiece.

III. Functional Assessment of Specific Rheumatic Disorders

A. Rheumatoid Arthritis

A number of physiologic abnormalities can accompany rheumatoid arthritis. These include (a) restrictive chest disease associated with interstitial pneumonitis and fibrosis (54), (b) airflow obstruction with or without bronchiolitis obliterans (55-57), (c) upper airway obstruction associated with laryngeal involvement (58), and (d) pulmonary hypertension associated with pulmonary vasculitis (59).

Restrictive chest disease is associated with reduced vital capacity, TLC, DL_{CO}, and arterial hypoxemia (5,54). These abnormalities may not be as severe as those that accompany systemic lupus erythematosus and scleroderma (Fig. 3) (60). Decreased DL_{CO} measurements may be present when patients with interstitial disease are asymptomatic and their chest roentgenograms are normal (5-7). Furthermore, heavy cigarette smoking may significantly reduce DL_{CO} in patients with rheumatoid arthritis, even without clinical or physiologic evidence of emphysema (6). Based on these observations, measurement of DL_{CO} during an initial assessment appears warranted, particularly if therapy with gold salts or methotrexate is planned.

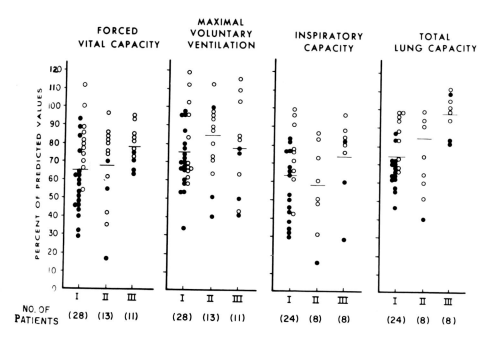

Figure 3 Pulmonary function measurements of patients with systemic lupus erythematosus (I), scleroderma (II), and rheumatoid arthritis (III). Patients were included with (●) and without (○) clinical evidence of pulmonary disease. (From ref. 60.)

Collins et al. have described reductions of maximal midexpiratory flow rates among smokers and nonsmokers with classic rheumatoid arthritis (55). This study only included one nonsmoker with mild airflow obstruction. Thus, cigarette smoking likely contributes substantially to airflow obstruction accompanying rheumatoid arthritis. The maximal midexpiratory flow rates of smokers with rheumatoid arthritis were lower than those of smokers with osteoarthritis, raising the question of pathogenetic synergism between cigarette smoke and rheumatoid arthritis.

Begin et al. described six nonsmokers with rheumatoid arthritis and lymphocytic exocrinopathy who had reduced expiratory flow rates and progressively increasing residual volume (57). Histopathologic examinations demonstrated bronchiolar and peribronchiolar lymphocytic inflammation.

Geddes et al. described airflow obstruction at low lung volumes and air trapping which accompanied progressive airway obliteration associated with rheumatoid arthritis (56). Penicillamine therapy was associated with three of six cases. Total lung capacity and residual volume measurements exceeded the predicted values. Spirometry did not improve with bronchodilators or corticosteroids. DL_{CO} was decreased, but DL_{CO} corrected for alveolar volume (DL/VA) was normal, differentiating this lesion from emphysema.

Computerized tomography of the neck has documented laryngeal involvement associated with rheumatoid arthritis (20,58). Maximal inspiratory and expiratory flow volume curves offer a practical method for the functional assessment and monitoring of cricoarytenoid involvement associated with rheumatoid arthritis.

Pulmonary hypertension has complicated rheumatoid arthritis (59). Measurements of pulmonary hemodynamics have been recorded (61), but the response to vasodilators remains undefined in this rare patient subset.

B. Systemic Lupus Erythematosus

Systemic lupus erythematosus (SLE) can produce both restrictive and obstructive abnormalities of pulmonary function. DL_{CO} abnormalities may occur in the absence of symptoms, signs, and abnormal chest roentgenograms (8,9).

Chest restriction is the most common pulmonary function abnormality associated with SLE (8,62,63). This may be related to pleuritis (9), interstitial pneumonitis (63), or diaphragmatic dysfunction (9). Forced vital capacity and TLC capacity are reduced proportionately (8). Reductions of DL_{CO} after correction for anemia have been reported to occur in 80% of an unselected group of patients with SLE (9,64). The restrictive defect was a major determinant of abnormally low DL_{CO} values in these patients. The alveolar-arterial PO_2 difference is often abnormally increased (63), and Vd/Vt may occasionally be increased (64).

Airflow obstruction rarely accompanies SLE (64,65). This abnormality may respond to corticosteroids but not to beta-agonists or theophylline (65).

Poor diaphragm excursion has been associated with SLE (9,62,63). Adhesions from pleuritis, pulmonary disease with decreased lung compliance, and diaphragm dysfunction may each contribute to reduced diaphragm excursion. Gibson et al. measured maximum inspiratory pressures in seven patients with chest restriction (9). They reported that inspiratory muscles were unable to generate normal pressures in six of the seven patients. Furthermore, maximal transdiaphragmatic pressures were considerably below normal. The authors suggested that either diaphragmatic adhesions or myopathy involving the diaphragm could explain these observations. Martens et al. extended these observations to include weakness of expiratory as well as inspiratory muscles (66).

Severe pulmonary hypertension also has been associated with SLE (67).

C. Progressive Systemic Sclerosis (Scleroderma)

A restrictive pattern of pulmonary function is the most common abnormality associated with scleroderma (68-72). Reductions of vital capacity and total lung capacity reflect decreased lung compliance due to pulmonary fibrosis rather than cutaneous restriction of the chest wall (70). Gas exchange abnormalities include decreased DL_{CO} (70,71) and abnormally increased P_AO_2-P_aO_2 during exercise. Ritchie reported that 7 of 22 patients with scleroderma had a lower DL_{CO} than normal, but 3 of the 7 were cigarette smokers (70). These lung function abnormalities do not correlate with the degree of cutaneous involvement and may precede skin changes (70).

Pulmonary hypertension frequently complicates the CREST variant of systemic sclerosis (1,71-73). Initially, pulmonary hypertension may not be detected by routine history, physical examination, and basic laboratory studies (73). Severe reduction of DL_{CO} may provide an early clue to the presence of pulmonary hypertension (1,71), but early diagnosis of pulmonary hypertension usually requires right heart catheterization (73). As pulmonary vascular injury evolves, pulmonary hypertension becomes severe and often proves fatal. It does not respond to vasodilators (1) even when titrated to high doses, as illustrated by a patient who was recently studied in our catheterization laboratory (Table 6).

In addition to restrictive pulmonary dysfunction and pulmonary hypertension, airflow obstruction may complicate scleroderma (60,71,72,74).

A number of investigators have studied the natural history of pulmonary function abnormalities associated with systemic sclerosis (75-78). Colp et al. measured serial PFTs over periods of 2-10 years and reported a very gradual decline in pulmonary function (75). Schneider et al. (76) and Peters-

Table 6 Hemodynamic Data Following "High Dose" Titration of Nifedipine: 48-Year-Old Female with CREST, Scleroderma, and Pulmonary Hypertension

Time	Condition	$\overline{PAP}$ (mmHg)	Qt (L/min)	HR (bpm)	PVR (wood units)	$\overline{AP}$ (mmHg)
1039	Baseline	58	2.80	88	18.9	91
1539	Nifedipine 100 mg PO cumulative dose at 20 mg/h PO	62	3.56	96	15.4	76

Abbreviations: $\overline{PAP}$, mean pulmonary artery pressure; Qt, cardiac output; HR, heart rate; PVR, pulmonary vascular resistance; $\overline{AP}$, mean systemic blood pressure.

Golden et al. (2) reported that the course of pulmonary function abnormalities associated with systemic sclerosis was variable, unlike that of idiopathic pulmonary fibrosis. The mean rate of change for FVC, TLC, and DL_{CO} did not differ from that of normal populations, although the DL_{CO} of patients with severe Raynaud's (digital ulcers or amputation) declined more rapidly. Spontaneous improvements of pulmonary function were observed as well as rare progressive airflow obstruction. Greenwald et al. (77) prospectively identified a greater than normal decline in lung volumes and DL_{CO} but also emphasized the variability of pulmonary function for individual patients. The influence of treatment on the natural history of pulmonary function studies remains obscured by this variability and the absence of prospectively randomized and controlled trials (2,75,78).

D. Dermatomyositis-Polymyositis

Interstitial lung disease, aspiration pneumonitis, and weakness of the ventilatory muscles represent common respiratory manifestations of polymyositis and dermatomyositis (79-81). One or more of these complications can account for the restrictive pattern of pulmonary function, decreased DL_{CO}, and increased $P_{A-a}O_2$ that has been associated with polymyositis (79-82).

Severe pulmonary hypertension due to disease of the small pulmonary arteries can accompany polymyositis and dermatomyositis (83,84).

E. Sjogren's Syndrome

Sjogren's syndrome can occur as a primary disorder or in association with other rheumatic diseases. A number of pulmonary function abnormalities have been associated with primary and secondary Sjogren's syndrome.

Vitali et al. (85) studied 20 nonsmokers with primary Sjogren's syndrome and 20 patients with Sjogren's syndrome and associated rheumatic disease ("secondary Sjogren's syndrome"). Most patients were asymptomatic, and those with symptoms complained of nonproductive cough and mild exertional dyspnea. The most common lung function abnormality was a reduced DL_{CO}. This abnormality was more pronounced with secondary Sjogren's and was more likely to occur when Raynaud's phenomenon was present. Bariffi et al. also found decreased DL_{CO} in 18 nonsmokers with Sjogren's syndrome (86). Both studies suggested that interstitial lymphocytic inflammation contributed to the abnormal DL_{CO}.

Newball described five nonsmokers with spirometric evidence of airflow obstruction unresponsive to bronchodilators (87). The authors suggested that lymphocytic infiltration of bronchioles caused airflow obstruction.

Although the aforementioned studies did not identify chest restriction, Strimlan et al. noted a restricted pattern in 18 patients (88). Because the majority of these patients had concomitant rheumatic diseases, the restriction may have resulted from these disorders rather than Sjogren's syndrome.

F. Mixed Connective Tissue Disease

Abnormalities of pulmonary function commonly accompany mixed connective tissue disease. Harmon et al. reported abnormal pulmonary function studies in 20 of 24 patients (89). Eight of 13 asymptomatic patients had abnormal pulmonary function. Abnormal reductions of DL_{CO} were uniformly present, and TLC was less often abnormally decreased. Derderian and associates confirmed these observations and also reported reductions of static lung compliance without abnormalities of respiratory muscle function (90).

Pulmonary hypertension has been associated with mixed connective tissue disease (91,92). The case reported by Guit et al. (92) exhibited moderate pulmonary hypertension, whereas the patient described by Jones et al. (91) had severe pulmonary hypertension which proved fatal.

G. Ankylosing Spondylitis

Because ankylosing spondylitis involves the chest wall as well as the lung, a number of investigations have examined the effects of limited chest expansion on pulmonary function (93-95). These studies have shown that even with severe ankylosis of the rib cage, abnormalities of pulmonary function are mild and cardiorespiratory failure does not occur.

Reductions of TLC are less severe than reductions of FVC. Mean percent of predicted TLC ranged from 92% (96) to 85% when maximum chest expansion was more limited (97). Reductions of mean percent of predicted FVC have ranged from 80% (95) to 72% (94). The difference between reductions in TLC and FVC reflects increased residual volume (93,98). Reductions of TLC and FVC correlate well with impaired thoracic mobility (96) while lung compliance remains normal (99) or mildly decreased (93,98). Limited expansion of the rib cage does not cause a ventilatory limitation to exercise (97), presumably because the chest wall is fixed at an increased lung volume and diaphragm excursion is preserved.

Consensus is lacking with respect to the effects of ankylosing spondylitis on pulmonary gas exchange. Renzetti et al. reported an increase in physiologic dead space and mild arterial hypoxia due to increased venous admixture (95). Gacad and Hamosh found normal arterial PO_2 in nonsmokers with advanced ankylosing spondylitis (93). Similarly, Miller and Sproule reported normal P_AO_2-P_aO_2 and dead space in nonsmokers with ankylosing spondylitis (94). Measurements of DL_{CO} also remain normal when indexed to alveolar volume (DL/VA) (97,99). Thus, in the absence of upper lobe fibrosis or concomitant pulmonary disease, pulmonary gas exchange is minimally affected by ankylosis of the thorax.

H. Systemic Vasculitides

Wegener's Granulomatosis

Wegener's granulomatosis can run the gamut of pulmonary function abnormalities from upper airway obstruction to abnormally increased DL_{CO} associated with diffuse pulmonary hemorrhage.

Rosenberg et al. examined the usefulness of pulmonary function testing in managing 22 patients with Wegener's granulomatosis (18). They noted that reduced lung volumes and DL_{CO} occurred frequently, but the most common abnormality was airflow obstruction (Fig. 4). Reduced lung volumes were associated with focal infiltrates, cavities, or masses. Reduction of FEV_1/ FVC detected focal large airway lesions, suggesting that spirometry is useful in evaluating laryngotracheal involvement by Wegener's granulomatosis.

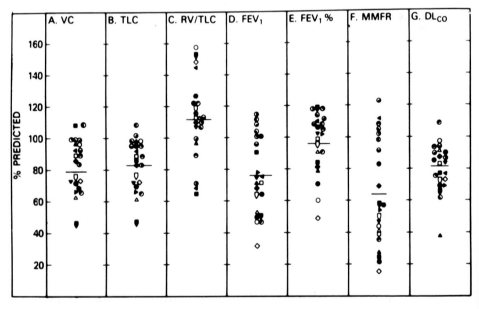

Figure 4   Lung volumes, expiratory flow rates, and DL_{CO} of patients with Wegener's granulomatosis. The normal range was 80-120% of predicted except for FEV_1, where normal was greater than or equal to 95% of predicted. (From ref. 18.)

Churg-Strauss Syndrome

Airflow obstruction that responds to bronchodilators characterizes pulmonary involvement associated with allergic granulomatosis and angiitis (Churg-Strauss syndrome). Patients with this disorder may have airflow obstruction that can prove fatal (101).

Relapsing Polychondritis

Relapsing polychondritis produces inflammation and destruction of cartilage in the trachea and bronchi. This process produces a pattern of upper airway obstruction, allowing differentiation from asthma or other pulmonary disorders.

IV. Strategies for the Respiratory Evaluation of Patients with Rheumatic Diseases

Guidelines for the respiratory evaluation of patients with rheumatic disorders remain difficult to define. The difficulties relate to (a) the reasons for respiratory evaluation, e.g., clinical vs. research; (b) the limited scope of published data, e.g., most studies describe small numbers of highly selected patients; (c) the sometimes conflicting reports of the relationships between physiologic observations, e.g., the relationship between single-breath DL_{CO} and exercise P_AO_2-P_aO_2; and (d) the interlaboratory variability in methodologies and interpretation of physiologic studies. This section acknowledges these difficulties and describes approaches to the physiologic assessment of the conducting airways, gas exchange surface, pulmonary circulation, and ventilatory muscles, based on current knowledge.

A. Airways

Since a number of rheumatic diseases can involve the trachea and larynx, functional evaluation of the upper airway may be necessary. The flow-volume loop, a plot of maximal forced expiratory and inspiratory flow over the range of vital capacity, provides definitive physiologic assessment of upper airway obstruction. Studies of patients with upper airway obstruction suggest that the ratio of maximum midinspiratory flow to maximum midexpiratory flow (MMIF/MMEF, or FIF_{25-75}/FEF_{25-75}) may differentiate upper airway obstruction from other conditions that cause airflow obstruction, e.g., emphysema. Normally, this ratio exceeds 1.5, and it is increased in patients with chronic obstructive pulmonary disease. In contrast, MMIF/MMEF is usually less than 1.0 when upper airway disease decreases airflow (102).

B. Small Airways

Hypoxemia associated with fibrotic lung diseases may result from abnormal ventilation of small (<2 mm) airways (103). These airways remain difficult to evaluate with standard physiologic studies—e.g., FEV_1/FVC or airways resistance. However, Fulmer et al. (103) have reported that measurements of dynamic compliance and analysis of maximal expiratory flow volume curves can predict histologic abnormalities of the small conducting airways in patients with idiopathic pulmonary fibrosis. These patients had normal measures of FEV_1/FVC and airway resistance. Measurement of MMEF rates (FEF_{25-75}) may also allow identification of subsets of patients with small airways disease (55,57). However, identification of disease of the small airways for an individual patient remains difficult because of the large variability in FEF_{25-75} in normal subjects (17).

C. Pulmonary Circulation

Definitive physiologic characterization of pulmonary vascular disease associated with rheumatic disorders requires right heart catheterization (32). When resting mean pulmonary artery pressures are normal, the pulmonary vascular tree can be stressed by the increased cardiac output that accompanies exercise. When mean pulmonary artery pressure is increased, pulmonary capillary wedge pressure must be measured in order to exclude pulmonary hypertension caused by disease of the left heart. Similarly, the evaluation is incomplete if pulmonary vascular resistance has not been calculated.

Although noninvasive studies may suggest pulmonary vascular disease, measurements of dead space to tidal volume ratio at rest and during exercise (32), measurements obtained from surface electrocardiograms, chest roentgenograms, and echocardiograms remain insensitive to the presence of hemodynamically significant pulmonary vascular disease associated with rheumatic disorders (104). Measurements of DL_{CO}, whether or not augmented by various stimuli, may be sensitive but nonspecific indicators of pulmonary vascular disease.

D. Gas Exchange Surface

Determination of the single-breath DL_{CO} represents a sensitive laboratory test for detection of disease involving the gas exchange surface of lung parenchyma. Conversely, abnormal reductions of DL_{CO} do not specify the underlying pathology. Emphysema, interstitial lung diseases, pulmonary vascular occlusion or obliteration, and pulmonary edema may reduce DL_{CO}. Therefore, specific diagnoses in patients with rheumatic diseases often require additional tests—e.g., spirometry to detect airflow obstruction. Nevertheless, because of its sensitivity, the DL_{CO} is often the first test used to detect impairment of the gas exchange surface (105).

When parenchymal pulmonary disease is strongly suspected and rheumatic joint involvement permits exercise, the changes in PaO_2 or P_AO_2-P_aO_2 that accompany exercise are also sensitive tools for the detection of disease involving the gas exchange surface of the lungs (44). These measurements are not widely applied clinically because they require arterial catheterization and additional expensive laboratory equipment. Nevertheless, available data suggest that the ratios of ΔP_AO_2-P_aO_2 to $\Delta \dot{V}O_2$ and ΔPaO_2 to $\Delta \dot{V}O_2$ provide strong correlation with morphologic measures of fibrosis (42).

Routine measurement of P_AO_2-P_aO_2 provides a fundamental evaluation of the resistance of the lung to the transfer of oxygen from the alveoli to capillary blood. Because P_AO_2-P_aO_2 depends on matching of ventilation to perfusion rather than on the gas exchange surface area, it complements the information provided by DL_{CO} measurements. Importantly, the P_AO_2-P_aO_2 at rest is often normal when fibrotic lung disease is present (106).

Clinicians commonly use the chest roentgenogram, vital capacity, TLC, DL_{CO}, and resting PaO_2 to monitor patients with fibrotic lung disease. These measurements may not correlate well with the degree of fibrosis measured on biopsy specimens (42,106). Fulmer and associates (42) reported that exercise changes in PaO_2 and P_AO_2-P_aO_2 were the most useful methods for staging and following alveolitis and fibrosis. However, these measures often have limited utility for patients with rheumatic disorders. Therefore, quantitative assessment of such patients may be best performed with composite clinical, radiographic, and physiologic scores (47). Such scores require adjustment for patients whose rheumatic joint or muscle disease precludes exercise.

E. Ventilatory Muscles

Assessment of ventilatory muscle function should be undertaken for patients with dyspnea and/or respiratory failure. The simplest method for clinical assessment involves a careful physical examination for evidence of accessory muscle recruitment. The scaleni, intercostals including parasternal intercostals, sternocleidomastoid, and abdominal muscle groups must each be examined. Active contraction of these muscle groups suggests an increased work of breathing and raises the possibility of ventilatory muscle fatigue or failure.

Laboratory assessment of ventilatory muscle function includes assessment of strength and endurance as well as evaluation of the pathophysiology of dysfunction (107). Measurement of maximal inspiratory and expiratory pressures, corrected for lung volume, confirms and quantitates the clinical impression of ventilatory muscle weakness. Measurement of maximal voluntary ventilation, a test of ventilatory muscle endurance, is limited by the confounding influences of airways resistance (108), patient effort, or malnutrition (109). Assessment of endurance with repetitive maximal inspiratory or expiratory contractions may obviate this problem (110).

References

1. Stupi, A. M., Steen, V. D., Owens, G. R., Barnes, E. L., Rodnan, G. P., and Medsger, T. A. (1986). Pulmonary hypertension in the CREST syndrome variant of systemic sclerosis. *Arthritis Rheum.* **29**:515-524.
2. Peters-Golden, M., Wise, R. A., Schneider, P., Hochberg, M., Stevens, M. B., and Wigley, F. (1984). Clinical and demographic predictors of loss of pulmonary function in systemic sclerosis. *Medicine* **63**(4):221-231.
3. Turner-Warwick, M., Burrows, B., and Johnson, A. (1980). Cryptogenic fibrosing alveolitis: Clinical features and their influence on survival. *Thorax* **35**:171-180.
4. Epler, G. R., McCloud, T. C., Gaensler, E. A., Minus, J. P., and Carrington, C. G. (1978). Normal chest roentgenograms in chronic diffuse interstitial lung disease. *N. Engl. J. Med.* **298**:934-939.
5. Frank, S. T., Weg, J. G., Harkleroad, L. E., and Fitch, R. F. (1973). Pulmonary dysfunction in rheumatoid arthritis. *Chest* **63**:27-34.
6. Davidson, C., Brooks, A. G. F., and Bacon, P. A. (1974). Lung function in rheumatoid arthritis. *Ann. Rheum. Dis.* **33**:293-297.
7. Popper, M. S., Bogdonoff, M. L., and Hughes, R. L. (1972). Interstitial rheumatoid lung disease. *Chest* **62**:243-450.
8. Huang, C., Hennigar, G. R., and Lyons, H. A. (1965). Pulmonary dysfunction in systemic lupus erythematosus. *N. Engl. J. Med.* **272**:288-293.
9. Gibson, G. J., Edmonds, J. P., and Hughes, G. R. V. (1977). Diaphragm function and lung involvement in systemic lupus erythematosus. *Am. J. Med.* **63**:926-932.
10. Smith, W., and Ball, G. V. (1980). Lung injury due to gold treatment. *Arthritis Rheum.* **23**:351-354.
11. Raghu, G. (1987). Idiopathic pulmonary fibrosis: A rational clinical approach. *Chest* **92**:148-154.
12. Owens, M. W., Kinasewitz, G. T., and Strain, D. S. (1986). Evaluating the effects of chronic therapy in patients with irreversible air-flow obstruction. *Am. Rev. Respir. Dis.* **134**:935-937.
13. Oren, A., Sue, D. Y., Hansen, J. E., Torrance, D. J., and Wasserman, K. (1987). The role of exercise testing in impairment evaluation. *Am. Rev. Respir. Dis.* **135**:230-235.

14. Renzetti, A. D. Jr., Bleeker, E. R., Epler, G. R., Jones, R. N., Kanner, R. E., and Repsher, L. H. (1986). Evaluation of impairment/disability secondary to respiratory disorders. *Am. Rev. Dis.* **133:**1205-1209.
15. Nelson, S. B. (1987). Commercially available spirometers: Performance evaluation. MS thesis, Department of Medical Informatics, University of Utah.
16. Gardner, R. M., Hankinson, J. L., Clausen, J. L., Crapo, R. O., Johnson, R. L. Jr., and Epler, G. R. (1986) Standardization of spirometry — 1987 update. *Am. Rev. Respir. Dis.* **136:**1285-1298.
17. Morris, A. H., Kanner, R. E., Crapo, R. O., and Gardner, R. M. (1984). *Clinical Pulmonary Function Testing: A Manual of Uniform Laboratory Procedures,* 2d ed. Intermountain Thoracic Society, Salt Lake City, UT.
18. Rosenberg, D. M., Weinberger, S. E., Fulmer, J. D., Flye, M. W., Fauci, A. S., and Crystal, R. G. (1980). Functional correlates of lung involvement in Wegener's granulomatosis. *Am. J. Med.* **69:**387-394.
19. Horns, J. W., O'Loughlin, B. J. (1962). Tracheal collapse in polychondritis. *A.J.R.* **87:**844-846.
20. Lawry, G., Finerman, M., Hanafee, W., Mancuso, A., Fan, P., and Bluestone, R. (1984). Laryngeal involvement in rheumatoid arthritis. *Arthritis Rheum.* **27:**873-882.
21. Kryger, M., Bode, F., Antic, R., and Anthonisen, N. (1976). Diagnosis of obstruction of the upper and central airways. *Am. J. Med.* **61:**85-93.
22. Forster, R. E., and Ogilvie, C. (1983). The single-breath carbon monoxide transfer 25 years on: A reappraisal. *Thorax* **38:**1-9.
23. Gelb, A. F., Gold, W. M., Wright, R. R., Bruch, H. R., and Nadel, J. A. (1973). Physiologic diagnosis of subclinical emphysema. *Am. Rev. Respir. Dis.* **107:**50-63.
24. Cotes, J. E. (1976). *Lung Function,* 4th ed. Blackwell Scientific Publications, London, p. 246.
25. Mohsenifar, Z., and Tashkin, D. P. (1979). Effect of carboxyhemoglobin on the single breath diffusing capacity: Derivation of an empirical correction factor. *Respiration* **87:**185-191.
26. Clausen, J., Crapo, R. O., and Gardner, R. M. (1984). Interlaboratory comparisons of pulmonary function testing [abstract]. *Am. Rev. Respir. Dis.* **129**(pt. 2):A37.
27. Morris, A. H., and Crapo, R. O. (1985). Standardization of computation of single-breath transfer factor. *Bull. Eur. Physiopathol. Respir.* **21:**183-189.
28. Crapo, R. O. (1986). DLCO reference equations: A perspective. *Am. Rev. Respir. Dis.* **134:**856.

29. Gray, G., Zamel, N., and Crapo. R. O. (1986). Effect of a simulated 3,048 meter altitude on the single-breath transfer factor. *Bull. Eur. Physiopathol. Respir.* **22**:429-431.
30. Kanner, R. E., and Crapo, R. O. (1986). The relationship between alveolar oxygen tension and the single-breath carbon monoxide diffusing capacity. *Am. Rev. Respir. Dis.* **133**:676-678.
31. Crapo, R. O. Personal communication.
32. Mohsenifar, Z., Tashkin, D. P., Vevy, S. E., Bjerje, R. D., Clements, P. J., and Furst, D. (1981). Lack of sensitivity of measurement of VD/VT at rest and during exercise in detection of hemodynamically significant pulmonary vascular abnormalities in collagen vascular disease. *Am. Rev. Respir. Dis.* **123**:508-512.
33. Wise, R. A., Wigley, F., Newball, H. H., and Stevens, M. B. (1982). The effect of cold exposure on diffusing capacity in patients with Raynaud's phenomenon. *Chest* **81**:695-698.
34. Miller, M. J. (1983). Effect of the cold pressor test on diffusing capacity: Comparison of normal subjects and those with Raynaud's disease and progressive systematic sclerosis. *Chest* **84**:264-266.
35. Fahey, P. J., Utell, M. J., Condemi, S. J., Green, R., and Hyde, R. W. (1984). Raynaud's phenomenon of the lung. *Am. J. Med.* **76**:263-269.
36. Ettinger, W. H., Wise, R. A., Stevens, M. B., and Wigley, F. M. (1983). Absence of positional change in pulmonary diffusing capacity in systematic sclerosis. *Am. J. Med.* **75**:305-311.
37. Ewan, P. W., Jones, H. A., Rhodes, C. G., and Hughes, J. M. B. (1976). Detection of intrapulmonary hemmorhage with carbon monoxide uptake. *N. Engl. J. Med.* **295**:1391-1396.
38. Jalowayski, A. A., Dawson, A., Zarins, L. P., and Clausen, J. L. (1982). *Pulmonary Function Testing: Guidelines and Controversies.* Academic Press, New York, pp. 115-163.
39. Barnhart, S., Hudson, L. D., Mason, S. E., Pierson, D. J., and Rosenstock, L. (1988). Total lung capacity: An insensitive measure of impairment in patients with asbestosis and chronic obstructive pulmonary disease? *Chest* **93**:299-302.
40. Austrian, R., McClement, J. H., Renzetti, A. D., Donald, K. W., Riley, R. L., and Cournand, A. (1951). Clinical and physiologic features of some types of pulmonary diseases with impairment of alveolar-capillary diffusion. *Am. J. Med.* **11**:667-685.
41. Crystal, R. G., Fulmer, J. D., Roberts, W. C., Moss, M. L., Fine, R. R., and Reynolds, H. Y. (1976). Idiopathic pulmonary fibrosis: Clinical, histologic, radiographic, physiologic, scintigraphic, cytologic, and biochemical aspects. *Ann. Intern. Med.* **85**:769-788.
42. Fulmer, J. D., Roberts, W. C., and Vongal, E. R. (1979). Morphologic-physiologic correlates of the severity of fibrosis and degree of cellularity in idiopathic pulmonary fibrosis. *J. Clin. Invest.* **63**:665-676.

43. Nadel, J. A., Gold, W. M., and Burgess, J. H. (1968). Early diagnosis of chronic pulmonary vascular obstruction. Value of pulmonary function tests. *Am. J. Med.* **44**:16-24.
44. Sue, D. Y., Oren, A., Hansen, J. E., and Wasserman, K. (1987). Diffusing capacity for carbon monoxide as a predictor of gas exchange during exercise. *N. Engl. J. Med.* **316**:1301-1306.
45. Ries, A. L., Fedullo, P. F., and Clausen, J. L. (1983). Rapid changes in arterial blood gas levels after exercise in pulmonary patients. *Chest* **83**:454-456.
46. Frye, M., Di Benedetto, R., Lain, D., and Morgan, K. (1988). Single arterial puncture vs. arterial cannula for arterial blood gas analysis after exercise. *Chest* **93**:294-298.
47. Watters, L. C., King, T. E., Schwarz, M. I., Waldron, J. A., Stanford, R. E., and Cherniack, R. M. (1986). A clinical, radiographic and physiologic scoring system for the longitudinal assessment of patients with idiopathic pulmonary fibrosis. *Am. Rev. Respir. Dis.* **133**:97-103.
48. Ries, A. L., Farrow, J. T., and Clausen, J. L. (1985). Accuracy of two ear oximeters at rest and during exercise in pulmonary patients. *Am. Rev. Respir. Dis.* **132**:685-689.
49. Risk, C., Epler, G. R., and Gaensler, E. A. (1984). Exercise alveolar-arterial oxygen pressure difference in interstitial disease. *Chest* **85**:69-74.
50. Owens, G. R., Rogers, R. M., Pennock, B. E., and Levin, D. (1984). The diffusing capacity as a predictor of arterial oxygen desaturation during exercise in patients with chronic obstructive pulmonary disease. *N. Engl. J. Med.* **310**:1218-1221.
51. D'Alonzo, G. E., Gianotti, L. A., Pohil, R. L., et al. (1987). Comparison of progressive exercise performance of normal subjects and patients with primary pulmonary hypertension. *Chest* **92**:57-62.
52. Jones, N. L. (1966). Physiologic dead space and alveolar gas pressure differences during exercise. *Clin. Sci.* **31**:19-29.
53. Black, L. F., and Hyatt, R. E. (1969). Maximal respiratory pressures: Normal values and relationship to age and sex. *Am. Rev. Respir. Dis.* **99**:696-702.
54. Walker, W. C., and Wright, V. (1968). Pulmonary lesions and rheumatoid arthritis. *Medicine* **47**:501-520.
55. Collins, R. L., Turner, R. A., Johnson, A. M., Whitley, N. O., and McLean, R. L. (1976). Obstructive pulmonary disease in rheumatoid arthritis. *Arthritis Rheum.* **19**:623-628.
56. Geddes, D. M., Corrin, B., Brewerton, D. A., Davies, R. J., and Turner-Warwick, M. (1977). Progressive airway obliteration in adults and its association with rheumatoid arthritis. *Q. J. Med.* **184**:427-444.
57. Begin, R., Masse, S., Cantin, A., Menard, H., and Bureau, M. (1982). Airway disease in a subset of non-smoking rheumatoid patients.

Characterization of the disease and evidence of an autoimmune pathogenesis. *Am. J. Med.* **1982**:743-749.

58. Baker, O. A., and Bywaters, E. G. L. (1957). Laryngeal stridor in rheumatoid arthritis due to crico-arytenoid joint involvement. *Br. Med. J.* **2**:140.
59. Gardner, D. L., Duthie, J. J. R., MacLeod, J., and Allan, W. S. A. (1957). Pulmonary hypertension in rheumatoid arthritis. *Scot. Med. J.* **2**:183-188.
60. Huang, C. T., and Lyons, H. A. (1966). Comparison of pulmonary function in patients with systemic lupus erythematosus, scleroderma, and rheumatoid arthritis. *Am. Rev. Respir. Dis.* **93**:865-875.
61. Jordan, J. D., and Snyder, C. H. (1964). Rheumatoid disease of the lung and cor pulmonale. *Am. J. Dis. Child.* **108**:174-180.
62. Hoffbrand, B. I., and Beck, E. R. (1965). Unexplained dyspnoea and shrinking lungs in systemic lupus erythematosus. *Br. Med. J.* **1**:1273-1277.
63. Eisenberg, H., Dubois, E. L., Sherwin, R. P., and Balchum, O. J. (1973). Diffuse interstitial lung disease in systemic lupus erythematosus. *Ann. Intern. Med.* **79**:37-45.
64. Gold, W. M., and Jennings, D. B. (1966). Pulmonary function in paients with systemic lupus erythematosus. *Am. Rev. Respir. Dis.* **93**:566-567.
65. Kinney, W. W., and Angellillo, V. A. (1982). Bronchiolitis in systemic lupus erythematosis. *Chest* **82**:646-648.
66. Martens, J., Dermedts, M., Vanmeenen, M. T., Dequeker, J. (1983). Respiratory muscle dysfunction in systemic lupus erythematosus. *Chest* **84**:170-175.
67. Nair, S. S., Askari, A. D., Popelka, C. G., and Kleinerman, J. F. (1980). Pulmonary hypertension and systemic lupus erythematosus. *Arch. Intern. Med.* **140**:109-111.
68. Baldwin, E., Cournand, A., and Richards, D. W. Jr. (1949). Pulmonary insufficiency. II: A study of 39 cause of pulmonary fibrosis. *Medicine* **28**:1-25.
69. Spain, D. M., and Thomas, A. G. (1950). The pulmonary manifestations of scleroderma: An anatomic-physiologic correlation. *Ann. Intern. Med.* **32**:152-161.
70. Ritchie, B. (1964). Pulmonary function in scleroderma. *Thorax* **19**:28-36.
71. Hughes, D. T. D., and Lee, F. I. (1963). Lung function in patients with systematic sclerosis. *Thorax* **18**:16-20.
72. Owens, G. R., Fina, G. L., Herbert, D. L., et al. (1983). Pulmonary function in progressive systemic sclerosis. *Chest* **84**:546-550.
73. Sackner, M. A., Akgun, N., Kimbel, P., and Lewis, D. H. (1964). The pathophysiology of scleroderma involving the heart and respiratory system. *Ann. Intern. Med.* **60**:611-630.
74. Guttadauria, M., Ellman, H., Emmanuel, G., Kaplan, D., and Dia-

mond, H. (1977). Pulmonary function in scleroderma. *Arthritis Rheum.* **20**:1071-1079.

75. Colp., C. R., Riker, J., and Williams, M. H. Jr. (1973). Serial changes in scleroderma and idiopathic interstitial lung disease. *Arch. Intern. Med.* **132**:506-515.
76. Schneider, P. D., Wise, R. A., Hochberg, M. C., and Wigley, F. M. (1982). Serial pulmonary function in systemic sclerosis. *Am. J. Med.* **73**:385-394.
77. Greenwald, G. I., Tashkin, D. P., Gong, H., et al. (1987). Longitudinal changes in lung function and respiratory symptoms in progressive systemic sclerosis. *Am. J. Med.* **83**:83-92.
78. Steen, V. D., Owens, G. R., Redmond, C., Rodnan, G. P., and Medsger, T. A. Jr. (1985). The effect of D-penicillamine on pulmonary findings in systemic sclerosis. *Arthritis Rheum.* **28(8)**:882-888.
79. Olsen, G. N., and Swensen, E. W. (1972). Polymyositis and interstitial lung disease. *Am. Rev. Respir. Dis.* **105**:611-617.
80. Camp, A. V., Lane, D. J., and Mowat, A. G. (1972). Dermatomyositis with parenchymal lung involvement. *Br. Med. J.* **1**:155-156.
81. Duncan, P. E., Griffin, J. P., Garcia, A., and Kaplan, S. B. (1974). Fibrosing alveolitis in polymyositis. *Am. J. Med.* **57**:621-626.
82. Frazier, A. R., and Miller, R. D. (1974). Interstitial pneumonitis in association with polymyositis and dermatomyositis. *Chest* **65**:403-407.
83. Caldwell, I. W., and Aitchison, J. D. (1956). Pulmonary hypertension in dermatomyositis. *Br. Heart J.* **18**:273-276.
84. Bunch, T. W., Tancredi, R. G., and Lie, J. T. (1981). Pulmonary hypertension in polymyositis. *Chest* **79**:105-107.
85. Vitali, C., Tavoni, A., Viegi, G., Begliomini, E., Agnesi, A., and Bombardieri, S. (1985). Lung involvement in Sjögren's syndrome: a comparison between patients with primary and with secondary syndrome. *Ann. Rheum. Dis.* **44**:455-461.
86. Bariffi, F., Pesci, A., Bertorelli, G., Manganelli, P., and Ambanelli, U. (1984). Pulmonary involvement in Sjogren's syndrome. *Respiration* **46**:82-87.
87. Newball, H. H., and Brahim, S. A. (1977). Chronic obstructive airway disease in patients with Sjogren's syndrome. *Am. Rev. Respir. Dis.* **115**:295-304.
88. Strimlan, C. V., Rosenow, E. C., Divertie, M. B., and Harrison, E. G. (1976). Pulmonary manifestations of Sjogren's syndrome. *Chest* **70**:354-361.
89. Harmon, C., Wolfe, F., Lillard, S., Held, C., Condon, R., and Sharp, G. C. (1976). Pulmonary involvement in mixed connective tissue disease (MCTD) [Abstract]. *Arthritis Rheum.* **19**:801.
90. Derderian, S. S., Tellis, C. J., Abbrecht, P. H., Welton, R. C., and Rajagopal, K. R. (1985). Pulmonary involvement in mixed connective tissue disease. *Chest* **88**:45-89.

91. Jones, M. B., Osterholm, R. K., Wilson, R. B., Martin, F. H., Commers, J. R., and Bachmayer, J. D. (1978). Fatal pulmonary hypertension and resolving immune-complex glomerulonephritis in mixed connective tissue diesease. *Am. J. Med.* **65**:855-863.

92. Guit, G. L., Shaw, P. C., Ehrlich, J., Kroon, H. M., and Oudkirk, M. (1985). Mediastinal lymphadenopathy and pulmonary arterial hypertension in mixed connective tissue disease. *Radiology* **154**:305-306.

93. Gacad, G., and Hamosh, P. (1975). The lung in ankylosing spondylitis. *Am. Rev. Respir. Dis.* **107**:286-289.

94. Miller, J. M., and Sproule, B. J. (1964). Pulmonary function in ankylosing spondylitis. *Am. Rev. Respir. Dis.* **90**:376-382.

95. Renzetti, A. D., Nicholas, W., Dutton, R. E., and Jivoff, L. (1960). Some effects of ankylosing spondylitis on pulmonary gas exchange. *N. Engl. J. Med.* **262**:215-218.

96. Feltelius, N., Hedenstrom, H., Hillerdal, G., and Hallgren, R. (1986). Pulmonary involvement in ankylosing spondylitis. *Ann. Rheumatol. Dis.* **45**:736-740.

97. Elliott, C. G., Hill, T. R., Adams, T. E., Crapo, R. O., Nietrzeba, R. M., and Gardner, R. M. (1985). Exercise performance of subjects with ankylosing spondylitis and limited chest expansion. *Bull. Eur. Physiopathol. Respir.* **21**:363-368.

98. Sharp, J. T., Sweany, S. K., Henry, J. P., et al. (1964). Lung and thoracic compliances in ankylosing spondylitis. *J. Lab. Clin. Med.* **63**:254-263.

99. Zorab, P. A. (1962). The lungs in ankylosing spondylitis. *Q. J. Med.* **31**:267-280.

100. Hauge, B. (1973). Diaphragmatic movements and spirometric volume in patients with ankylosing spondylitis. *Scand. J. Respir. Dis.* **54**:38-44.

101. Ehrlich, J. C., and Romanoff, A. (1951). Allergic granuloma of lung: Clinical and anatomic findings in a patient with bronchial asthma and eosinophilia. *Arch. Intern. Med.* **87**:259-268.

102. Shim, C., Corro, P., Park, S. S., and Williams, M. H. (1972). Pulmonary function studies in patients with upper airway obstruction. *Am. Rev. Respir. Dis.* **106**:233-238.

103. Fulmer, J. D., Roberts, W. C., Von Gal, E. R., and Crystal, R. G. (1977). Small airways in idiopathic pulmonary fibrosis. *J. Clin. Invest.* **60**:595-610.

104. Reeves, J. T., and Groves, B. M. (1984). In *Pulmonary Hypertension* Edited by Weir, E. K., and J. T. Reeves, Futura, Mount Kisco, N.Y.

105. Wilson, R. J., Rodnan, G. P., and Robin, E. D. (1964). An early pulmonary physiologic abnormality in progressive systemic sclerosis. *Am. J. Med.* **36**:361-369.

106. Crystal, R. G., Fulmer, J. D., Roberts, W. C., Moss, M. L., Line, B. R., and Reynolds, H. Y. (1976). Idiopathic pulmonary fibrosis: Clinical, histologic, radiographic, physiologic, scintigraphic, cytologic, and biochemical aspects. *Ann. Intern. Med.* **85:**769-788.
107. Rochester, D. F. (1988). Clinics in chest medicine. Respiratory muscles: Function in health and disease. *Tests Respir. Muscle Funct.* **9:**249-263.
108. Aldrich, T. K., Arora, N. S., and Rochester, D. F. (1982). The influence of airway obstruction and respiratory muscle strength on maximal voluntary ventilation in lung disease. *Am. Rev. Respir. Dis.* **126:**195-199.
109. Arora, N. S., and Rochester, D. F. (1982). Respiratory muscle strength and maximal voluntary ventilation in undernourished patients. *Am. Rev. Respir. Dis.* **126:**5.
110. McKenzie, D. K., and Gandevia, S. C. (1986). Strength and endurance of inspiratory, expiratory, and limb muscles in asthma. *Am. Rev. Respir. Dis.* **134:**999-1004.

4

Chest Radiography and Other Imaging Techniques

IRENA M. TOCINO

University of Utah and LDS Hospital
Salt Lake City, Utah

The collagen vascular diseases and the angiitis-granulomatosis syndromes comprise a complex group of maladies displaying a rich spectrum of clinical and radiographic pulmonary manifestations. The diverse susceptibility of each organ system often results in a characteristic set of radiographic findings peculiar to each of these disorders. Similar pulmonary radiographic manifestations, such as interstitial infiltrates, honeycombing, and pleural effusion, may occur in several of the collagen vascular diseases. However, integrating these findings with the clinical presentation and other associated radiographic chest observations, such as skeletal abnormalities or esophageal dilatation, will usually differentiate an individual disease. On the other hand, a broad overlap of radiographic findings occurs in the angiitis-granulomatosis syndromes. For example, ill-defined alveolar infiltrates and nodules progressing to cavity formation are present in most of the vasculitides. In this group of diseases a specific diagnosis may not be possible from the radiograph.

The present discussion will review the radiographic manifestations of the so-called classic collagen vascular diseases (1) which include rheumatoid arthritis, systemic lupus erythematosus, progressive systemic sclerosis, dermatomyositis, and Sjögren's syndrome. In the angiitis-granulomatosis group, discussion will be limited to the two most common diseases, Wegener's granulomatosis and lymphomatoid granulomatosis. The radiographic manifestations of these groups of diseases have been recently reviewed by Feigin (2) and provide a valuable source of current information.

I. Rheumatoid Arthritis

In contrast to the higher incidence of rheumatoid arthritis (RA) in females, pleuropulmonary manifestations are more common in males (3). By the time pulmonary involvement manifests, the patient usually has a long history of arthritis. Occasionally, however, pleuritis and pleural effusion may be the first clinical manifestation of the disease in patients with positive serology but without joint complaints (4,5). The radiographic findings can be separated into those affecting the pleura and those involving the lung parenchyma (Table 1).

A. Pleural Involvement

Pleuritis and pleural effusions are the most common radiographic abnormalities. Pleurisy has been described in 21% of patients with RA, but pleural thickening and adhesions are found in as many as 50% of RA patients at autopsy (1). The pleural effusions are often unilateral and commonly become

Table 1   Chest Radiograph Findings in Collagen Vascular Diseases

Findings	RA/SJ	SLE	PSS/DM	AS
Pleural effusions	Very common	Very common	No	Very common
Small irregular shadows	Basilar	Uncommon	Basilar, very common	No
Honeycombing	Common	Rare	Very common	No
Apical bullae	No	No	No	Very common
Nodules	Often	Rare	No	No
Cavitation	Often	Very rare	No	Apical
Pulmonary hypertension	Rare	Rare	Common	No

RA, rheumatoid arthritis; SLE, systemic lupus erythematosus; PSS, progressive systemic sclerosis; DM, dermatomyositis; AS, ankylosing spondylitis; SJ, Sjogren's syndrome.

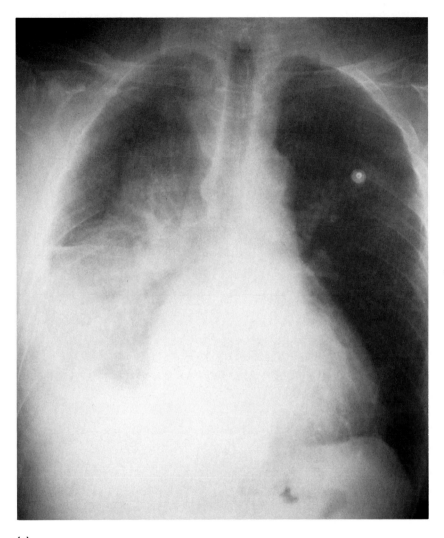

(a)

Figure 1 Rheumatoid arthritis. (a) Large pleural effusion loculated within the major fissure. No visible underlying parenchymal disease (the round density in the left upper lung field is an artifact). (b) Spontaneous pneumothorax loculated within the major fissure. Note air-fluid level (arrowheads).

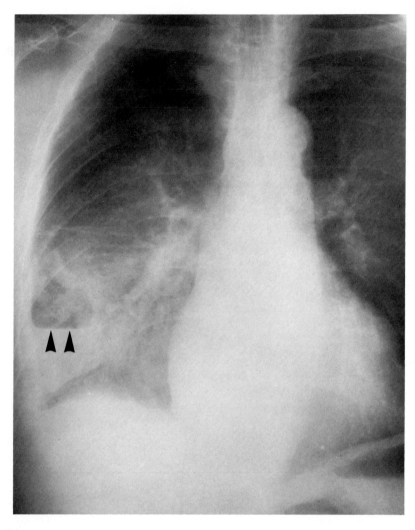

(b)

loculated (6) (Fig. 1a). Although loculations may develop from simple adhesions, empyema should always be strongly suspected, since these patients often are placed on chronic steroid therapy. An air-fluid level from rupture of subpleural blebs or frank pneumothorax from rupture of necrobiotic nodules causing bronchopleural fistula formation may further complicate pleural effusions (7) (Fig. 1b). The effusions remain chronic or tend to recur (8), occasionally requiring thoracentesis or, more rarely, sclerotherapy.

B. Parenchymal Involvement

Some parenchymal involvement, most commonly necrobiotic nodules, will occur in almost a third of patients with pleural effusions. Multiple round nodules, histologically similar to those present in periarticular subcutaneous tissue, develop subpleurally in RA patients. The subpleural nodules often cavitate, yielding a spectrum of cavities varying from thick irregular walls to very thin, well-defined walls in the same patient (Fig. 2). A solitary pulmonary nodule may be the only manifestation of parenchymal disease. Nodule size can change rapidly, a variability that often corresponds to the activity of the arthritis (9,10).

The combination of a subpleural location and the tendency to excavate can cause a pneumothorax to develop in an otherwise asymptomatic pulmonary nodule. In up to 50% of RA patients, necrobiotic nodules may be associated with diffuse interstitial lung disease, although the radiographic findings may be subtle. In patients with severe interstitial fibrosis, the nodules may be obscured completely by the parenchymal infiltrates on chest films and may be detectable only by computerized tomography (11).

Diffuse Interstitial Lung Disease

Interstitial lung disease in RA patients correlates with the joint disease severity, ranging from an incidence of just 1% in mild RA to a 30-40% association in patients with severe joint deformity. Furthermore, a significant number of patients with abnormal pulmonary function tests may have a normal chest radiograph (12) (see also Chap. 3). Interstitial infiltrates are depicted radiographically as small, irregular "shadows" or opacities located predominantly in the lung bases (Fig. 3). This term, borrowed by Felson (13) from the UICC/Cincinnati classification of pneumoconiosis, very precisely describes the early radiographic changes of interstitial lung disease in patients with collagen vascular disease and other processes such as interstitial pneumonias. Other terms used to describe this appearance include "reticular and reticulonodular densities," "ground glass densities," and "increased interstitial markings." Thickened interlobular septa, called Kerley A and B lines, are often present on the radiograph in association with small irregular shadows.

Eventually the infiltrates extend to the upper lung fields. The ensuing interstitial fibrosis is defined radiographically by areas of honeycombing. Honeycombing indicates the presence of round or polygonal air cysts with a well-defined wall measuring less than 5 mm in diameter (13) (Fig. 4). Thin-section CT is able to detect these small air cysts and surrounding small irregular shadows, offering a better definition of the extent of the disease (11). The cysts may eventually become confluent, forming large, destructive cavities

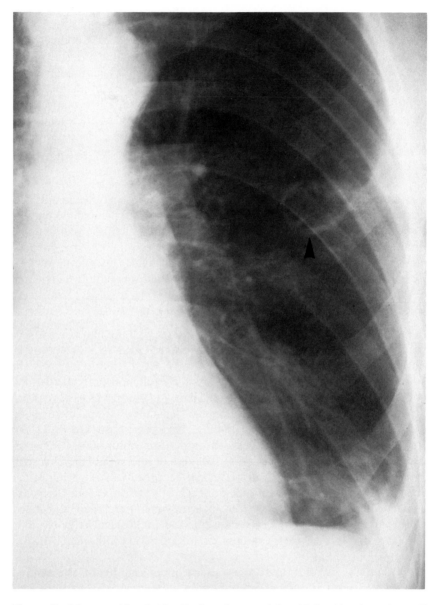

Figure 2 Rheumatoid arthritis. Cavitary lung nodule with knobby, irregular wall in left upper lobe (arrowhead). Ill-defined nodule and small pleural effusion in left costophrenic angle.

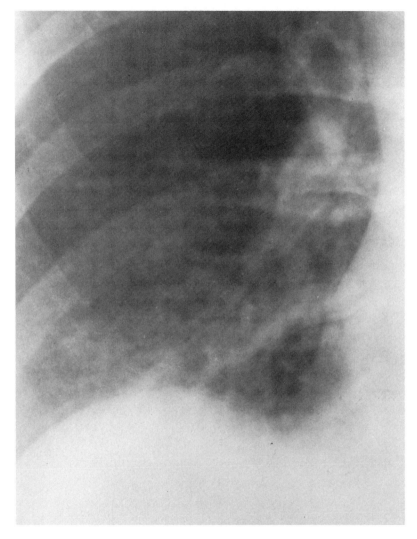

Figure 3 Rheumatoid arthritis. Small irregular shadows are present in the lung base, obscuring lower lobe vascular structures and contour of the diaphragm.

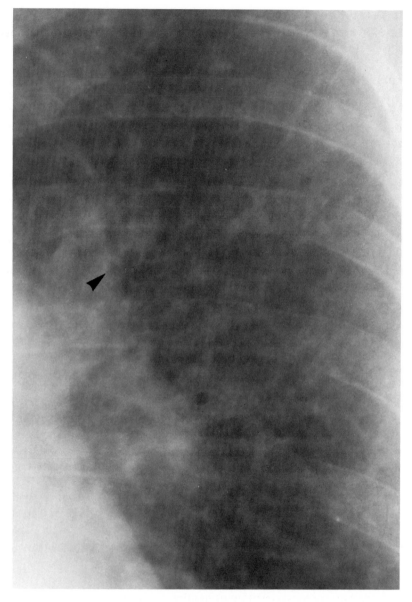

Figure 4   Rheumatoid arthritis. Diffuse lung involvement with small irregular shadows and areas of honeycombing representing lung fibrosis (arrowhead).

in the subpleural space. If rupture occurs, pneumothorax often results. Severe interstitial lung disease is invariably associated with progressive volume loss and elevation of the diaphragm.

In patients with both RA and a heavy smoking history, the honeycombing of the lung can be associated with extensive emphysema. Rather than the typical contraction of lung volume by interstitial fibrosis, hyperinflation of the lung with depressed diaphragms will be present. Marked hyperinflation and abnormal pulmonary function tests indicating airway obstruction also suggest the diagnosis of bronchiolitis obliterans in RA patients,* particularly if penicillamine has been administered (see Chap. 14).

In a small percentage of patients receiving gold therapy, a diffuse perihilar alveolar infiltrate similar to that seen in acute pulmonary edema may be a first sign of gold toxicity. The infiltrates resolve rapidly after discontinuing the drug (14) (see also Chap. 14).

Parenchymal infiltrates in the lung bases may be a sign of aspiration pneumonia in patients with involvement of arytenoid cartilages. Lobar or segmental consolidation in RA patients is undoubtedly the result of infectious pneumonia; an opportunistic infection should be suspected in patients receiving corticosteroids.

Caplan's Syndrome

Also referred to as rheumatoid pneumoconiosis, Caplan's syndrome was first described in coal miners in Wales. The initial radiographic description reported the combination of simple pneumoconiosis and superimposed round opacities. In contrast to the opacities of progressive massive fibrosis (PMF), these lesions are well defined, round, and peripheral in location, and they can change rapidly in size or even disappear spontaneously (1). They are located in the upper lobes and may become coalescent as in PMF but do not have the associated scarring, retraction, or central migration characteristic of PMF.

The lesions may cavitate; when solitary, they may be indistinguishable from a cavitated neoplasm or tuberculosis. A broader definition of Caplan's syndrome has been proposed to include other pulmonary manifestations of RA such as diffuse interstitial lung disease in patients with pneumoconiosis (15).

C. Pulmonary Hypertension

A radiographic pattern consisting of multiple nodules, representing enlarged pulmonary vessels viewed end on, occurs in those patients with RA and severe

---

*Editors note: Bronchiolitis can also cause pulmonary function abnormalities consistent with lung restriction.

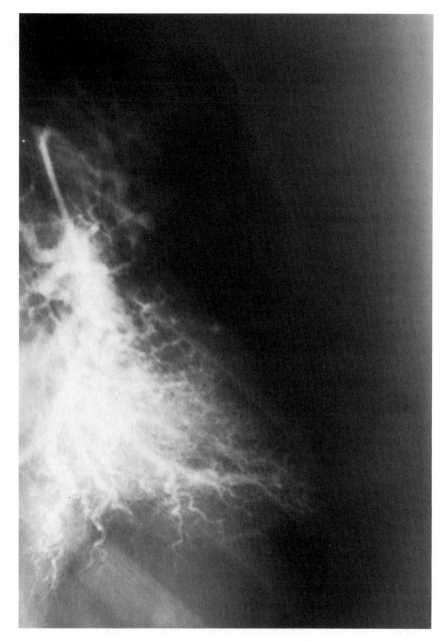

Figure 5 Rheumatoid arthritis. Pulmonary arteriogram left lower lobe. Corkscrew appearance of pulmonary arteries and severe "pruning" of vascular tree. Crowding of the vessels by volume loss. Severe vasculitis demonstrated at autopsy.

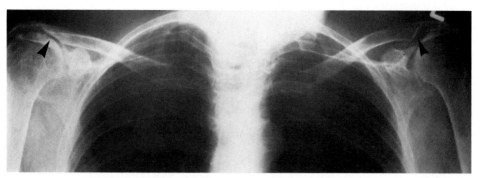

Figure 6 Rheumatoid arthritis. Severe osteoporosis and resorption of distal ends of clavicles bilaterally (arrowheads).

vasculitis (16). Detection of main pulmonary artery enlargement may be prevented by obliteration of hilar contours by the diffuse parenchymal disease. We have encountered two cases in whom the pulmonary vasculature mimicked nodular disease, causing a granulomatous infection to be suspected. A lung biopsy revealed almost complete obliteration of small-size arterioles but no parenchymal nodules (Fig. 5). Overall, pulmonary hypertension occurs infrequently in RA (16).

D. Skeletal Changes

Marked osteoporosis is a constant radiographic finding in RA patients. Resorption of the distal ends of the clavicles (Fig. 6) or, less commonly, of the proximal ends of the clavicles is virtually pathognomonic of RA and is one additional manifestation of the erosive changes occurring elsewhere, particularly in the peripheral skeleton. Close examination of the clavicles for these features should be prompted by the presence of honeycombing on the chest radiograph.

II. Progressive Systemic Sclerosis

Within the group of collagen vascular diseases, scleroderma has the highest incidence of pulmonary parenchymal involvement. Interstitial fibrosis is present at autopsy in the majority of patients (1). The radiographic findings, however, may be subtle or absent, with detectable diffuse interstitial lung disease and honeycombing present only in the more severe forms of the disease (Table 1). Initially, bilateral and symmetrical small irregular shadows are found in the lung bases on the chest film (Figs. 7, 8a). It remains uncertain

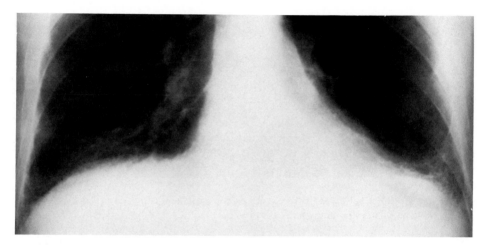

Figure 7 Scleroderma. Coned-down view of the lung bases shows small irregular shadows with shaggy heart borders and diaphragmatic contours.

whether these infiltrates represent the early stages of interstitial lung fibrosis or represent repeated episodes of aspiration pneumonia secondary to an esophageal motility disorder. The presence of a dilated esophagus without an air fluid level indicates esophageal dysfunction. According to Mahrer et al., an abnormal esophagus can be identified on the chest film in 62% of patients with scleroderma (17) (Fig. 8b,c). As the disease advances, the interstitial infiltrates migrate to peripheral zones of the lungs with progressive honeycomb formation and subsequent breakdown into large confluent air cysts (2) that may lead to pneumothorax (18). Progressive lung volume loss manifested by a serially diminishing diameter between the lung apex and the diaphragm can be readily observed on sequential chest radiographs (2) (Fig. 8).

In contrast to rheumatoid arthritis, pleural effusion does not develop in progressive systemic sclerosis, but pleural thickening may be recognized occasionally. Alveolar cell carcinoma can complicate all diseases having pulmonary fibrosis and has been described in patients with scleroderma (19). Pulmonary hypertension may develop in patients with scleroderma with progressive increase in size of the central pulmonary arteries detectable in sequential chest radiographs.

III. Polymyositis/Dermatomyositis

Radiographically, the pulmonary manifestations of polymyositis and dermatomyositis are similar to those seen in patients with scleroderma (Fig. 9a).

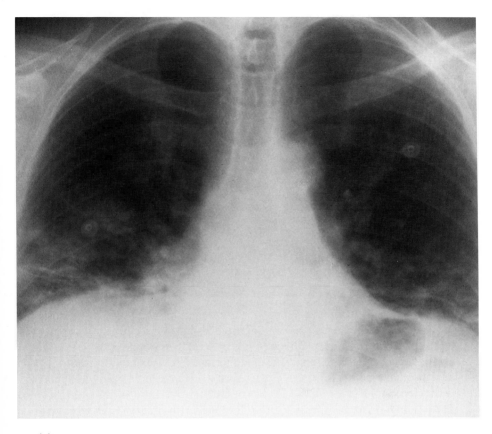

(a)

Figure 8 Scleroderma. (a, b) Diffuse parenchymal infiltrates (small irregular shadows and honeycombing) are apparent in the posteroanterior (a) and lateral (b) views. While the disease involves the lung bases most severely, infiltrates are also present in the upper lung fields. A generalized decrease in lung volume is also apparent (the rounded densities in the left upper and right lower lung field are artifacts). (c) A dilated esophagus visible on the lateral view (arrowheads) is confirmed by barium swallow.

Esophageal motility disorders in patients with dermatomyositis lead to repeated episodes of aspiration pneumonia commonly resulting in diffuse bibasilar alveolar infiltrates on the chest films (2). The involvement of pharyngeal muscles and ineffective cough due to weakness of chest wall muscles aggravates the tendency of these patients to aspirate (2). In the presence of diffuse interstitial fibrosis as represented by honeycombing radiographically,

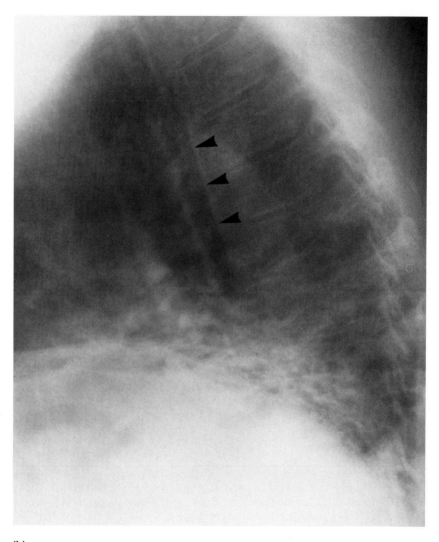

(b)
Figure 8 (continued)

alveolar cell cancer may develop (19). Therefore, a focal, slow-growing infiltrate or bilateral indolent alveolar infiltrates should elicit the differential
diagnosis of infection or alveolar cell carcinoma (Fig. 9b). Finally, in patients receiving methotrexate treatment, a hypersensitivity pneumonitis with
bilateral parenchymal infiltrates and pleural effusions may occur, which is

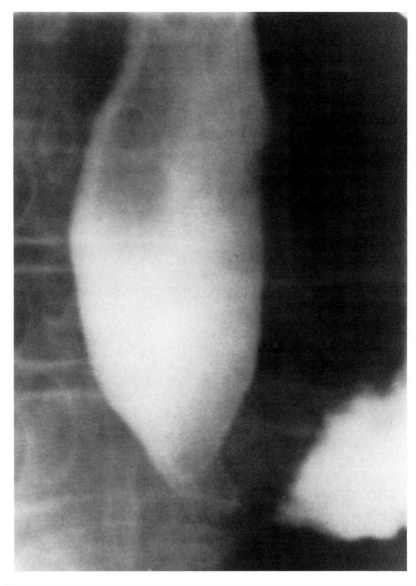

(c)

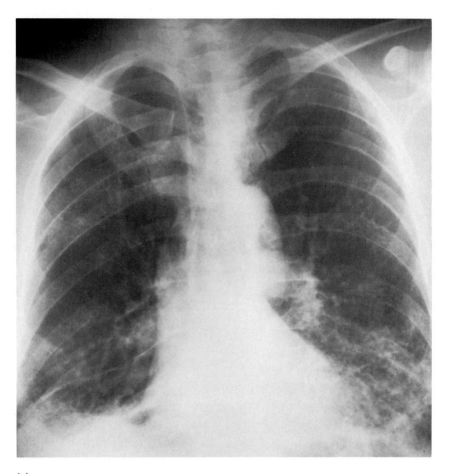

(a)

Figure 9 Dermatomyositis. (a) After a 4-year history of dermatomyositis this patient has bilateral lower lung infiltrates with honeycombing and volume loss. (b) A
localized alveolar infiltrate and right pleural effusion developed during the subsequent year. A transbronchial biopsy revealed alveolar cell carcinoma.

often easily reversible after discontinuation of the therapy with this drug
(see Chap. 14).

IV. Sjögren's Syndrome

Because of the common association of Sjögren's syndrome with RA, most
of the pulmonary manifestations of rheumatoid disease apply to Sjögren's

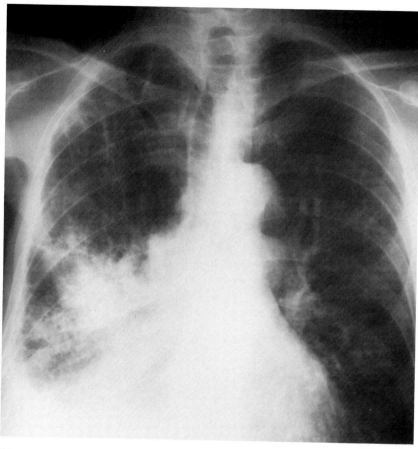

(b)

syndrome. In particular, diffuse interstitial parenchymal infiltrates progressing to honeycombing commonly develop in Sjögren's syndrome. Pulmonary parenchymal involvement was detected in 9% and pleural effusion in 16% of 31 patients studied by Strimlan et al. (21). Sjögren's syndrome is particularly distinguished by the prevalence of pulmonary lymphoproliferative disorders. There exists a spectrum ranging from the benign infiltrates of lymphocytic interstitial pneumonitis (LIP) (Fig. 10) and pseudolymphma to the malignant infiltrates of true lymphoma (1). The radiographic findings do not differentiate among the lymphoproliferative disorders. They all share a nonspecific pattern of diffuse alveolar infiltrates and ill-defined nodules. A masslike presentation is more often seen in pseudolymphoma; pleural

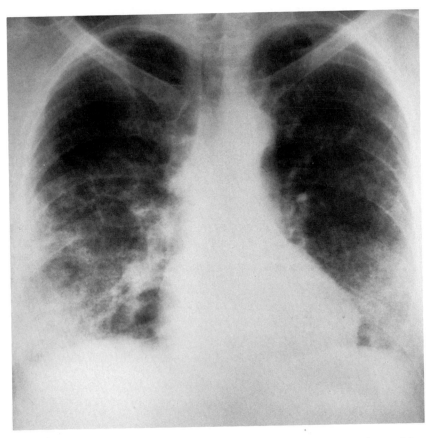

Figure 10   Lymphocytic interstitial pneumonia (LIP) in Sjögren's syndrome. Note diffuse peripheral alveolar infiltrates superimposed on background of honeycombing, which was found to represent LIP at autopsy.

effusions may be more common in patients with lymphoma. Amyloidosis has also been reported in association with Sjögren's syndrome and can present with ill-defined nodules on a background of interstitial lung disease.

V. Systemic Lupus Erythematosus (SLE)

Pines et al. recently reviewed the pleuropulmonary manifestations of SLE (22). The incidence of radiographic abnormalities approached 70% if complications such as infectious pneumonia were included. Most commonly, pleural effusion and pleural thickening occur in 50-75% of SLE patients

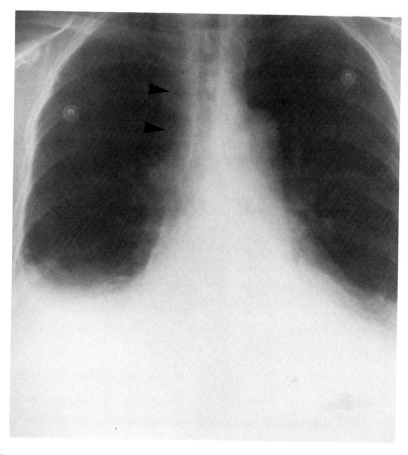

Figure 11 Systemic lupus erythematosus. Bilateral subpulmonic pleural effusions and enlargement of cardiopericardial silhouette by pericardial effusion. Also wide mediastinum caused by fat deposition following steroid treatment (arrowheads). Linear atelectasis present in lung bases bilaterally.

(23,24) (Table 1). Pericardial effusion is often concomitant. A characteristic appearance of small lung volumes often signals the SLE patient. The decreased lung volumes in part reflect compression by bilateral subpulmonic pleural effusions (Fig. 11). In addition, elevation of the diaphragms may result from diaphragmatic dysfunction often present in those SLE patients with generalized muscle involvement. Often the cause of dyspnea in the supine position, diaphragmatic dysfunction is a reversible condition (25).

Parenchymal abnormalities of SLE can be classified as follows:

A. Atelectasis

Atelectasis associated with decreased lung volume often presents as transient, linear densities at lung bases. Atelectasis occurs most commonly in patients with pleural effusions and diaphragmatic dysfunction (Fig. 11). In other SLE patients pulmonary infarctions can result in linear scars that tend to resolve more slowly than atelectasis (2).

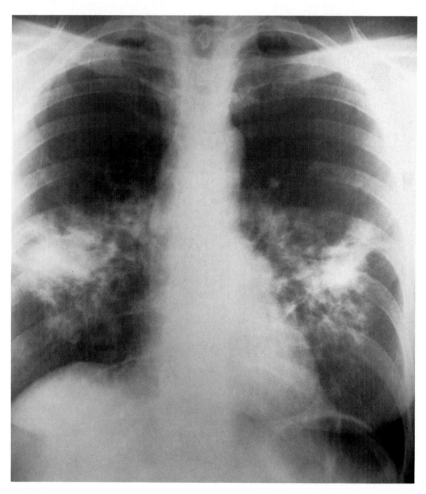

Figure 12 Systemic lupus erythematosus. Bilateral perihilar alveolar infiltrates in this patient resolved rapidly after steroid treatment. The infiltrates were considered to represent lupus pneumonitis.

B. Lupus Pneumonitis

Lupus pneumonitis presents radiographically as bilateral basilar alveolar infiltrates and clinically as pneumonia (Fig. 12). However, lupus pneumonitis can be diagnosed only after exclusion of microbial infection, which occurs frequently in SLE patients. Lupus may also present as nodules that tend to

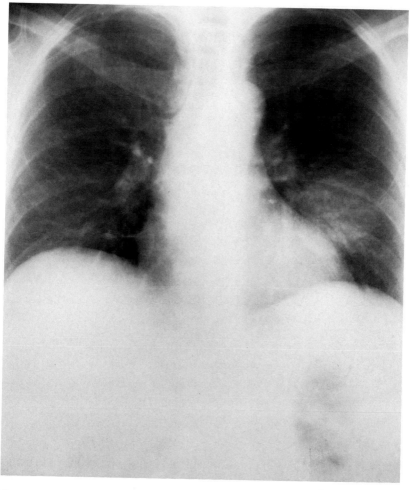

(a)

Figure 13 Systemic lupus erythematosus. (a, b) Pleural-based round mass in posteroanterior (a) and lateral (b) chest radiographs. (c) Chest CT prior to percutaneous biopsy of lesion shows a lucent, necrotic center. Needle aspirate yielded *Nocardia*.

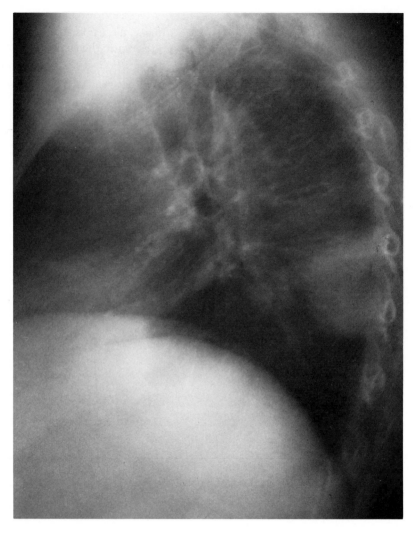

(b)

Figure 13 (continued)

cavitate. For this variety of lupus, opportunistic infection and septic emboli should first be excluded. The rapid clearing of the infiltrates after cortico-steroid treatment supports the diagnosis of lupus pneumonitis (26).

C. Diffuse Interstitial Disease

In a small percentage of patients, a pattern of diffuse, small, irregular shad-ows similar to those found in RA has been reported in patients with SLE (27).

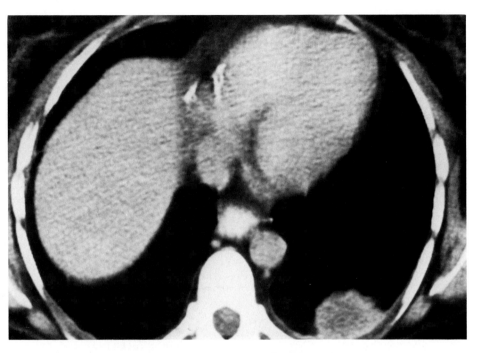

(c)

Lymphoproliferative disorders present as diffuse parenchymal infiltrates or localized pulmonary masses in SLE patients as in Sjögren's syndrome. Parenchymal infiltrates related to drug toxicity in patients treated with cyclophosphamide and azathioprine (Chap. 14) may be diffuse or localized.

D. Acute Alveolar Infiltrates

Bacterial pneumonia causes most alveolar infiltrates in SLE patients, and aggressive search for organisms is mandatory (Fig. 13). Pulmonary edema caused by renal failure should be considered if bilateral perihilar infiltrates are noted. Mediastinal contour changes indicating pericardial effusion or enlargement of the superior vena cava and the azygos vein provide excellent additional evidence of fluid overload from renal failure. Pulmonary hemorrhage, although uncommon, may be responsible for the acute onset of diffuse alveolar infiltrates in SLE (24,28).

A pleural-based parenchymal infiltrate having a round or triangular shape and associated with a pleural effusion strongly suggests a pulmonary infarction, a common event in patients with SLE (22). The phenomena responsible for the thromboembolic disease probably cause the pulmonary hypertension in SLE (29).

E. Mediastinal Abnormalities

Mediastinal widening with a double contour of the superior vena cava and aortic knob is often due to fat deposition in patients treated with corticosteroids (Fig. 11, arrowheads).

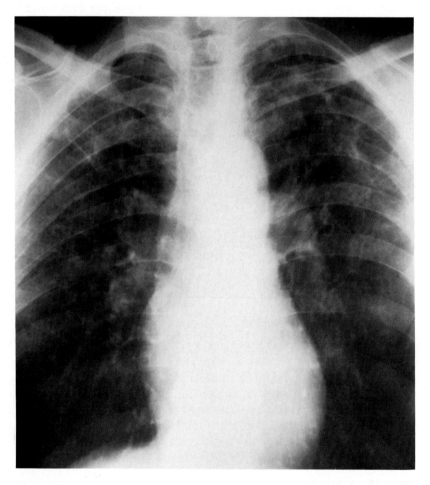

Figure 14 Ankylosing spondylitis. Note fibronodular lesions in both upper lobes with retraction of the hila toward the apices.

VI. Ankylosing Spondylitis (AS)

The classic skeletal manifestations of AS on the chest radiograph include ossification of the spinal ligaments and fusion of vertebral bodies. In addition, a small number of patients (less than 5%) have lung involvement (Fig. 14). Rosenow et al. reported an incidence of 1.3% among 2,080 subjects with AS (30). The most common finding in that series was apical fibrobullous changes that initially affected one lung but eventually involved both upper lobes symmetrically (Fig. 15). Pleural thickening in the apices may be an early manifestation of AS but cannot be distinguished from a similar-appearing nonspecific abnormality that occurs in the normal population. Superinfection

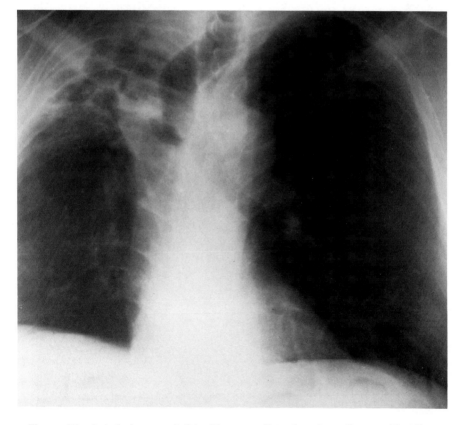

Figure 15 Ankylosing spondylitis. Observe unilateral cavitary disease with collapse of the right upper lobe. Also note tracheal displacement caused by the right upper lobe volume loss and fibrosis.

of the bullae with aspergillus results in formation of the so-called fungus ball, a round structure freely mobile within the bullae. Pneumothorax occurs but is not a common complication, even in the presence of large bullae.

Pleural effusions and empyema are rare; however, if a thoracotomy has been performed, bronchopleural fistula and empyema may be more common than in the overall population. A dilated ascending aorta due to aortitis and aortic insufficiency may be recognized on the chest radiograph of these patients.

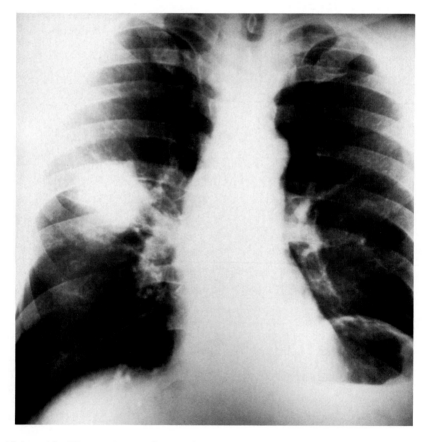

Figure 16 Wegener's granulomatosis. Note the solitary round alveolar opacification in the right midlung, which eventually cavitated.

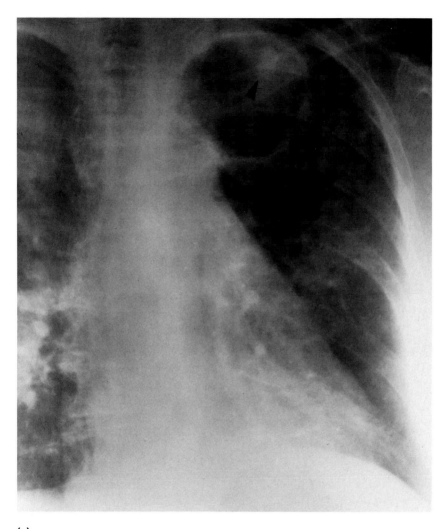

(a)

Figure 17 Wegener's granulomatosis. (a) There is a large cavitary lesion in left upper lobe with a small nodule attached to inner surface of its irregularly thickened wall
(arrowhead). (b) Complete resolution of the lesion following 3 weeks of steroid treatment.

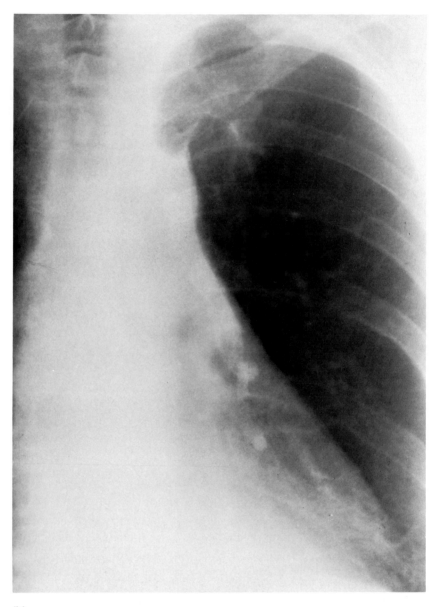

(b)

Figure 17 (continued)

VII. Wegener's Granulomatosis

Pleural and parenchymal involvement in Wegener's granulomatosis is usually preceded by a long history of upper respiratory tract involvement. Chronic sinusitis and rhinitis are reported as the earliest manifestations in 95% of patients (2,31). Even when the presenting clinical manifestation relates to the upper respiratory tract, the lungs are usually involved in patients with Wegener's granulomatosis (31).

The parenchymal disease is characterized by round alveolar opacities (Fig. 16) with a tendency to cavitate and by ill-defined alveolar infiltrates that are often transient in nature (1,2). Single or multiple pulmonary nodules may progress to cavities with thick, irregular walls. Less commonly, the cavities are thin-walled (Fig. 17). Both the infiltrates and the cavities can regress spontaneously and then subsequently reappear (32).

Endobronchial lesions are rare, but they can result in lobar collapse (33). Hilar and mediastinal nodes have been reported but remain a very rare manifestation of Wegener's granulomatosis (Table 2). Diffuse alveolar disease as a result of pulmonary hemorrhage may progress to acute respiratory failure.

We have observed a patient presenting clinically with acute pleuritis and radiographically with pleural effusions and pleural-based, wedge-shaped parenchymal infiltrates of pulmonary infarction (Fig. 18). Pleural effusions have been described in 25% of patients with Wegener's granulomatosis (2) (see also Chap. 2).

Table 2 Chest Radiograph Findings in Wegener's and Lymphomatoid Granulomatosis

Findings	Wegener's granulomatosis	Lymphomatoid granulomatosis
Alveolar nodules	Very common	Very common
Cavitation	Common	Less common
Interstitial infiltrate	No	May occur
Pulmonary infarction	Common	Common
Pleural disease	May occur	May occur

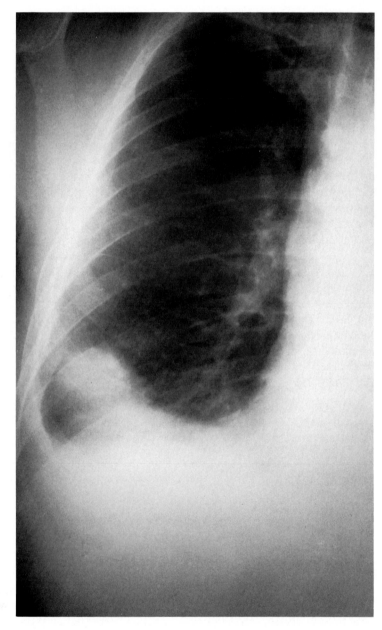

Figure 18 Wegener's granulomatosis. Right pleural effusion and a solitary parenchymal infiltrate simulating a pulmonary infarction both clinically and radiographically.

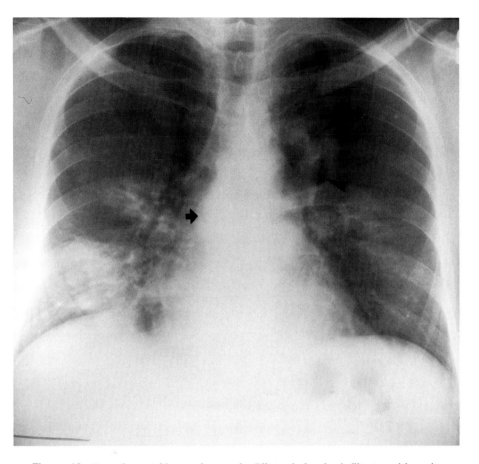

Figure 19 Lymphomatoid granulomatosis. Bilateral alveolar infiltrates with cavitation in some of lesions (arrowheads). Subcarinal nodal enlargement also detectable (small arrow).

VIII. Lymphomatoid Granulomatosis

Radiographic findings of lymphomatoid granulomatosis very closely mimic those of Wegener's granulomatosis (34) (Table 2). Just as in Wegener's, the lungs are virtually always involved in this disease. Multiple nodules with poorly defined borders occurred in 88% of patients reported by Wechsler et al. (35). These nodular infiltrates showed evidence of cavitation in 29% of patients (Fig. 19). Pleural effusion was present in 25% of patients, most

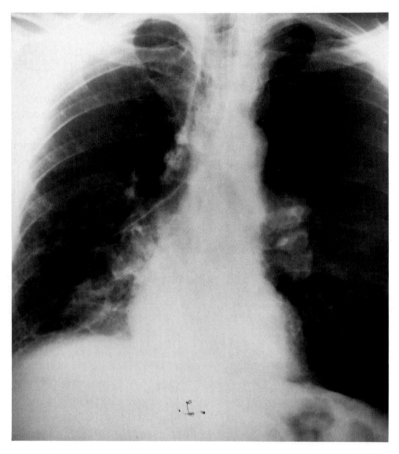

Figure 20 Lymphomatoid granulomatosis. Note right lower lobe parenchymal infiltrate and bilateral hilar node enlargement.

likely related to the pleural reaction secondary to pulmonary infarction that
occurs commonly in patients with vasculitis. A diffuse reticular nodular
pattern was present in three patients with lymphomatoid granulomatosis, a
pattern very seldom seen in patients with Wegener's granulomatosis. Lymphomatoid granulomatosis may also present as a parenchymal infiltrate with
or without hilar adenopathy (Fig. 20). An association of lymphomatoid granulomatosis and lymphoma has been described in 12% of patients (36). Unilateral or bilateral large pulmonary masses measuring more than 10 cm in
size very often signal the presence of lymphoma in patients with lymphomatoid granulomatosis (37).

References

1. Hunninghake, G. W., and Fauci, A. (1979). Pulmonary involvement in the collagen vascular diseases. *Am. Rev. Respir. Dis.* **119**:471-503.
2. Feigin, D. S. (1988). Vasculitis in the lung. *J. Thorac. Imag.* **3**:33-48.
3. Gordon, D. A., Stein, J. L., and Broder, I. (1973). The extra-articular features of rheumatoid arthritis, a systemic analysis of 127 cases. *Am. J. Med.* **54**:445-452.
4. Stretton, T. B., and Seeming, J. T. (1964). Diffuse interstitial pulmonary fibrosis in patients with a positive sheep cell agglutination test. *Thorax* **19**:79-84.
5. Ward, R. (1961). Pleural effusion and rheumatoid disease. *Lancet* **2**: 1336-1338.
6. Martel, W., Abell, M. R., and Mikkelsen, W. M. (1968). Pulmonary and pleural lesions in rheumatoid disease. *Radiology* **90**:641-653.
7. Eraut, D., Evans, J., and Caplin, M. (1978). Pulmonary necrobiotic nodules without rheumatoid arthritis. *Br. J. Dis. Chest.* **72**:301-306.
8. Walker, W. G., and Wright, V. (1967). Rheumatoid pleuritis. *Ann. Rheum. Dis.* **26**:467-474.
9. Burrows, F. G. O. (1967). Pulmonary nodules in rheumatoid disease: A report of two cases. *Br. J. Radiol.* **40**:256.
10. Morgan, W. K. C., and Wolfel, D. A. (1966). The lungs and pleura in rheumatoid arthritis. *A.J.R.* **98**:334.
11. Steinberg, D. L., and Webb, W. R. (1984). CT appearances of rheumatoid lung disease. *J. Comput. Assist. Tomogr.* **8**:881-884.
12. Frank, S. T., Weg, J. G., Harkleroad, L. E., and Fitch, R. F. (1973). Pulmonary dysfunction in rheumatioid disease. *Chest* **63**:27-34.
13. Felson, B. (1973). *Chest Roentgenology.* W.B. Saunders, Philadelphia, pp. 314-349.
14. Reed, C. E., and De Shazo, R. (1982). Immunologic aspects of granulomatous and interstital lung diseases. *J.A.M.A.* **248**:2683-2691.
15. Caplan, A., Payne, R. B., and Withey, J. L. (1962). A broader concept of Caplan's syndrome related to rheumatoid factors. *Thorax* **17**:205-212.
16. Gardiner, D., Duthie, J. J. R., Macleod, J., and Allan, W. S. A. (1957). Pulmonary hypertension in rheumatoid arthritis: Report of a case with intimal sclerosis of the pulmonary digital arteries. *Scot. Med. J.* **2**:183-188.
17. Mahrer, P. R., Evans, J. A., and Steinberg, I. (1954). Scleroderma: Relation of pulmonary changes to esophageal disease. *Ann. Intern. Med.* **40**:97-101.
18. Gondos, B. (1960). Roentgen manifestations in progressive systemic sclerosis (diffuse scleroderma). *A.J.R.* **84**:235-247.

19. Spain, D. M. (1957). The association of terminal bronchiolar carcinoma with chronic interstitial inflammation and fibrosis of the lungs. *Am. Rev. Tuberc.* **76**:559-567.
20. Frazier, A. R., and Miller, R. D. (1974). Interstitial pneumonitis in association with polymyositis and dermatomyositis. *Chest* **65**:403-407.
21. Strimlan, C. V., Rosenow, E. C., Divertie, M. B., and Harrison, E. G. (1976). Pulmonary manifestations of Sjogren's syndrome. *Chest* **70**:354-361.
22. Pines, A., Kaplinsky, N., Olchovsky, D., et al. (1985). Pleuro-pulmonary manifestations of systemic lupus erythematosus: Clinical features of its subgroups, prognostic and therapeutic implications. *Chest* **88**: 129-135.
23. Dubois, E. L., and Tuffanelli, D. L. (1964). Clinical manifestations of systemic lupus erythematosus, computer analysis of 520 cases. *J.A.M.A.* **190**:104-111.
24. Turner-Stokes, L., and Turner-Warwick, M. (1982). Intrathoracic manifestations of SLE. *Clin. Rheum. Dis.* **8**:229-242.
25. Martens, J., Demedts, M., Vanmeenen, M. T., and Dequeker, J. (1984). Respiratory muscle dysfunction in systemic lupus erythematosus. *Chest* **84**:170-175.
26. Matthay, R. A., Schwartz, M. I., Petty, T. L., Stanford, R. E., Gupta, R. C., Sahn, S. A., and Steigerwald, J. C. (1975). Pulmonary manifestations of systemic lupus erythematosus. *Medicine* **54**:397-409.
27. Eisenberg, H., Dubois, E. L., Sherwin, R. P., and Balchum, O. J. (1973). Interstitial lung disease in systemic lupus erythematosus. *Ann. Intern. Med.* **79**:37-45.
28. Marion, C. T., and Pertschuk, L. P. (1981). Pulmonary hemorrhage in systemic lupus erythematosus. *Arch. Intern. Med.* **141**:201-203.
29. Asherson, R. A., Mackworth-Young, C. G., Boey, M. L., Hughes, G. R. V., Hull, R. G., Saunders, A., Gharavi, A. E., and Hughes, G. R. (1983). Pulmonary hypertension in systemic lupus erythematosus. *Br. Med. J.* **287**:1024-1025.
30. Rosenow, E. C., Sttimlam, C. V., Muhm, J. R., and Ferguson, R. H. (1977). Pleuropulmonary manifestations of ankylosing spondylitis. *Mayo Clin. Proc.* **52**:641-649.
31. Fauci, A. S., Haynes, B. F., Katz, P., and Wolff, S. M. (1983). Wegener's granulomatosis: Prospective clinical and therapeutic experience with 85 patients for 21 years. *Ann. Intern. Med.* **98**:76-85.
32. Landman, S., and Burgener, F. (1974). Pulmonary manifestations of Wegener's granulomatosis. *A.J.R.* **122**:750-757.
33. Maguire, R., Fauci, A. S., Doppman, J. L., and Wolff, S. M. (1978). Unusual radiographic features of Wegener's granulomatosis. *A.J.R.* **130**:233-238.

34. Dee, P. M., Arora, N. S., and Innes, D. J. Jr. (1982). The pulmonary manifestations of lymphomatoid granulomatosis. *Radiology* **143**:613-618.
35. Wechsler, R. J., Steiner, R. M., Israel, H. L., and Patchefsky, A. S. (1984). Chest radiograph in lymphomatoid granulomatosis: Comparison with Wegener's granulomatosis. *A.J.R.* **142**:79-83.
36. Katzenstein, A. A., Carrington, C. B., and Liebow, A. A. (1979). Lymphomatoid granulomatosis. A clinicopathologic study of 152 cases. *Cancer* **43**:360-373.
37. Fauci, A. S., Haynes, B. F., Costa, J., Katz, P., and Wolff, S. M. (1982). Lymphamatoid granulomatosis: Prospective clinical and therapeutic experience over 10 years. *N. Engl. J. Med.* **306**:68-74.

5

Lung Biopsy, Bronchoalveolar Lavage, and Gallium Scanning

MARK R. ELSTAD

University of Utah
Salt Lake City, Utah

I. Introduction

The rheumatic diseases, also referred to as collagen-vascular diseases, are systemic disorders that affect the lung function by involvement of the ventilatory muscles, airways, blood vessels, and alveolar structures. Large amounts of connective tissue, abundant vasculature, and the potential ability to generate immune complexes in situ make the lung vulnerable to immune-mediated injury (1,2). The interstitial lung diseases are a group of disorders characterized by chronic inflammation in the lower respiratory tract (reviewed in 3). These disorders exhibit common clinical, radiographic, and physiologic features as discussed below. The association of interstitial lung disease with the rheumatic diseases is well established (1) and accounts for approximately 1600 deaths per year, or 2% of deaths from all respiratory diseases (4). Although interstitial lung disease is most commonly seen in progressive systemic sclerosis (PSS) and rheumatoid arthritis (RA), it may occur in association with any of the rheumatic diseases (1).

The pathogenesis of the interstitial lung diseases is discussed in detail in Chapter 1. Briefly, interstitial lung disease develops following an initial insult to the alveolus, delivered by either the capillaries or the airways, that causes the accumulation of immune effector cells in the alveolar walls and air spaces ("alveolitis"). The total number of immune effector cells and the relative number of individual cell types (macrophages, lymphocytes, neutrophils, etc.) vary according to the individual disease process and its stage. These cells release mediators that directly injure the lung, recruit additional inflammatory cells, and alter the function of other lung cells (e.g., fibroblasts) or groups of cells (e.g., vessels or airways). Although the alveolitis may distort air space anatomy and cause abnormal gas exchange, it is potentially reversible. If the inflammatory process continues in an unregulated fashion, an irreversible accumulation and disordering of connective tissue ("pulmonary fibrosis") occurs (3).

The mechanisms of alveolar injury in the rheumatic diseases are not well understood. Circulating or locally generated immune complexes have been implicated in the pathogenesis of interstitial lung disease associated with RA and systemic lupus erythematosis (SLE) (2,5,6). Other proposed mechanisms for alveolar injury include a lymphocytic proliferative response in Sjogren's syndrome (SS) (7), direct vascular injury in PSS (8), and cell-mediated immune damage in polymyositis/dermatomyositis (PM/DM) (9). Lung injury in a given patient may involve more than one mechanism or different mechanisms at different stages of disease. Further, the histopathologic features of interstitial lung disease associated with RA, SLE, PSS, and PM/DM may be indistinguishable from each other and from idiopathic fibrosis. Unfortunately, present methods have not allowed us to directly relate the pathophysiology of lung injury to the observed immunologic abnormalities in the rheumatic diseases. This is currently an area of active investigation.

II. Clinical Features of Interstitial Lung Disease in Patients with Collagen-Vascular Diseases

The clinical features of interstitial lung disease in patients with rheumatic diseases are similar to idiopathic pulmonary fibrosis (3). Systemic manifestations of the rheumatic disease tend to dominate the clinical picture and are usually, but not invariably, present prior to the onset of pulmonary symptoms. The "typical patient" presents with an insidious onset (months to years) of dyspnea, exercise limitation, and nonproductive cough. Crackles (end-inspiratory "Velcro" rales) are the most common sign. Tachypnea, decreased chest wall expansion, and clubbing may also be present. Laboratory abnormalities related to the rheumatic disease (e.g., high titers of rheumatoid factor or antinuclear antibody) are frequently present. The chest radiograph

Table 1 Common Causes of Pulmonary Infiltrates in Rheumatic Disease Patients

---

A. *Direct pulmonary involvement*
   Interstitial lung disease (alveolitis,[a] fibrosis)
   Pulmonary vasculitis
   Diffuse alveolar hemorrhage

B. *Secondary to extrapulmonary disease*
   Aspiration pneumonia (noninfectious, infectious)
   Atelectasis
   Uremic pneumonitis

C. *Miscellaneous*
   Infectious pneumonia
   Drug reaction
   Pulmonary emboli
   Unrelated lung disease secondary to smoking, pneumoconiosis, etc.

---

[a]Alveolitis may present insidiously or with symptoms and radiographic manifestations. It causes radiographic and clinical manifestations alone or in association with fibrosis and may occasionally have a fulminant toxic presentation. "Lupus pneumonitis" appears to be an example of the latter phenomenon. An acute presentation of alveolar injury may also occur in other collagen-vascular diseases (see text).

shows small irregular shadows that are most prominent at the bases ("diffuse interstitial infiltrates"), as discussed in Chapter 4. Pulmonary function testing reveals a restrictive ventilatory defect and impaired gas exchange (Chap. 3). Exceptions to the "typical" manifestations are common, as discussed below.

Other disease processes may cause pulmonary infiltrates in these patients (Table 1). The differential diagnosis may be narrowed by consideration of the underlying disease, the clinical course, and the radiographic pattern; however, accurate diagnosis frequently requires the collection of specimens for histologic, cytologic, and microbiologic examination, as discussed below.

III. Techniques Used to Evaluate Alveolar Injury and Interstitial Lung Disease

A. General Considerations

Proper management of patients with interstitial lung disease requires objective data for diagnosis, staging, predicting the prognosis and potential for response to therapy, and monitoring disease activity. These data have traditionally been obtained from physical examination, chest radiography, pulmonary function testing, and open lung biopsy. Radiographic and pulmonary function abnormalities tend to parallel the histopathologic severity of disease (14). However, with the possible exception of volume-pressure relationships as a predictor of fibrosis in idiopathic pulmonary fibrosis, these studies do not provide specific information regarding the relative contributions of alveolitis and fibrosis to the overall pathologic process (14). Studies of patients evaluated with open lung biopsies suggest that it is the relative amounts of irreversible scarring and active inflammation that determine disease activity and prognosis in idiopathic pulmonary fibrosis (10) and interstitial lung disease associated with rheumatic diseases (11-13). This suggests that differentiating alveolitis from fibrosis may have clinical utility.

B. Lung Biopsy

Histopathology, based on examination of specimens obtained by open lung biopsy, remains the "gold standard" for diagnosing and staging chronic infiltrative lung diseases (15). In a review of 15 series, open lung biopsy gave "diagnostic results" in 94% of the cases (15). The size of the open biopsy specimen allows adequate assessment of both the fibrotic and the inflammatory components. I routinely freeze tissue at the time of biopsy to use for immunologic marker or immune complex studies if they are indicated following initial histologic examination. Most authors feel that it is best to avoid the most abnormal regions of lung, as they are likely to show "end-stage disease of unrecognizable origin" (15). It has frequently been stated that the dependent portions of the lingula and right middle lobe are not appropriate biopsy sites because they commonly show nonspecific inflammatory changes, fibrosis, and vascular thickening (15,16). This is supported by one study that compared the histopathology of small autopsy specimens (1×2 cm) from the lingula and the left lower and right upper lobes (17). However, other studies have failed to demonstrate greater or nonspecific involvement of these sites (18,19). In the setting of an appropriate chest radiograph, it has been the experience of myself and others (Chap. 6) that biopsy specimens of adequate size (e.g., 3×3 cm) from the lingula and right middle lobe yield representative histopathology.

Transbronchial biopsy through the fiberoptic bronchoscope is the other technique commonly used to obtain histologic specimens (20). Although it has not been rigorously examined, four to six biopsy specimens from several different sites may provide a representative sample of alveolar tissue in diffuse lung disease (21). It must be remembered that certain histologic diagnoses, such as "interstitial pneumonia," "chronic inflammation," "nonspecific reaction," or "fibrosis," may be unreliable or misleading when based on transbronchial biopsy specimens (22).

C. Bronchoalveolar Lavage

Bronchoalveolar lavage (BAL) allows one to examine the cellular and non-cellular elements present on the epithelial surface of the alveolar space (23). BAL does not truly sample the lung parenchyma; however, in the few studies that have been performed there has been a good correlation between the type and number of inflammatory cells obtained by BAL and those obtained by digesting lung biopsy tissue from both normal and diseased (sarcoidosis and idiopathic pulmonary fibrosis) lungs (reviewed in 23). Thus, it is felt that analysis of BAL fluid components provides an assessment of inflammatory activity in the lower respiratory tract. In the clinical setting, BAL has proved to be of great practical value in the diagnosis of infections in immunocompromised hosts (24,25). A preliminary study suggests that BAL fluid cell analysis may influence clinical management of patients with a variety of interstitial lung diseases (26).

The value of BAL as a clinical tool depends in part on its reproducibility, which is in turn dependent on technique. My method (27) is similar to that described by other investigators (reviewed in 23). In diffuse disease, BAL is performed in the right middle lobe or the lingula because of technical ease. Fluid recovery from these areas is greater than from the lower lobes, although the cell counts, cell differentials, and protein concentrations are similar (28). There is no evidence that nonspecific inflammatory changes are seen in BAL specimens from the right middle lobe or lingula (see open-biopsy discussion above). I routinely lavage two separate areas because BAL cell differentials may exhibit large interlobar variation in patients with diseased lungs (29). Following routine inspection of the airways, a seal is obtained by "wedging" the bronchoscope into the desired third- or fourth-generation bronchus. Sterile buffered saline is instilled in four 50-ml aliquots that are withdrawn into the syringe by gentle hand suction. The first aliquot of fluid recovered, which is a small volume "bronchial" sample (30), is discarded, and the remaining fractions are pooled for analysis. Differential evaluation of the "bronchial" and "alveolar" samples may be useful in evaluating inflammatory airway disease; this possibility is under active evaluation.

The cells and extracellular molecules present in BAL fluid are then studied in the laboratory. Unsatisfactory specimens should be identified, as they provide misleading data (27,31). Although a complete discussion of BAL fluid analysis is beyond the scope of this manuscript, a few general comments are appropriate. To date there is no consensus as to what constitutes a "routine" analysis of BAL fluid. Total and differential cell counts, frequently with identification of T-lymphocyte subsets by monoclonal antibody techniques, are usually performed. BAL fluid from a nonsmoker normally contains 85-90% macrophages, 7-12% lymphocytes, and 0-1% neutrophils (23,27).

Patients may be classified as having neutrophil alveolitis or a lymphocyte alveolitis based on an increase in the percent neutrophils or lymphocytes, respectively. A neutrophil alveolitis is commonly seen in idiopathic pulmonary fibrosis, histiocytosis X, and cigarette smokers; a lymphocyte alveolitis is commonly seen in sarcoidosis, hypersensitivity pneumonitis, and granulomatous infections. It must be remembered that there is considerable overlap in the BAL findings associated with these disorders. Microscopic evaluation of Papanicolaou-stained cytocentrifuge preparations is also performed. When the Papanicolaou-stained slides demonstrate unusual features, or when the clinical situation dictates, other studies may be appropriate (e.g., immuno-staining, microbiological cultures, electron microscopy). Numerous molecules can be identified in the cell-free supernatant of BAL fluid. I freeze an aliquot of the supernatant for future study; however, I do not currently quantitate any of the soluble components, as there are no data to support the use of these markers in clinical decisions.

A variety of abnormal BAL findings have been described in patients with rheumatic diseases (Table 2). BAL cell analysis has most commonly revealed an increase in neutrophils, lymphocytes or both. Thus, these results are similar to those reported from patients with idiopathic pulmonary fibrosis. A number of factors make these studies difficult to interpret and apply to the clinical setting. Results from patients with different types of rheumatic diseases have frequently been combined, and patients have often been heterogeneous with respect to factors that independently alter BAL results, such as severity of clinical disease, smoking habits, and use of anti-rheumatic drugs.

D. Gallium Scanning

Lung scanning with gallium-67 has been recommended as a means of assessing pulmonary inflammation (32,33). Gallium-67 is injected intravenously and images are quantitated by one of several methods (33). At 48 hours, the gallium-67 activity in normal lungs is low. Gallium-67 uptake is increased in a variety of inflammatory and neoplastic pulmonary disorders. The increased uptake appears to result primarily from concentration of gallium in activated alveolar macrophages (34). Gallium-67 uptake has been statistically correlated with the percentage of BAL lymphocytes in sarcoidosis (35) and a histologic score of alveolar inflammation in idiopathic pulmonary fibrosis (36). However, others have failed to confirm this finding in sarcoidosis (37). It is generally felt that gallium scanning provides a sensitive but nonspecific assessment of pulmonary inflammation in idiopathic pulmonary fibrosis and other interstitial lung diseases (reviewed in 38). Its use in the clinical evaluation of patients with rheumatic diseases remains to be defined (see below).

Table 2 Major Bronchoalveolar Lavage Findings in Patients with Rheumatic Diseases[a]

Reference	Rheumatic disease (number of patients)	BAL findings
44	PSS (20) SS (9) RA (6) PM/DM (4) MCTD (3)	1. Abnormal BAL cell differentials common in asymptomatic patients (increased lymphocytes in 16%, neutrophils in 22%, both lymphocytes and neutrophils in 22%) 2. Similar findings in patients with clinical ILD[b] 3. Evidence for spontaneous activation of alveolar macrophages from asymptomatic patients
45	PSS (3) SLE (1) RA (1) MCTD (1)	1. Similar BAL findings in IPF[c] and rheumatic disease-associated ILD 2. Lymphocyte alveolitis (initial BAL) predicted clinical response to prednisone 3. Cyclophosphamide therapy associated with a fall in BAL eosinophils
46	RA (18) SLE (8) PSS (4) PM/DM (3) MCTD (2)	1. Progressive ILD associated with abnormal BAL cell differential 2. Lymphocyte alveolitis associated with response to prednisone
30	RA (4) MCTD (1)	1. Clinical ILD associated with neutrophil alveolitis 2. Large interlobar variation of BAL cell differentials in patients with clinical lung disease
47	SS (25) SLE (11) PSS (10) MCTD (8) RA (4)	1. Lymphocyte alveolitis common in asymptomatic patients with SS (11 of 25) and SLE (3 of 11) 2. Neutrophil alveolitis common in asymptomatic patients with PSS (16 of 10), RA (1 of 4), PM/DM (1 of 3), and MCTD (3 of 8)

(continues)

Table 2 Continued

Reference	Rheumatic disease (number of patients)	BAL findings
		3. Neutrophil alveolitis correlated with progressive deterioration in lung function
48	RA (6) SLE (3) SS (2) MCTD (2)	1. BAL T-lymphocyte subset analysis useful to differentiate IPF from rheumatic disease-associated ILD
5	RA (10) PSS (3) SLE (2)	1. Neutrophil alveolitis common in ILD 2. Immune complex concentrations higher in patients than controls 3. Corticosteroid therapy caused a decrease in BAL neutrophils and immune complex concentrations
49	PSS (6) RA (3) PM/DM (3) SLE (2)	1. Increased BAL neutrophils (mean 13%) in patients with both IPF and rheumatic disease-associated ILD 2. BAL lymphocyte counts higher in rheumatic disease-associated ILD (13%) than in IPF (6%) 3. Greater than 11% BAL lymphocytes correlated with corticosteroid response
50	PSS (14)	1. Clinical ILD associated with increased BAL neutrophils and eosinophils
51	PSS (11)	1. Increased BAL neutrophils and eosinophils correlated with clinical ILD 2. Macrophages from patients spontaneously released more fibronectin and alveolar macrophage-derived growth factor than control macrophages
52	PSS (25)	1. Lymphocyte alveolitis correlated with radiographic and pulmonary function abnormalities 2. Penicillamine therapy associated with lower BAL lymphocyte counts

(continues)

Table 2 Continued

Reference	Rheumatic disease (number of patients)	BAL findings
53	PSS (20)	1. Neutrophil or lymphocyte alveolitis (greater than 20% of total BAL cells) associated with fall in diffusing capacity 2. BAL fluid collagenase activity inversely correlated with pulmonary function
54	PSS (19)	1. Increase in BAL neutrophils and/or eosinophils common (58%) 2. Neutrophil counts correlated with radiographic and pulmonary function evidence of ILD
55	PSS (1)	1. Prednisone response of a PSS patient with ILD associated with normalization of neutrophil/eosinophil alveolitis
56	RA (24)	1. BAL fluid from patients with ILD capable of attracting and activating blood neutrophils 2. Myeloperoxidase and neutrophil elastase elevated in patients with ILD
57	RA (24)	1. Lymphocyte alveolitis common in asymptomatic patients and neutrophil alveolitis common in patients with clinical ILD 2. IgM detectable in BAL fluid from patients with abnormal cell differential 3. BAL T-lymphocyte helper/suppressor ratios were lower in patients with clinical ILD
58	RA (12)	1. In asymptomatic patients with normal pulmonary function, lymphocyte alveolitis associated with minimal basilar infiltrates on the chest radiograph
59	SS (29)	1. Lymphocyte (11 of 29) or lymphocyte/neutrophil alveolitis common in patients with no clinical evidence of ILD

[a]See text for discussion.
[b]Interstitial lung disease.
[c]Idiopathic pulmonary fibrosis.

IV. Diagnosis, Staging, and Management of Alveolar Injury and Interstitial Lung Disease

A. Rheumatoid Arthritis

Ellman and Ball first described the association between RA and interstitial lung disease 40 years ago (39). The reported incidence of interstitial lung disease in RA varies between 2% and 40%, depending on the method used for detection (1). Pulmonary symptoms (dyspnea and nonproductive cough) typically occur within 5 years of the onset of arthritis. Symptoms are usually associated with diffuse interstitial infiltrates and a restrictive ventilatory defect, as described for the typical patients with idiopathic pulmonary fibrosis (see above). Open lung biopsy is felt to provide the best specimen for diagnosis of chronic infiltrative lung disease (15,40). The interstitial lung disease of RA is associated with a wide spectrum of histologic lesions, as reviewed in Chapter 6.

Staging and determining the prognosis of interstitial lung disease in patients with RA are difficult. The disease varies from mild pulmonary involvement with slow progression to a severe and fulminant form (41). Experience with other interstitial lung disease suggests that conventional clinical assessment (symptoms, chest radiographs, and pulmonary function tests) is insensitive and potentially misleading when compared with pathologic activity (42). The prognosis depends on the maturity of the fibrotic component, which is presumed to be irreversible (11). The finding that the histologic pattern of usual interstitial pneumonitis is a poor prognostic feature (associated with death due to progressive pulmonary disease) supports this concept (12). The response rate to corticosteroids is not known (41); however, two studies suggest that prednisone responsiveness is associated with cellular histology (11, 43). Thus, histopathology observed on lung biopsy specimens appears to provide the most accurate staging and the best estimate of prognosis and potential for therapeutic response.

As discussed above, identification of the cellular constituents of BAL fluid may allow quantification of inflammatory events occurring in the pulmonary parenchyma. Abnormal BAL cell differentials have been reported in patients with RA (Table 2). Both a neutrophil alveolitis and, more commonly, a lymphocyte alveolitis have been observed (5,30,44,46,56,57). Unfortunately, these are nonspecific abnormalities and do not make the diagnosis of RA-associated interstitial lung disease. In idiopathic pulmonary fibrosis and sarcoidosis, it has been suggested that the BAL cell differential provides an estimate of the intensity of alveolitis and useful staging and prognostic information (3). A subgroup of RA patients has been found to have a lymphocyte alveolitis (44,56-58), spontaneously activated alveolar macrophages (44), and no clinical evidence of pulmonary disease. The prognostic significance of a lymphocyte alveolitis is unknown, and it is not clear if these patients should be considered to have interstitial lung "disease" or if therapy is indicated. A neutrophil alveolitis is commonly reported in patients with clinical, radiographic, and physiologic evidence of pulmonary disease (45, 46,48,56). Thus, preliminary evidence suggests that lymphocytes predominate in the early stage of disease and that an influx of neutrophils is associated with later, more severe pulmonary dysfunction. An increase in BAL lymphocytes has been associated with prednisone responsiveness in patients with idiopathic pulmonary fibrosis (49). Whether these data can be applied to patients with RA remains to be seen.

The greatest value of BAL may be for following the clinical response to therapy and for deciding when it is appropriate to discontinue treatment (60). A recent study that included a subgroup of patients with rheumatic disease-associated idiopathic pulmonary fibrosis demonstrated an association between a clinical response to prednisone and a decrease in BAL neutrophils (45). Although it is not yet rigorously proved, it may be reasonable to follow the BAL cell profile as therapy is discontinued. An increase in BAL neutrophils may signal impending relapse and call for an alteration in therapy. The clinical utility of such an approach has yet to be determined.

Abnormal pulmonary uptake of gallium-67 has been described in a study of 36 patients with interstitial lung disease, including 18 with RA (46). Seventeen of 20 patients with progressive dyspnea and none of 16 nonprogressive patients had abnormal pulmonary uptake of gallium-67. Although abnormal gallium-67 uptake was a specific finding for clinical disease in the chest, it did not predict mortality or response to steroids. Further, subclinical alveolitis that was present by BAL fluid cellular analysis was not detected. The use of gallium-67 scanning for following therapy in this group of patients has yet to be determined.

Based on these data I manage patients with RA and suspected interstitial lung disease as outlined in Figure 1. Patients are followed for the development of pulmonary symptoms and/or changes in the chest radiograph or lung function tests. Bronchoscopy with transbronchial biopsies and BAL is performed on most patients with abnormal or deteriorating pulmonary function. If the biopsies suggest idiopathic pulmonary fibrosis and there is no evidence of malignancy, infection, or granulomatous disease, an empiric trial of corticosteroids is given with a presumptive diagnosis of interstitial lung disease associated with RA. In atypical patients, as well as patients who fail to respond to empiric corticosteroids, open lung biopsy may be performed in an attempt to determine a specific diagnosis. The risk vs. benefit for this procedure in the individual patient must be carefully considered. Patients undergoing therapy are followed by clinical evaluation, chest radiographs, and lung function tests. BAL fluid analysis may be useful for following pa-

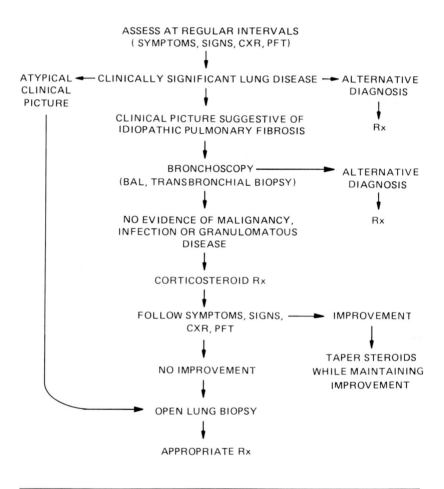

Figure 1 Clinical approach to the rheumatic disease patient with suspected interstitial lung disease.

tients in the future; however, controlled trials are needed. In addition to cell differential counts, other data derived from BAL such as characterization of alveolar macrophage activation may provide clinically useful information (44). I do not routinely use gallium-67 scans in the management of these patients.

This approach demands careful and critical evaluation of the individual patient, and exceptions must be made frequently. For example, in a patient with classic RA (positive serology, typical joint involvement, etc.), clinical, radiographic, and physiologic features suggestive of typical idiopathic pulmonary fibrosis, and no other reason to have interstitial lung disease, a tentative diagnosis of RA-associated interstitial lung disease may be made without histologic confirmation. Conversely, an atypical clinical presentation or rapid disease progression may warrant an aggressive diagnostic approach that includes open lung biopsy as the initial procedure.

B. Progressive Systemic Sclerosis

The incidence of interstitial lung disease associated with PSS ranges from 14% to 90% in clinical studies and from 60% to 100% in autopsy studies (41). The interstitial lung disease may be mimicked by chronic aspiration (to be discussed) or metastatic cancer and may be masked by pulmonary hypertension. The clinical, radiographic, and physiologic manifestations resemble the typical case of idiopathic pulmonary fibrosis as described above. A gradual deterioration in pulmonary function is usually seen. Clinical and pulmonary function parameters are unreliable predictors of prognosis, although patients with severe Raynaud's phenomenon and smokers appear to be at high risk for rapid deterioration (61). Case reports have demonstrated occasional benefit from corticosteroid therapy, and preliminary studies suggest that penicillamine slows disease progression (41). Mortality secondary to pulmonary fibrosis ranges from 5% to 17% (41). As discussed in Chapter 6, the major histopathology occurs in the interstitium and the blood vessel walls. The relationship of histopathology to prognosis in PSS-associated interstitial lung disease has not been established.

BAL cell differential counts have been reported to show a normal distribution as well as neutrophil or, less commonly, a lymphocyte predominance (Table 2). No BAL finding is specific for the diagnosis of interstitial lung disease associated with PSS. Wallaert et al. have used BAL to address the issue of subclinical alveolar inflammation in patients with PSS (44). A neutrophil alveolitis was observed in five of seven patients with no symptoms and normal chest radiographs. No patient developed symptoms or radiographic abnormalities over 12 months; however, all four untreated patients with neutrophil alveolitis deteriorated by at least one pulmonary function parameter. The two patients with normal BAL cell differentials and the single corticosteroid-treated patient with a neutrophil alveolitis remained stable.

Four studies have correlated clinical lung dysfunction with a neutrophil or a neutrophil/eosinophil alveolitis (50,51,53,54). The one study reporting a lymphocyte predominance (52) failed to provide normal values for their laboratory and defined greater than 10% lymphocytes, a value many consider normal (23), as abnormal. Thus, preliminary evidence suggests that a neutrophil alveolitis is common in both subclinical and symptomatic patients with PSS. The case report of a patient in whom corticosteroid therapy resulted in rapid normalization of both pulmonary function and BAL neutrophil predominance (55) supports the concept that pulmonary inflammation in PSS is potentially reversible. The clinical importance of BAL fluid analysis in these patients has yet to be determined.

Increased gallium-67 uptake in the lungs of patients with PSS and clinical interstitial lung disease has been reported, suggesting the presence of an ongoing inflammatory process (46,50-52,62,63). However, no correlation with clinical, radiographic, or physiologic evidence of disease has been demonstrated (54,62). There are no data to support the use of gallium-67 scanning as a means of detecting subclinical pulmonary inflammation in these patients.

My current approach to PSS patients with possible interstitial lung disease is the same as outlined for patients with RA (see above; Fig. 1). The use of BAL and gallium-67 scanning data for staging and therapeutic decisions should still be considered investigational.

C. Systemic Lupus Erythematosis

It has been stated that pleuropulmonary manifestations occur more frequently in SLE than in other rheumatic diseases (1). Pulmonary infiltrates in SLE may be associated with clinical manifestations that range from the "acute lupus pneumonitis syndrome" to subacute or chronic forms. Acute lupus pneumonitis typically presents with fever, tachypnea, dyspnea, cough, and pulmonary infiltrates (Chap. 9). It must be remembered that infectious pneumonia is much more common than lupus pneumonitis in SLE patients (41). Therefore, pneumonia must be excluded as the cause of this clinical presentation, particularly in immunocompromised patients (e.g., corticosteroid therapy, renal insufficiency). If examination of expectorated sputum does not yield a specific diagnosis, I will usually perform bronchoscopy with BAL and transbronchial biopsies. If examination of these specimens does not reveal an infectious etiology, it seems reasonable to initially treat for presumed lupus pneumonitis with high-dose corticosteroids. Although BAL has been shown to be an effective procedure for diagnosing opportunistic infections in other patient populations (24,25), its utility in this setting has not been studied.

Chronic interstitial lung disease is felt to be uncommon in SLE. However, coexisting pleuropulmonary abnormalities make physiologic testing difficult to interpret and may obscure the true incidence. Many investigators believe that interstitial lung disease associated with SLE represents the end stage of a process that initially manifests as acute lupus pneumonitis (41).

The clinical, radiographic, and physiologic features are similar to the other forms of interstitial lung disease described above. Although there are no controlled trials, interstitial lung disease in SLE is generally felt to be poorly responsive to corticosteroid therapy (41). A number of histologic patterns may be associated with this disorder, and the histopathologic findings of acute lung injury, such as diffuse alveolar damage and alveolar hemorrhage, may coexist with chronic changes (Chap. 6).

As shown in Table 2, both a normal BAL cell differential count and a lymphocyte predominance have been described in SLE patients with (48) and without (47,64) clinical or radiologic evidence of lung disease. I am unaware of studies that define the usefulness of BAL data for estimating prognosis, following the course of disease, or following the response to therapy in the chronic interstitial lung disease. As discussed above and below, BAL may be a useful tool for diagnosing pulmonary infections and differentiating pneumonia from acute lupus pneumonitis.

Eight patients with SLE and pulmonary symptoms were included in a study that examined the value of gallium-67 scanning for predicting clinical outcome and response to therapy in patients with rheumatic diseases (46). The specific data with respect to patients with SLE, other than a lack of gallium-67 uptake in the lungs of the three "nonprogressive" patients, are not presented. Thus, the diagnostic and prognostic value of gallium-67 scans in this setting is unknown.

I follow the same approach to the management of chronic interstitial lung disease in patients with SLE as described above and outlined in Figure 1.

D. Polymyositis/Dermatomyositis

Interstitial lung disease associated with PM/DM is thought to occur in approximately 10% of patients (41). An interesting and unique feature of the interstitial disease in PM/DM is its association with autoantibodies directed against aminoacyl-tRNA synthetases (Chap. 11). The clinical features are similar to idiopathic pulmonary fibrosis. In addition to the typical chronic form, an acute presentation of lung injury may be seen. Determining the precise nature of lung involvement in PM/DM is made particularly difficult by the high incidence of lung disease caused by muscle weakness (aspiration, atelectasis, and secondary infection), therapeutic complications (opportunistic infections and drug-induced lung disease), and associated malignancies. The natural history of interstitial lung disease in patients with PM/DM is not well described; however, the response rate to corticosteroids, which may be up to 50% (65), is higher than is seen in other rheumatic diseases.

The lung histopathology is similar to that of other interstitial lung diseases. Usual interstitial pneumonitis is typically seen on open lung biopsy specimens (13), and bronchiolitis obliterans with organizing pneumonia has been described (65). Corticosteroid responses have been associated with cellular histology (13,65).

A study of BAL fluid from three patients with no evidence of clinical disease described both a neutrophil (two of three) and a lymphocyte (one of three) predominance (47; Table 2). The relationship of BAL abnormalities to clinical disease has not been established, and its usefulness for staging and following therapy is unknown. BAL fluid analysis may allow diagnosis of other lung diseases that mimic PM/DM-associated interstitial lung disease (e.g., opportunistic infections, aspiration, and malignancy). The clinical use of gallium-67 scanning has not been studied in these patients.

As with the other syndromes described above, patients with PM/DM and lung involvement are selected for invasive diagnostic evaluation based on the severity of lung function impairment, the rapidity of disease progression, and the possible presence of complicating lung diseases that may require specific therapy (Fig. 1). The roles for BAL and gallium-67 scanning have yet to be determined.

E. Sjogren's Syndrome

Diffuse interstitial lung disease is probably the most common respiratory manifestation of primary SS (SS with no evidence of another rheumatic disease; 41). The clinical, radiographic, and physiologic features are indistinguishable from those of idiopathic pulmonary fibrosis, as described above. Interstitial disease associated with lymphocytic interstitial pneumonitis, a common histopathologic finding, may resolve or may progress to fibrosis or malignant lymphoma. Corticosteroids improve clinical disease in some patients; however, there have been no controlled studies (39).

Examination of open lung biopsy specimens allows a precise determination of histopathology (Chap. 6). Lymphocytic interstitial pneumonitis, lymphoid hyperplasia, pseudolymphoma, lymphoma, and bronchiolitis obliterans with organizing pneumonia have all been described. Biopsy tissue should be frozen for immune marker studies to help differentiate malignant from benign lymphoproliferation. In certain cases of secondary SS (SS associated with another rheumatic disease), the lesions of SS can be differentiated from those of the associated disorder.

The most common BAL finding in asymptomatic patients with SS is a lymphocyte alveolitis (44,57,59; see Table 2). The relationship of BAL findings to histopathology and clinical variables has not been described. The diagnosis of lymphoma, a potential complication of SS, by cellular analysis of BAL fluid has recently been reported (66).

Abnormal lung uptake of gallium-67 in 10 of 12 patients with SS has been reported (67). Sixty percent of the patients in this study had dyspnea on exertion, and all had "essentially normal" chest radiographs. The significance of this finding is unknown.

My clinical approach to the patient with SS and suspected ILD is the same as described for RA (see above, Fig. 1). If a patient with lymphocytic interstitial pneumonitis worsens, it may be due to progression of the initial pathology or due to occurrence of a different histologic lesion, such as lymphoma. In this situation I perform bronchoscopy with BAL and transbronchial biopsies as the initial diagnostic procedure. These specimens are routinely examined for immunologic markers suggestive of lymphoma. If these studies are nondiagnostic, I proceed to open-lung biopsy.

F. Mixed Connective Tissue Disease

One third of patients with mixed connective tissue disease (MCTD) have chest radiographs suggestive of interstitial lung disease at time of diagnosis, and up to 82% will have pulmonary involvement during the course of their disease (68). Severe pulmonary hypertension from primary vascular involvement may mask the symptoms and gas exchange abnormalities of interstitial lung disease. Further, 80% of patients with MCTD have esophageal dysmotility, a condition that may cause chronic aspiration pneumonitis and lead to pulmonary fibrosis. The natural history of interstitial lung disease in patients with MCTD has not been well described, although most authors consider it to be a long-term disabling disease (68). Clinical remission in up to 38% of patients in response to steroids and cyclophosphamide has been reported (68).

The most common histopathologic pattern is usual interstitial pneumonia (Chap. 6). This may be overshadowed by intimal proliferation and medial muscular hypertrophy involving the pulmonary arterioles (68). There is little information available on BAL and gallium-67 scanning in MCTD patients. A lymphocytic alveolitis has been reported in three asymptomatic patients (44). Abnormal gallium-67 lung scans have been reported (46,68); however, no significant correlation with pulmonary function or clinical status was found (68).

My approach to the management of patients with MCTD and suspected interstitial lung disease is outlined in Figure 1. In selected cases, right heart catheterization may help delineate the relative contributions of pulmonary hypertension and interstitial lung disease to pulmonary function abnormalities.

V. Use of Bronchoalveolar Lavage to Evaluate Related Clinical Problems

A. Pulmonary Infections

The pathogenesis and clinical features of pulmonary infections are discussed in detail in Chapter 7. Rheumatic diseases predispose to pneumonia by direct impairment of lung defenses and by extrapulmonary organ system involvement. Aspiration syndromes caused by esophageal dysmotility and pharyngeal muscle dysfunction are examples of the latter. Impaired cough and hypoventilation, resulting from respiratory muscle dysfunction, predispose to atelectasis and complicating bacterial pneumonia. Finally, renal disease, corticosteroids, and cytotoxic drugs impair host defense mechanisms and may result in opportunistic infection. Pneumonia causes 15-19% of the deaths in RA patients, and infectious pneumonias greatly outnumber episodes of acute lupus pneumonitis in patients with SLE (41).

In the absence of obvious immune suppression due to corticosteroid therapy, cytotoxic drug therapy, or renal insufficiency, I approach the rheumatic disease patient with productive cough, fever, and pulmonary infiltrates in the same manner as a typical outpatient. Sputum is obtained for Gram stain and culture, and initial therapy is based on the stain results. Fiberoptic bronchoscopy with BAL and transbronchial biopsy is performed on immunocompromised or severely ill patients with nondiagnostic sputum. Open lung biopsy is done if BAL findings are not diagnostic and clinical deterioration occurs. Although this approach has not been critically evaluated in patients with rheumatic diseases, it has been studied in other clinical settings. BAL has been shown to be a safe and effective diagnostic procedure in patients with opportunistic (24,25,69) and bacterial (70) infections.

B. Antirheumatic Drug Reactions

Pulmonary reactions to antirheumatic drugs are discussed in detail in Chapter 14. Both cytotoxic and noncytotoxic drugs used in the therapy of rheumatic diseases may cause lung injury. The most common clinical syndromes are chronic pneumonitis/fibrosis, hypersensitivity pneumonitis, and noncardiogenic pulmonary edema (71). Treatment requires early recognition of the problem and withdrawal of the drug, with a role for corticosteroids in selected cases. If the diagnosis is not made on clinical grounds, supportive evidence can be obtained from open-lung biopsy specimens. Histopathology, which may vary, typically shows endothelial cell damage and epithelial cell abnormalities (type I pneumocyte desquamation and type II cell dysplastic changes; 71). The utility of transbronchial biopsies in diagnosing cytotoxic drug-induced pulmonary disease has not been rigorously examined. One would anticipate that this procedure might provide useful information, particularly for drugs that cause hypersensitivity reactions manifested histologically by granulomas or interstitial eosinophilic infiltration.

BAL has not been very helpful in making a specific diagnosis of drug-induced pulmonary disease. Bronchial and alveolar cell atypia, BAL findings suggestive of drug toxicity, were present in only 6 of 15 cases in a study of immunocompromised patients with pulmonary infiltrates (24). A lymphocyte predominance has been described in methotrexate lung disease (72). Currently, the major value of BAL in the evaluation of suspected drug-induced pulmonary disease is to exclude infection.

My approach to the rheumatic disease patient with a suspected pulmonary reaction to an antirheumatic drug is as follows. The drug is discontinued and the patient's condition is followed by clinical evaluation, chest radiographs, and pulmonary function testing. Bronchoscopy with BAL and transbronchial biopsy is performed initially if an opportunistic infection is being considered. If there is no improvement following discontinuation of the drug, a therapeutic trial of corticosteroids is given. In cases of severe or progressive pulmonary dysfunction, an open lung biopsy is performed in an attempt to secure the diagnosis.

C. Aspiration

The aspiration of gastric contents is associated with several clinical syndromes including chemical pneumonitis, infectious pneumonia, and "recurring pneumonia syndrome" (73). Esophageal dysmotility is present in up to 80% of patients with PSS, PM/DM, and MCTD. Patients with PM/DM also have disordered swallowing reflexes due to oropharyngeal muscle involvement and an impaired cough secondary to respiratory muscle dysfunction. Occult aspiration may occur, with the patient noting only a chronic productive cough and intermittent fevers or episodic dyspnea and wheezing, suggestive of airway obstruction. Chronic aspiration may occasionally cause pulmonary fibrosis and mimic interstitial pulmonary involvement.

The diagnosis of an aspiration syndrome is based on history and clinical findings (73). It is frequently missed (74), at least in part owing to inadequate diagnostic tests (75). The clinical diagnosis can be supported by documentation of gastroesophageal reflux, direct radiographic evidence of barium aspiration, or open lung biopsy showing interstitial involvement with a granulomatous and fibrotic response. However, the only abnormality that unequivocally establishes the diagnosis of aspiration is the finding of food particles in the airway.

Despite a lack of data, it has frequently been stated that the appearance of lipid-laden macrophages in respiratory tract secretions is diagnostic of the aspiration of gastric contents. Corwin and Irwin prospectively evaluated macrophages obtained by BAL from patients with gastric aspiration and other parenchymal lung diseases for the presence of lipid (75). Intracellular lipid was present in macrophages from patients with all types of parenchymal lung disease examined; however, the use of a semiquantitative "lipid-laden alveolar macrophage index" was helpful in excluding aspiration as the cause of parenchymal lung disease. This study must be confirmed in other centers before BAL can be recommended as clinically useful in the diagnosis of gastric aspiration. The bronchoscopic demonstration of food particles in the airway is diagnostic, as mentioned above.

D. Alveolar Hemorrhage

Alveolar hemorrhage occurs in association with many immunologic disorders, including the rheumatic diseases (76). Pulmonary hemorrhage is most common in patients with active SLE (76) and has been reported in RA (77), PSS (78), and MCTD (79). The findings of hemoptysis, alveolar infiltrates, new or worsened anemia, and hypoxemia are strongly suggestive of alveolar hemorrhage.

Differentiating alveolar hemorrhage from other alveolar filling processes, particularly infection and edema, may be difficult. Correlation of sequential hemoglobins with chest radiographs and measurement of lung uptake of carbon monoxide ("diffusing capacity") are useful techniques for making these distinctions (76). Finding either frank blood or hemosiderin-laden macrophages in BAL fluid strongly suggests alveolar hemorrhage. It must be remembered that hemosiderin may not appear in BAL macrophages for 2 days following an acute hemorrhage and that it is generally cleared within 2 weeks (80). Kahn et al. studied the efficacy of BAL in diagnosing pulmonary hemorrhage (81). Severe pulmonary hemorrhage was diagnosed in 14 cases. In patients that had either lung biopsy or autopsy, the BAL macrophage "hemosiderin score" was closely correlated with the degree of hemorrhage seen in the histologic specimens.

Thus, BAL fluid analysis appears to be useful for the diagnosis of alveolar hemorrhage. Close consideration must be given to nonimmune causes of alveolar hemorrhage (e.g., necrotizing infections, hemorrhagic pulmonary edema, and severe coagulopathies) that can coexist in patients with CVD. BAL is particularly useful when both infection and alveolar hemorrhage are being considered (24).

VI. Conclusion

The clinical assessment of alveolar injury and interstitial lung disease in patients with rheumatic diseases is a difficult task. Both "traditional" (chest radiography, pulmonary function testing, and open lung biopsy) and "modern" (BAL and gallium-67 scanning) methods have failed to provide adequate data for optimal patient management. Fortunately, as detailed in Chapters 1 and 2, investigative efforts are beginning to unravel the mechanisms of pulmonary inflammation and fibrosis. To date the most promising technique for repetitively studying pulmonary inflammatory processes in humans is BAL. A greater understanding of basic mechanisms should allow us to focus our evaluation of lavage specimens on clinically relevant parameters. Finally, insights gained from basic investigation may allow the development of novel approaches to the clinical assessment of interstitial lung disease.

Acknowledgments

The author would like to thank Dr. Guy A. Zimmerman for helpful discussion and review of this manuscript and Linda Jara for assistance with its preparation.

References

1. Hunninghake, G. W., and Fauci, A. S. (1979). Pulmonary involvement in the collagen vascular diseases. *Am. Rev. Respir. Dis.* **119**:471-503.
2. Daniele, R. P., Henson, P. M., Fantone, J. C. III, Ward, P. A., and Dreisin, R. B. (1981). Immune complex injury of the lung. *Am. Rev. Respir. Dis.* **124**:738-755.
3. Crystal, R. G., Bitterman, P. B., Rennard, S. I., Hance, A. J., and Keogh, B. A. (1984). Interstitial lung diseases of unknown cause: Disorders characterized by chronic inflammation of the lower respiratory tract. *N. Engl. J. Med.* **310**:154-166, 235-244.
4. Black, L. F., and Katz, S. (1977). Respiratory diseases: Task force on prevention, control, education. National Heart and Lung Institute, Washington, DHEW Publication No. NIH, 77-1248.
5. Jansen, H. M., Schutte, A. J. H., Elema, J. D., et al. (1984). Local immune complexes and inflammatory response in patients with chronic interstitial pulmonary disorders associated with collagen vascular diseases. *Clin. Exp. Immunol.* **56**:311-320.
6. Decker, J. L., Steinberg, A. D., Reinertsen, J. L., Plotz, P. H., Balow, J. E., and Klippel, J. H. (1979). Systemic lupus erythematosis: Evolving concepts. *Ann. Intern. Med.* **91**:587-604.
7. Waellert, B., Prin, L., Hatron, P. Y., Ramon, P., Tonnel, A. B., and Voisin, C. (1987). Lymphocyte subpopulations in bronchoalveolar lavage in Sjogren's syndrome: Evidence for an expansion of cytotoxic/suppressor subset in patients with alveolar neutrophilia. *Chest* **92**:1025-1031.
8. Kahaleh, M. B., Sherer, G. K., and LeRoy, E. C. (1979). Endothelial injury in scleroderma. *J. Exp. Med.* **149**:1326-1335.
9. Currie, S., Saunders, M., Knowles, M., and Brown, A. E. (1971). Immunological aspects of polymyositis. *Q. J. Med.* **40**:63-84.
10. Carrington, C. B., Gaensler, E. A., Coutu, R. E., FitzGerald, M. X., and Gupta, R. G. (1978). Natural history and treated course of usual and desquamative interstitial pneumonia. *N. Engl. J. Med.* **298**:801-809.

11. Doctor, L., and Snider, G. L. (1962). Diffuse interstitial pulmonary fibrosis associated with arthritis: With comments on the definition of rheumatoid lung disease. *Am. Rev. Respir. Dis.* **85**:413-422.
12. Yousem, S. A., Colby, T. V., and Carrington, C. B. (1985). Lung biopsy in rheumatoid arthritis. *Am. Rev. Respir. Dis.* **131**:770-777.
13. Duncan, P. E., Griffin, J. P., Garcia, A., and Kaplan, S. B. (1974). Fibrosing alveolitis in polymyositis: A review of histologically confirmed cases. *Am. J. Med.* **57**:621-626.
14. Keogh, B. A., and Crystal, R. G. (1980). Clinical significance of pulmonary function tests: Pulmonary function testing in interstitial pulmonary disease—what does it tell us? *Chest* **78**:856-865.
15. Gaensler, E. A., and Carrington, C. B. (1980). Open biopsy for chronic diffuse infiltrative lung disease: Clinical, roentgenographic and physiological correlations in 502 patients. *Ann. Thorac. Surg.* **30**:411-426.
16. Ray, J. F. III, Lawton, B. R., Myers, W. O., et al. (1976). Open pulmonary biopsy: Nineteen-year experience with 416 consecutive operations. *Chest* **69**:43-47.
17. Newman, S. L., Michel, R. P., and Wang, N. (1985). Lingular lung biopsy: Is it representative? *Am. Rev. Respir. Dis.* **132**:1084-1086.
18. Wetstein, L. (1986). Sensitivity and specificity of lingular segmental biopsies of the lung. *Chest* **90**:383-386.
19. Miller, R. R., Nelems, B., Müller, N. L., Evans, K. G., and Ostrow, D. N. (1987). Lingular and right middle lobe biopsy in the assessment of diffuse lung disease. *Ann. Thorac. Surg.* **44**:269-273.
20. Levin, D. C., Wicks, A. B., and Ellis, J. H. Jr. (1974). Transbronchial lung biopsy via the fiberoptic bronchoscope. *Am. Rev. Respir. Dis.* **110**: 4-12.
21. Reynolds, H. Y. (1988). Staging and follow-up of disease activity. In *Interstitial Lung Disease.* Edited by Schwartz, M. I., and T. E. King Jr. B.C. Decker, Toronto, pp. 15-26.
22. Wall, C. P., Gaensler, E. A., Carrington, C. B., and Hayes, J. A. (1981). Comparison of transbronchial and open biopsies in chronic infiltrative lung diseases. *Am. Rev. Respir. Dis.* **123**:280-285.
23. Reynolds, H. Y. (1987). Bronchoalveolar lavage. *Am. Rev. Respir. Dis.* **135**:250-263.
24. Stover, D. E., Zaman, M. B., Hajdu, S. I., Lange, M., Gold, J., and Armstrong, D. (1984). Bronchoalveolar lavage in the diagnosis of diffuse pulmonary infiltrates in the immunosuppressed host. *Ann. Intern. Med.* **101**:1-7.
25. Rizzo, T., Rollins, R. J., Fairfax, W. R., Elstad, M. R., Weiss, R. L., and Schumann, G. B. (1988). Bronchoalveolar lavage (BAL) cytology allows rapid and accurate diagnosis of cytomegalovirus (CMV) and

Pneumocystis carinii pneumonia (PCP) in organ transplant patients. *Acta Cytol. 32*:7656.

26. Stoller, J. K., Rankin, J. A., and Reynolds, H. Y. (1987). The impact of bronchoalveolar lavage cell analysis on clinicians' diagnostic reasoning about interstitial lung disease. *Chest* **92**:839-843.

27. Elstad, M. R., and Schumann, G. B. (1989). Bronchoalveolar lavage cytology. (Submitted.)

28. Pingleton, S. K., Harrison, G. F., Stechschulte, D. J., Wesselius, L. J., Kerby, G. R., and Ruth, W. E. (1983). Effect of location, pH, and temperature of instillate in bronchoalveolar lavage in normal volunteers. *Am. Rev. Respir. Dis.* **128**:1035-1037.

29. Garcia, J. G. N., Wolven, R. G., Garcia, P. L., and Keogh, B. A. (1986). Assessment of interlobar variation of bronchoalveolar lavage cellular differentials in interstitial lung diseases. *Am. Rev. Respir. Dis.* **133**:444-449.

30. Tonnel, A. B., Voisin, C., Lafitte, J. J., et al. (1979). Variations des populations cellulaires recullies par lavage bronchoalveolaire en fonction de la topographie des lesions et de l'etage explore. *Inserm* **84**:271-280.

31. Chamberlain, D. W., Braude, A. C., and Rebuck, A. S. (1987). A critical evaluation of bronchoalveolar lavage: Criteria for identifying unsatisfactory specimens. *Acta Cytol.* **31**:599-605.

32. Staab, E. V., and McCartney, W. H. (1978). Role of gallium 67 in inflammatory disease. *Semin. Nucl. Med.* **8**:219-234.

33. Siemsen, J. K., Grebe, S. F., and Waxman, A. D. (1978). The use of gallium-67 in pulmonary disorders. *Semin. Nucl. Med.* **8**:235-249.

34. Hunninghake, G. W., Line, B. R., Szapiel, S. V., and Crystal, R. G. (1981). Activation of inflammatory cells increases the localization of gallium-67 at sites of disease. *Clin. Res.* **29**:171A (abstract).

35. Line, B. R., Hunninghake, G. W., Keogh, B. A., Jones, A. E., Johnston, G. S., and Crystal, R. G. (1981). Gallium-67 scanning to stage the alveolitis of sarcoidosis: Correlation with clinical studies, pulmonary function studies, and bronchoalveolar lavage. *Am. Rev. Respir. Dis.* **123**:440-446.

36. Line, B. R., Fulmer, J. D., Reynolds, H. Y., et al. (1978). Gallium-67 citrate scanning in the staging of idiopathic pulmonary fibrosis: Correlation with physiologic and morphologic features and bronchoalveolar lavage. *Am. Rev. Respir. Dis.* **118**:355-365.

37. Beaumont, D., Herry, J. Y., Sapene, M., Bourguet, P., Larzul, J. J., and De la Garthe, B. (1982). Gallium-67 in the evaluation of sarcoidosis: Correlations with serum angiotensin-converting enzyme and bronchoalveolar lavage. *Thorax* **37**:11-82.

38. King, T. E. Jr. (1988). Idiopathic pulmonary fibrosis. In *Interstitial Lung Disease*. Edited by Schwartz, M. I., and T. E. King Jr. B.C. Decker, Toronto, pp. 139-169.
39. Ellman, P., and Ball, R. E. (1948). "Rheumatoid disease" with joint and pulmonary manifestations. *Br. Med. J.* **2**:816-820.
40. Wall, C. P., Gaensler, E. A., Carrington, C. B., and Hayes, J. A. (1981). Comparison of transbronchial and open biopsies in chronic infiltrative lung diseases. *Am. Rev. Respir. Dis.* **123**:280-285.
41. King, T. E. Jr., and Dunn, T. L. (1988). Connective tissue disease. In *Interstitial Lung Disease*. Edited by Schwartz, M. I., and T. E. King Jr. B.C. Decker, Toronto, pp. 139-169.
42. Niden, A. H., Mishkin, F. S., and Khurana, M. M. L. (1976). 67-Gallium citrate lung scans in interstitial lung disease. *Chest* **69(s)**:266-268.
43. Turner-Warwick, M., and Evans, R. C. (1977). Pulmonary manifestations of rheumatoid disease. *Clin. Rheum. Dis.* **3**:549-564.
44. Wallaert, B., Bart, F., Aerts, C., et al. (1988). Activated alveolar macrophages in subclinical pulmonary inflammation in collagen vascular diseases. *Thorax* **43**:24-30.
45. Turner-Warwick, M., and Haslam, P. (1987). The value of serial bronchoalveolar lavages in assessing the clinical progress of patients with cryptogenic fibrosing alveolitis. *Am. Rev. Respir. Dis.* **135**:26-34.
46. Greene, N. B., Solinger, A. M., and Baughman, R. P. (1987). Patients with collagen vascular disease and dyspnea: The value of gallium scanning and bronchoalveolar lavage in predicting response to steroid therapy and clinical outcome. *Chest* **91**:698-703.
47. Wallaert, B., Hatron, P. Y., Grosbois, J. M., Tonnel, A. B., Devulder, B., and Voisin, C. (1986). Subclinical pulmonary involvement in collagen-vascular diseases assessed by bronchoalveolar lavage: Relationship between alveolitis and subsequent changes in lung function. *Am. Rev. Respir. Dis.* **133**:574-580.
48. Nagai, S., Fujimura, N., Hirata, T., and Izumi, T. (1985). Differentiation between idiopathic pulmonary fibrosis and interstitial pneumonia associated with collagen vascular diseases by comparison of the ratio of OKT4 + cells and OKT8 + cells in BALF T lymphocytes. *Eur. J. Respir. Dis.* **67**:1-9.
49. Haslam, P. L., Turton, C. W. G., Lukoszek, A., et al. (1980). Bronchoalveolar lavage fluid cell counts in cryptogenic fibrosing alveolitis and their relation to therapy. *Thorax* **35**:328-339.
50. Owens, G. R., Paradis, I. L., Gryzan, S., et al. (1986). Role of inflammation in the lung disease of systemic sclerosis: Comparison with idiopathic pulmonary fibrosis. *J. Lab. Clin. Med.* **107**:253-260.

51. Rossi, G. A., Bitterman, P. B., Rennard, S. I., Ferrans, V. J., and Crystal, R. G. (1985). Evidence for chronic inflammation as a component of the interstitial lung disease associated with progressive systemic sclerosis. *Am. Rev. Respir. Dis.* **131**:612-617.

52. Edelson, J. D., Hyland, R. H., Ramsden, M., et al. (1985). Lung inflammation in scleroderma: Clinical, radiographic, physiologic and cytopathological features. *J. Rheum.* **12**:957-963.

53. König, G., Luderschmidt, C., Hammer, C., Adelmann-Grill, B. C., Braun-Falco, O., and Fruhmann, G. (1984). Lung involvement in scleroderma. *Chest* **85**:318-324.

54. Silver, R. M., Metcalf, J. F., Stanley, J. H., and LeRoy, E. C. (1984). Interstitial lung disease in scleroderma: Analysis by bronchoalveolar lavage. *Arthritis Rheum.* **27**:1254-1262.

55. Kallenberg, C. G. M., Jansen, H. M., Elema, J. D., and The, T. H. (1984). Steroid-responsive interstitial pulmonary disease in systemic sclerosis: Monitoring by bronchoalveolar lavage. *Chest* **86**:489-492.

56. Garcia, J. G. N., James, H. L., Zinkgraf, S., Perlman, M. B., and Keogh, B. A. (1987). Lower respiratory tract abnormalities in rheumatoid interstitial lung disease: Potential role of neutrophils in lung injury. *Am. Rev. Respir. Dis.* **136**:811-817.

57. Garcia, J. G. N., Parhami, N., Killam, D., Garcia, P. L., and Keogh, B. A. (1986). Bronchoalveolar lavage fluid evaluation in rheumatoid arthritis. *Am. Rev. Respir. Dis.* **133**:450-454.

58. Tishler, M., Grief, J., Fireman, E., Yaron, M., and Topilsky, M. (1986). Bronchoalveolar lavage—a sensitive tool for early diagnosis of pulmonary involvement in rheumatoid arthritis. *J. Rheumatol.* **13**:547-550.

59. Hatron, P.-Y., Wallaert, B., Gosset, D., et al. (1987). Subclinical lung inflammation in primary Sjögren's syndrome: Relationship between bronchoalveolar lavage cellular analysis findings and characteristics of the disease. *Arthritis Rheum.* **30**:1226-1231.

60. Thomas, P. D., and Hunninghake, G. W. (1987). Current concepts of the pathogenesis of sarcoidosis. *Am. Rev. Respir. Dis.* **135**:747-760.

61. Peters-Golden, M., Wise, R. A., Schneider, P., Hochberg, M., Stevens, M. B., and Wigley, F. (1984). Clinical and demographic predictors of loss of pulmonary function in systemic sclerosis. *Medicine* **63**:211-231.

62. Baron, M., Geiglin, D., Hyland, R., Urowitz, M. B., and Shiff, B. (1983). 67-Gallium lung scans in progressive systemic sclerosis. *Arthritis Rheum.* **26**:969-974.

63. Furst, D. E., Davis, J. A., Clements, P. J., Chopra, S. K., Theofilopoulos, A. N., and Chia, D. (1981). Abnormalities of pulmonary vascular dynamics and inflammation in early progressive systemic sclerosis. *Arthritis Rheum.* **24**:1403-1408.

64. Wallaert, B., Aerts, C., Bart, F., et al. (1987). Alveolar macrophage dysfunction in systemic lupus erythematosus. *Am. Rev. Respir. Dis.* **136**:.293-297.
65. Schwartz, M. I., Matthay, R. A., Sahn, S. A., Stanford, R. E., Marmorstein, B. L., and Scheinhorn, D. J. (1976). Interstitial lung disease in polymyositis and dermatomyositis: Analysis of six cases and review of the literature. *Medicine* **55**:89-104.
66. Davis, W. B., and Gadek, J. E. (1987). Detection of pulmonary lymphoma by bronchoalveolar lavage. *Chest* **91**:787-790.
67. Collins, R. D. Jr., Ball, G. V., and Logic, J. R. (1984). Gallium-67 scanning in Sjögren's syndrome: Concise communication. *J. Nucl. Med.* **25**:299-302.
68. Sullivan, W. D., Hurst, D. J., Harmon, C. E., et al. (1984). A prospective evaluation emphasizing pulmonary involvement in patients with mixed connective tissue disease. *Medicine* **63**:92-107.
69. Springmeyer, S. C., Hackman, R. C., Holle, R., et al. (1986). Use of bronchoalveolar lavage to diagnose acute diffuse pneumonia in the immunocompromised host. *J. Infect. Dis.* **154**:604-611.
70. Kahn, F. W., and Jones, J. M. (1987). Diagnosing bacterial respiratory infection by bronchoalveolar lavage. *J. Infect. Dis.* **155**:862-869.
71. Cooper, J. A. D. Jr., White, D. A., and Matthay, R. A. (1986). Drug-induced pulmonary disease. Part 1: Cytotoxic drugs; Part 2: Noncytotoxic drugs. *Am. Rev. Respir. Dis.* **133**:321-340, 488-505.
72. Akoun, G. M., Mayaud, C. M., Touboul, J.-L., and Denis, M. (1986). Methotrexate-induced pneumonitis: Diagnostic value of bronchoalveolar lavage cell data. *Arch. Intern. Med.* **146**:804 (letter).
73. Zimmerman, G. A. (1987). Syndromes caused by the aspiration of gastric contents. In *Current Therapy in Critical Care Medicine.* Edited by Parillo, J. E., B.C. Decker, Toronto, pp. 178-184.
74. Volk, B. W., Nathanson, L., Losner, S., Slade, W. R., and Jacobi, M. (1951). Incidence of lipoid pneumonia in a survey of 389 chronically ill patients. *Am. J. Med.* **10**:316-324.
75. Corwin, R. W., and Irwin, R. S. (1985). The lipid-laden alveolar macrophage as a marker of aspiration in parenchymal lung disease. *Am. Rev. Respir. Dis.* **132**:576-581.
76. Leatherman, J. W. (1987). Immune alveolar hemorrhage. *Chest* **91**: 891-897.
77. Smith, B. S. (1966). Idiopathic pulmonary haemosiderosis and rheumatoid arthritis. *Br. Med. J.* **1**:1403-1404.
78. Kallenbach, J., Prinsloo, I., and Zwi, S. (1977). Progressive systemic sclerosis complicated by diffuse pulmonary haemorrhage. *Thorax* **32**: 767-770.

79. Germain, M. J., and Davidman, M. (1984). Pulmonary hemorrhage and acute renal failure in a patient with mixed connective tissue disease. *Am. J. Kidney Dis.* **3**:420-424.

80. Sherman, J. M., Winnie, G., Thomassen, M. J., Abdul-Karim, F. W., and Boat, T. F. (1984). Time course of hemosiderin production and clearance by human pulmonary macrophages. *Chest* **86**:409-411.

81. Kahn, F. W., Jones, J. M., and England, D. M. (1987). Diagnosis of pulmonary hemorrhage in the immunocompromised host. *Am. Rev. Respir. Dis.* **136**:155-160.

6

Lung Pathology

THOMAS V. COLBY

Mayo Clinic
Rochester, Minnesota

I. Introduction

There are a number of problems that arise in assessing the pulmonary pathology associated with collagen vascular diseases. In the first place, clinical definitions of collagen vascular diseases are somewhat arbitrary; the pathologist is at the mercy of the clinical diagnosis, and it may not always be possible to correlate histologic changes with specific collagen vascular diseases. Second, there is the possibility that pulmonary abnormalities may be coincidental in a patient who also has collagen vascular disease. Determinations of real associations are also somewhat arbitrary; however, it is generally agreed that many collagen vascular diseases are associated with a number of pulmonary conditions, which are included in the following discussion.

Clinical and functional evaluations of asymptomatic patients with a variety of collagen vascular diseases have shown the presence of minor but identifiable pulmonary deficits in a significant percentage (1-4). Because these patients have subclinical abnormalities, their histologic correlate is often not known. In addition, among patients who are symptomatic, there are usually several different histologic patterns that can produce a similar clinical picture; rarely does one have a one-to-one association between a morphologic lesion and a clinical syndrome.

The pathogenesis of lung disease in collagen vascular diseases is not well understood, and in relatively few instances is there good correlation. Acute interstitial lung disease and/or alveolar hemorrhage in patients with systemic lupus erythematosis is thought to be immune complex mediated (5-11); however, the mere identification of immune complexes is not always synonomous with disease, and they may be absent in patients who have overt pulmonary disease, and present in patients who have pulmonary disease caused by other problems (such as pulmonary edema). Recent bronchoalveolar lavage findings have shown a subclinical "alveolitis" in patients with collagen vascular diseases (3,4), and the significance of this remains to be shown; however, data of this type may help elucidate the pathogenesis of the pathologic findings associated with collagen vascular diseases.

There are also secondary and treatment-related conditions that may be identical in their clinical and even their histologic presentation to the lesions known to be associated with collagen vascular diseases. These can be broadly divided into secondary effects of the disease itself and consequences of its treatment. The former include systemic amyloidosis with lung involvement in patients with chronic rheumatoid arthritis, the development of bronchoalveolar carcinoma in patients with interstitial fibrosis associated with progressive systemic sclerosis (12), and pulmonary emboli in patients with lupus anticoagulant (13,14). Among the latter are immunosuppression with opportunistic infections and toxic and idiosyncratic drug reactions.

Table 1 shows an overview of the pulmonary pathologic changes found in the collagen vascular diseases.

II. Rheumatoid Arthritis

The major pathologic changes in the lungs of patients with rheumatoid arthritis (RA) are represented by pleural, interstitial, and nodular disease; airway lesions and vascular changes are less common (7,8,15-24). Presentation with lung disease may precede the articular findings by months or years.

Pleural fibrosis is almost universal at autopsy and is indicative of a previous active pleuritis which may occasionally be seen in biopsy material. The fibrotic reaction is generally quite nonspecific and may resemble the hyaline pleural plaques seen in patients with asbestos exposure. The active pleuritis is usually also nonspecific; however, occasionally it is sufficiently distinct to allow the pathologist to consider RA (Fig. 1). It is almost as if a rheumatoid nodule has been marsupialized onto the pleural surface: there is a fibrinous pleuritis with fibrinoid material surrounded by palisaded cells, as seen in a rheumatoid nodule. Clinically, this may produce a sterile empyema.

Table 1 Pulmonary Pathology in the Collagen Vascular Disease[a]

	Rheumatoid arthritis	Juvenile rheumatoid arthritis	Systemic lupus erythematosus	Progressive systemic sclerosis	Polymyositis dermatomyositis	Mixed connective tissue disease	Sjögren's syndrome	Ankylosing spondylitis	Behçet's disease
Pleural inflammation, fibrosis, effusions	X	X	X	X					
Airway disease, inflammation, obstruction, lymphoid hyperplasia	X	X	X	X			X		
Interstitial disease	X	X	X	X	X	X	X		
Acute (+/−) hemorrhage)	X	X	X	X					
Subacute/organizing (BOOP)	X		X	X	X		X		
Chronic cellular	X		X				X		
Chronic cellular and fibrosing	X	X	X	X	X	X	X		
Eosinophilic infiltrates	X								
Vascular disease Hypertension/ vasculitis	X	X	X	X		X	X		X
Parenchymal nodules	X	X							
Apical fibrobullous disease	X							X	
Lymphoid proliferations							X		

[a]Modified from reference 15.

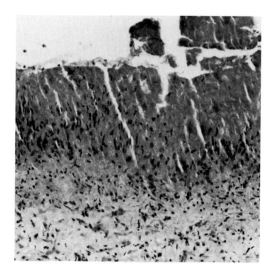

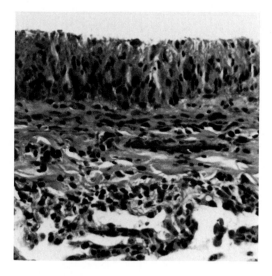

Figure 1 Aseptic rheumatoid empyema associated with fibrinous debris in the pleural space which is lined by a layer of palisaded histiocytes reminiscent of a rheumatoid nodule.

The interstitial lung disease associated with RA comprises a broad spectrum that includes both acute and chronic histologic lesions (24). Patterns include cellular interstitial infiltrates without significant fibrosis, interstitial fibrosing pneumonias resembling usual interstitial pneumonia (UIP; synonym = idiopathic pulmonary fibrosis), desquamative interstitial pneumonia, and lymphocytic interstitial pneumonia (Figs. 2-4). In addition, a significant

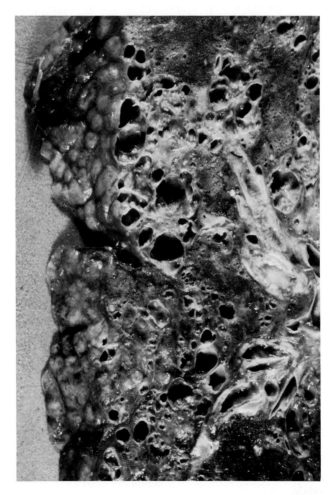

Figure 2 Gross findings at autopsy from a patient with RA and chronic fibrosing interstitial lung disease leading to honeycombing. Note the honeycomb spaces lined by gray fibrotic walls and the knobby, contracted pleural surface.

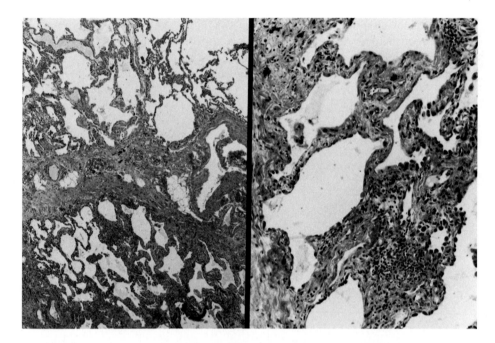

Figure 3 Chronic fibrosing interstitial pneumonia in RA associated with patchy septal and alveolar wall scarring. Note the absence of involvement of some alveolar walls. Involved alveolar walls (right) show fibrosis and a modest chronic inflammatory infiltrate.

number of cases show subacute features with abundant organizing granulation tissue within air spaces, producing the pattern of bronchiolitis obliterans organizing pneumonia (BOOP). Occasional cases manifest only as lymphoid hyperplasia along lymphatic routes (along bronchovascular structures in the septa and the pleura). Lymphoid hyperplasia along the airways has led to the descriptive designations of follicular bronchitis or follicular bronchiolitis. The histologic picture of chronic eosinophilic pneumonia is sometimes seen in RA (18,19,24). Acute interstitial lung disease with the histologic features of diffuse alveolar damage is also occasionally seen (24). Rheumatoid nodules may be found on biopsies done for radiographic evidence of interstitial lung disease (24).

    Combinations of patterns frequently occur in RA, and precise classification may prove difficult, requiring designation of two or more patterns (24). The prognosis of interstitial lung disease in RA is correlated with the amount of irreversible scarring and honeycombing (24). Thus, patients who lack much fibrosis even though they may have an impressive degree of cellular

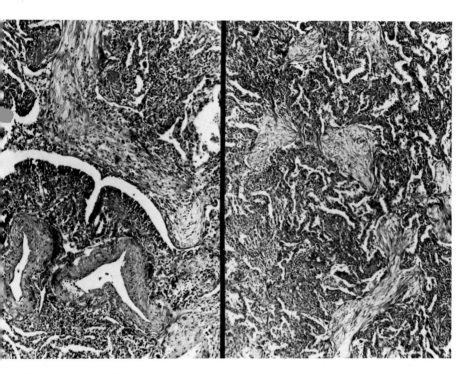

Figure 4 Bronchiolitis obliterans organizing pneumonia in RA. There is organizing granulation tissue within bronchiolar lumens (left) with extension into distal parenchyma, particularly alveolar ducts (right). There are pale, evenly spaced plugs of edematous connective tissue with intervening lung parenchyma showing interstitial thickening with a chronic inflammatory infiltrate. There is relative preservation of the lung architecture.

infiltrates and lymphoid proliferation have a better prognosis; patients with abundant airspace organization fare better than those with interstitial scarring and honeycombing. Since the drugs used to treat rheumatoid arthritis, particularly methotrexate (Fig. 5) and gold, may produce a number of similar histologic patterns (21,25), they should always be considered in the differential diagnosis, and in most cases a drug reaction cannot be excluded on histologic grounds alone.

Patients with rheumatoid nodules in the lung usually have subcutaneous rheumatoid nodules and active joint disease. Rarely, rheumatoid nodules in the lung are discovered in the absence of articular manifestations (17). The histologic findings in the lung are similar to rheumatoid nodules in the subcutaneous tissue (Fig. 6), and their distribution in a pleural and septal location is

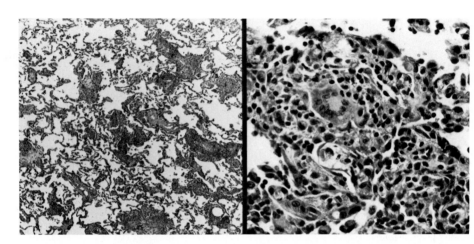

Figure 5 Interstitial pneumonia due to a low-dose methotrexate therapy in RA. There is a patchy inflammatory process associated with prominent perivenular infiltrates as well as small foci of organization with a chronic inflammatory infiltrate. Small clusters of epithelioid histiocytes with giant cells (granulomas) were found.

helpful in the differential diagnosis. Centrally there is fibrinoid debris surrounded by palisaded histiocytes. Giant cells are occasionally seen although not prominent, and sarcoidlike, noncaseating granulomas are unusual. The central necrosis may contain neutrophils and basophilic debris but is more often eosinophilic and fibrinoid in character.

Caplan's syndrome represents the development of rheumatoid arthritis in patients with established silicosis (8). The fibrotic silicotic nodules undergo fibrinoid degeneration, sometimes with conglomeration of nodules and extensive scarring. Tuberculosis should also be considered in the differential diagnosis.

Although uncommon, airway involvement in rheumatoid arthritis may be rapidly fatal (20,21). Mild airway changes, including peribronchial and peribronchiolar lymphoid infiltrates and/or fibrosis with lymphoid hyperplasia (germinal centers), are relatively common and may not be associated with much symptomatology. Bronchiolitis obliterans affecting small airways without involvement of adjacent lung parenchyma (and hence a distinguishing feature from BOOP) is a rare but devastating problem that is associated with progressive airway obstruction and usually leads to death over a period of months (Fig. 7). This rare form of pure bronchiolitis obliterans with obstruction has been seen in patients on penicillamine therapy as well as in patients who have not had penicillamine (21). The histologic changes may be relatively subtle since only the smaller airways are affected, and one may

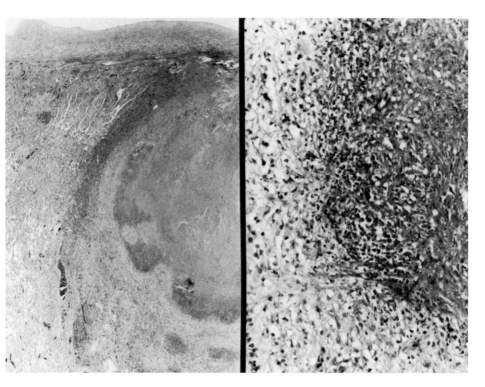

Figure 6 Rheumatoid nodules are generally pleural or septal in distribution and associated with central fibrinoid necrosis surrounded by a rim of fibrous tissue, palisaded histiocytes, and chronic inflammatory cells. This lesion is subpleural (left), and there are both fibrinoid material and agranular neutrophilic debris (right) in the necrotic center.

need to examine multiple sections at various levels to demonstrate the occlusive lesions in the small airways which may be focal and segmental. The use of elastic tissue stains is extremely valuable in recognizing these lesions.

Pulmonary arterial and venous thickening and intimal sclerosis are common in any widespread fibrosing lung disease and are almost universal in rheumatoid patients with extensive interstitial fibrosis. This is a secondary phenomenon related to the fibrosis and rarely associated with clinically significant pulmonary vascular disease other than the cor pulmonale that develops in patients with extensive interstitial fibrosis. Pulmonary hypertension in the absence of extensive interstitial disease occurs rarely in rheumatoid arthritis, and the characteristic medial and intimal thickening, as with any case of pulmonary hypertension, is seen histologically. When pulmonary

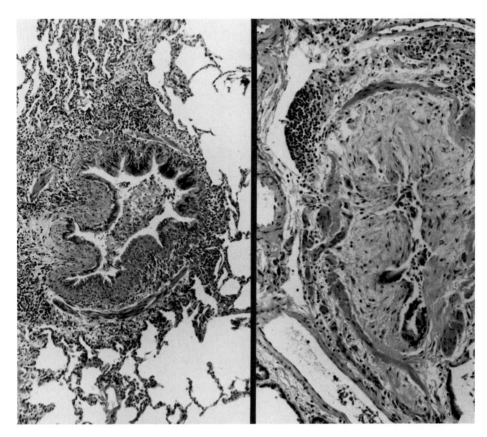

Figure 7 Progressive fatal bronchiolitis obliterans associated with progressive airway obstruction in RA. There are varying degrees of submucosal scarring, inflammation, and luminal compromise; the bronchiole at right is almost entirely obliterated.

hypertension is severe, necrotizing arteritis may develop superimposed on the hypertensive changes (Fig. 8). Primary vasculitis affecting pulmonary arteries and/or veins in the lungs of patients with rheumatoid arthritis also occurs.

Patients with rheumatoid arthritis who develop pulmonary complications are often said to have "rheumatoid lung." From the pathologist's point of view this designation is incomplete without a histologic modifier to subclassify the lesion, which, as can be seen from the table, can assume a variety of histologic patterns with quite variable prognoses.

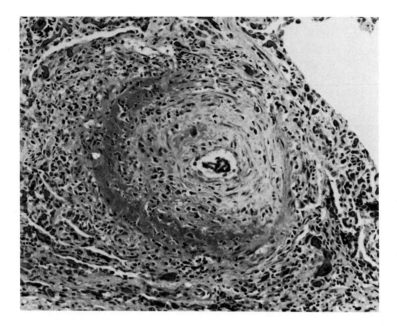

Figure 8 Pulmonary hypertension with secondary necrotizing vasculitis in a patient with long-standing RA. This patient had a 4-year history of pulmonary hypertension with terminal rapid deterioration. Open lung biopsy prior to death and autopsy showed a necrotizing arteritis with fibrinoid necrosis involving arterial walls superimposed on changes of chronic pulmonary hypertension with medial hypertrophy and intimal thickening.

III. Juvenile Rheumatoid Arthritis (JRA)

A number of lesions have been described clinically in patients with juvenile rheumatoid arthritis, but histologic documentation is incomplete (23,26-29). One patient had evidence of pulmonary disease 7 years prior to the development of JRA (23). In another report, abnormal pulmonary function tests were found in 50% of patients (28). The histologic lesions described include organizing pleuritis, pleural adhesions, lymphoid hyperplasia and follicular bronchiolitis (Fig. 9), interstitial infiltrates with or without fibrosis, pulmonary hypertension with arteritis, and siderosis indicative of prior alveolar hemorrhage.

IV. Sjogren's Syndrome

Since a number of patients with Sjögren's syndrome also have rheumatoid arthritis, any of the changes described in RA may occur in Sjögren's syndrome.

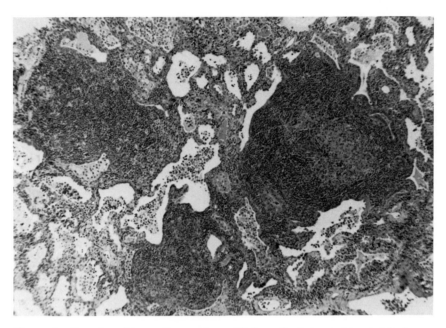

Figure 9   Open lung biopsy from patient with juvenile rheumatoid arthritis showing pulmonary lymphoid hyperplasia with prominent lymphoid follicles containing
germinal centers associated with secondary nonspecific accumulations of macrophages
within airspaces and a mild alveolar wall infiltrate.

However, pulmonary involvement is also relatively frequent in patients with
Sjögren's syndrome who do not have RA; the changes mainly include interstitial lung disease and airway disease with involvement of the small airways,
upper airway desiccation due to minor salivary gland atrophy, and large airway obstruction (8,15,20,30-33).

   Histologic changes associated with the airways disease include a secondary tracheobronchitis due to atrophy of the submucosal glands which
shows lymphoid infiltrates similar to those in the major and minor salivary
glands. The airways may also show peribronchial and peribronchiolar infiltrates with or without fibrosis and/or lymphoid hyperplasia (Fig. 10) and
bronchiolitis obliterans either as granulation tissue plugs or as fibrotic obliteration or stenosis. The histologic spectrum of interstitial disease includes
BOOP, nonspecific cellular interstitial infiltrates, which may become sufficiently dense to make the label lymphocytic interstitial pneumonia (LIP)
appropriate (Fig. 11), and fibrosing interstitial pneumonias resembling usual
interstitial pneumonia. A distinctive lesion in Sjögren's syndrome is a dense
but sometimes patchy lymphoid infiltrate associated with large numbers of

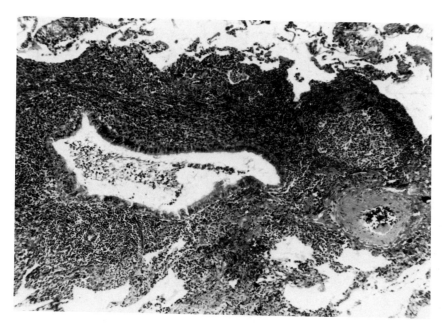

Figure 10 Follicular bronchiolitis in Sjögren's syndrome. There is marked lymphoid hyperplasia with germinal center formation along the small airways. Some compromise of the airway function is noted by the presence of mucostasis and cells within the bronchiolar lumen.

histiocytes aggregating into granulomas, as well as giant cells either singly or in clusters. While granulomas are characteristic of Sjögren's syndrome, their presence should lead to an exclusion of infection (Fig. 12), particularly in patients who have been on steroids. As in rheumatoid arthritis, more than one histologic pattern may be present, and precise characterization may prove difficult.

Patients with Sjögren's syndrome are prone to develop lymphoproliferative lesions in a number of sites, and the lung is no exception (8). The term pseudolymphoma has often been used, but a number of these lesions have been found to be monoclonal and hence low-grade lymphomas. Thus, lymphoma is a possibility in any patient with Sjögren's syndrome with dense lymphoid infiltrates, either nodular or diffuse. At the time of biopsy, consideration should be given to freezing tissue for immunologic marker studies.

V. Systemic Lupus Erythematosus (SLE)

The major histologic lesions seen in SLE include pleuritis or pleural fibrosis, acute interstitial lung disease, chronic interstitial lung disease, and pulmonary

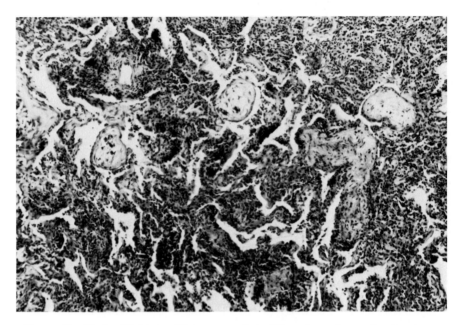

Figure 11   Unclassified interstitial pneumonia in Sjögren's syndrome showing dense alveolar wall infiltrates resembling lymphocytic interstitial pneumonia associated with pale tufts of organizing granulation tissue (organizing pneumonia) within air spaces.

hypertension (5-8,10,13-15,24,34-40). Since patients with SLE have frequently been on immunosuppressive therapy, the possibility of secondary pulmonary lesions such as infectious pneumonias and pulmonary edema should be considered, and, in fact, numerically these are more common causes of lung pathology at autopsy (35).

The pleural changes include an acute and/or organizing fibrinous pleuritis, pleural fibrosis (Fig. 13), and the presence of hematoxylin bodies in cytologic preparations of pleural effusions (Fig. 14). Hematoxylin bodies are rarely seen in biopsy specimens.

Acute interstitial lung disease in SLE takes the form of edema, diffuse alveolar damage (Figs. 15, 16), or alveolar hemorrhage (Fig. 17); the term "lupus pneumonitis" has often been used for the last two. If frozen tissue is examined, immune complexes are frequently demonstrated. The diffuse alveolar damage varies from a diffuse mild interstitial pneumonia with prominent type 2 cells and hyaline membranes to a diffuse organizing lesion dominated by intraalveolar and alveolar wall fibroplasia. A distinctive, though nonspecific, feature of diffuse alveolar damage in SLE is the presence of basophilic edematous widening of the alveolar septa. A finding in some cases

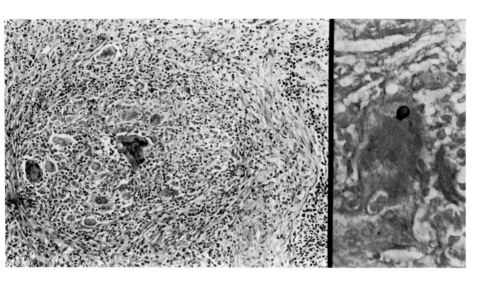

(a)

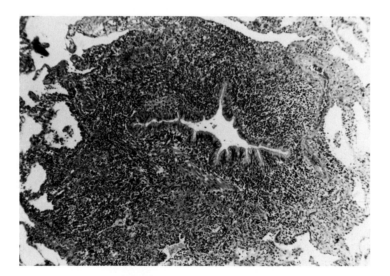

(b)

Figure 12 A patient with Sjögren's syndrome on steroids developed a localized infiltrate. (a) There is granulomatous inflammation (left), and rare yeast forms on silver stain (right). Culture grew *Blastomyces*. (b) Airways at some distance away showed a cellular bronchiolitis typical of Sjogren's syndrome.

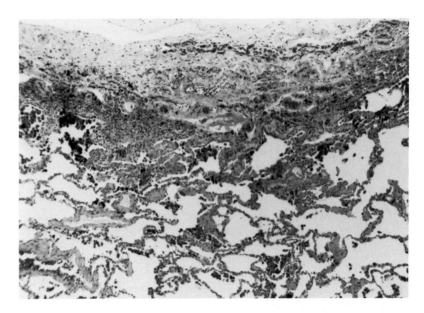

Figure 13 Open lung biopsy from a patient with long-standing SLE with a history of recurrent pleuritis and effusions. There are pleural fibrosis and adhesions indicative of a healed pleuritis. The subpleural parenchyma shows a mild inflammatory infiltrate of the interstitium with accumulations of macrophages in airspaces which appear dark because of the presence of hemosiderin. The findings were interpreted as evidence of recurrent pulmonary hemorrhage leaving a residue of hemosiderin-filled macrophages.

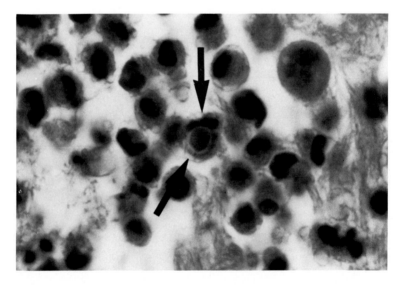

Figure 14 Cell block preparation from a pleural effusion in SLE. Numerous hematoxylin bodies (center) were identified.

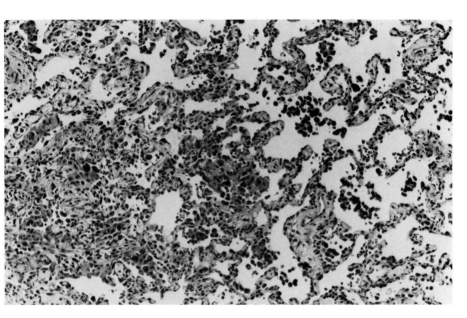

Figure 15 Steroid-responsive acute interstitial pneumonia in SLE. There is uniform mild edematous widening of alveolar walls with a modest inflammatory infiltrate and a mild to moderate alveolar space infiltrate of macrophages, some of which contain hemosiderin and red blood cells.

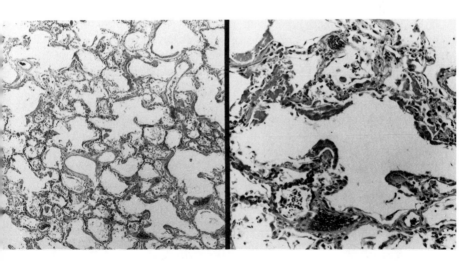

Figure 16 Diffuse alveolar damage with hyaline membrane formation at autopsy in patient with SLE. No other cause for the diffuse alveolar damage was identified, and it was presumed (by exclusion) to be due to SLE.

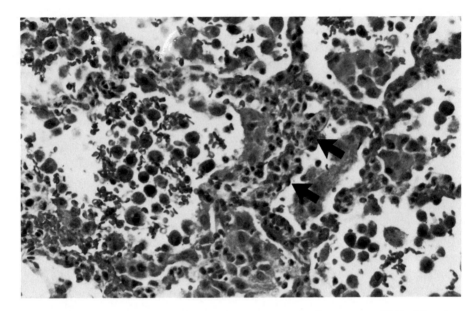

Figure 17   Acute pulmonary hemorrhage in lupus. The air spaces are filled with red blood cells and macrophages, many of which contain hemosiderin, indicative of recent and old hemorrhage. The capillary wall (arrows) shows an infiltrate of neutrophils (capillaritis), and immune complexes were demonstrated by immunofluorescence.

is capillaritis (39), a neutrophilic infiltrate limited to the capillary wall with little associated air space accumulation (which would be typical of a bacterial pneumonia). This is probably a histologic correlate of immune complex deposition. Capillaritis is nonspecific and may be seen with infections and other vasculidities, and in its absence the hemorrhage and diffuse alveolar damage of SLE are quite nonspecific.

The chronic interstitial lung disease seen in SLE (Fig. 18) includes the patterns of nonspecific cellular interstitial infiltrates, usual interstitial pneumonia, BOOP, and a mild nonspecific interstitial fibrosis associated with marked increase in hemosiderin-filled macrophages (hemosiderosis), representing the residue of prior and/or recurrent pulmonary hemorrhage, which may or may not have been clinically evident.

The vascular changes in SLE include pulmonary hypertension with or without an associated secondary necrotizing vasculitis when the hypertension is severe; the histologic features in such cases are nonspecific, being identical to those seen in idiopathic plexogenic arteriopathy (primary pulmonary hypertension). Primary pulmonary vasculitis is described in SLE, and this may overlap with the capillaritis in acute interstitial disease or show the pattern of a lymphocytic vasculitis (Fig. 19).

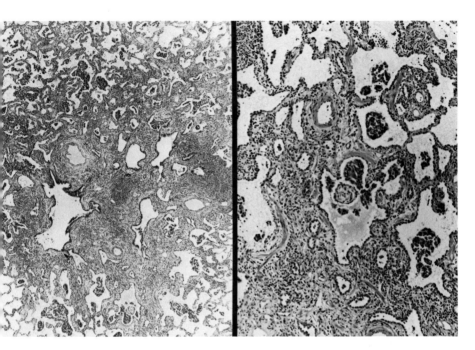

Figure 18 Chronic cellular and fibrosing interstitial pneumonia in SLE. There are both a lymphoid hyperplasia and an interstitial infiltrate of chronic inflammatory cells with interstitial fibrosis. Such a case is probably best classified as interstitial pneumonia with features of UIP associated with lymphoid hyperplasia.

Bronchial and bronchiolar inflammation, sometimes with germinal centers (follicular bronchitis or follicular bronchiolitis), has been described in SLE, as has a pure form of bronchiolitis obliterans with airway obstruction (36). Patients with circulating lupus anticoagulant may develop chronic and/or recurrent pulmonary emboli (Fig. 20) with the associated changes of pulmonary infarction and/or pulmonary hypertension (13,14).

The term "lupus pneumonitis" has been applied to a number of lesions and should not be used without an appropriate modifier. Most frequently, lupus pneumonia appears to have referred to the acute hemorrhage or acute interstitial pneumonia (diffuse alveolar damage).

VI. Progressive Systemic Sclerosis (PSS)

Asymptomatic patients with abnormal chest radiographs and/or abnormal pulmonary functions are relatively common in PSS and outnumber those that have significant pulmonary abnormalities clinically (1,2). Pulmonary

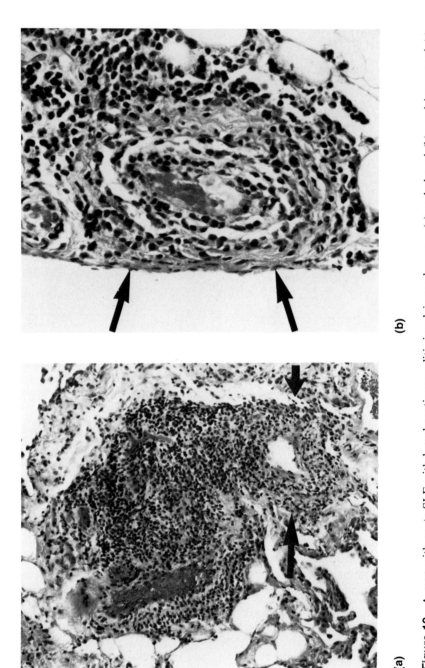

(a)

(b)

Figure 19 A man with acute SLE with lymphocytic vasculitis involving pulmonary (a), subpleural (b), and intercostal (c) veins (arrows) and a large intercostal artery (d).

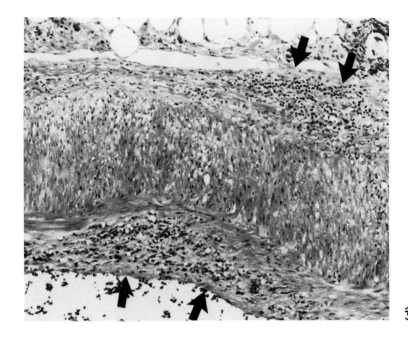

(d)

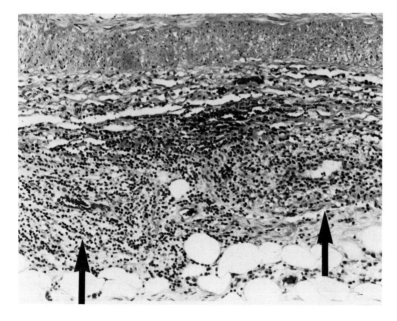

(c)

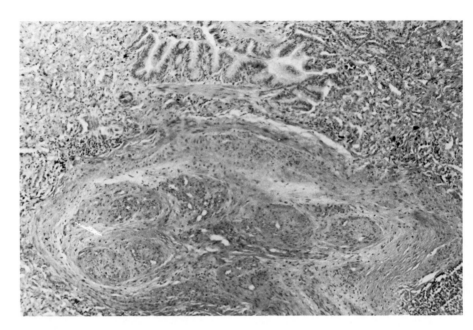

Figure 20 Biopsy from a patient with lupus anticoagulant and recurrent pulmonary emboli. The pulmonary artery in the lower two thirds of the field is occluded by an organized embolus.

involvement is much more common in patients with PSS than in those with localized scleroderma. Two main lesions are recognized, and they may co-exist but are probably separate and progress at different rates (41). Histologically, these include interstitial lung disease and pulmonary vascular disease with pulmonary hypertension (1,41-45). Interstitial lung disease typically has the pattern of usual interstitial pneumonia (Fig. 21); subpleural honeycombing is characteristic, and the rate of progression may be slower than in idiopathic UIP. Rarely a more fulminant acute interstitial lung disease or subacute BOOP may be seen in PSS. The vascular changes associated with pulmonary hypertension are characteristic, with edematous onion-skin proliferation in the intima of pulmonary arteries and arterioles, associated with marked medial thickening (Fig. 22).

Pleural fibrosis has been described in patients with PSS (42). Secondary bronchoalveolar carcinoma arising in the fibrotic lungs of PSS patients has also been described (12). Recurrent aspiration from esophageal involvement by PSS may be a complicating factor and associated with fibrosis, bronchitis/bronchiolitis, and recurrent pneumonias (8).

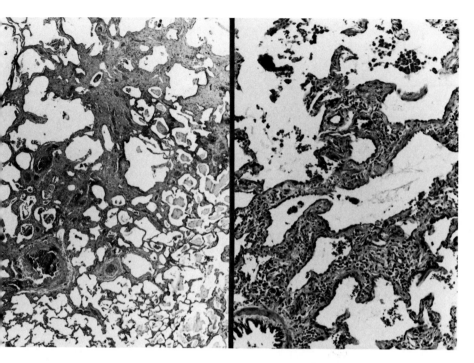

Figure 21 Chronic fibrosing interstitial pneumonia with features of UIP in sclero-derma. There are interstitial fibrosis and microhoneycombing in a patchy distribution with some preservation of alveolar walls.

VII. Mixed Connective Tissue Disease

The pathologic changes in the lungs of patients with mixed connective tissue disease include pulmonary hypertension and interstitial lung disease (Fig. 23) with the pattern of usual interstitial pneumonia (8,15,46-49); in one series the patients with pulmonary hypertension fared much worse (49).

VIII. Dermatomyositis/Polymyositis

Pulmonary involvement may precede the clinical myositis, and interstitial lung disease has usually been described (8,15,50-55). It has the pattern of BOOP (Figs. 24, 25) or usual interstitial pneumonia (Fig. 26), with the prognosis response to steroids being worse in the latter. Rarely, a fulminant acute

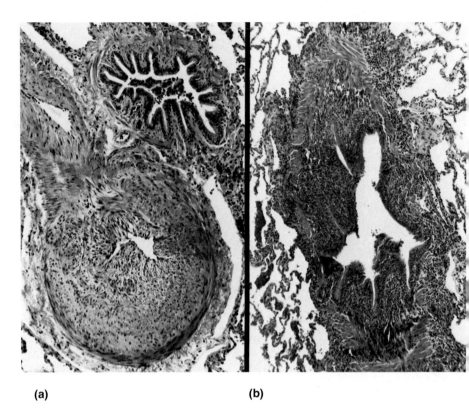

(a)   (b)

Figure 22 Pulmonary hypertension in scleroderma with intimal hypertrophy and marked intimal proliferation with severe luminal compromise. Such an "onion-skinning" intimal proliferation is characteristic of scleroderma. Some airways in this case (right) showed a mild cellular (subclinical) bronchiolitis.

interstitial lung disease with histologic features of diffuse alveolar damage occurs (Fig. 27). Pulmonary hypertension has also been described.

IX. Ankylosing Spondylitis

The apical fibrobullous disease associated with ankylosing spondylitis is of unknown cause and is rarely seen pathologically (8,56). By description the appearance is nonspecific with parenchymal destruction and replacement by

Figure 24 Bronchiolitis obliterans organizing pneumonia in polymyositis. There is granulation tissue in the small airways (left), which extends to involve alveolar ducts in the more distal parenchyma (right). Though the degree of organization and inflammation is quite marked (right), there is relative architectural preservation, and many of the alveolar walls can be discerned.

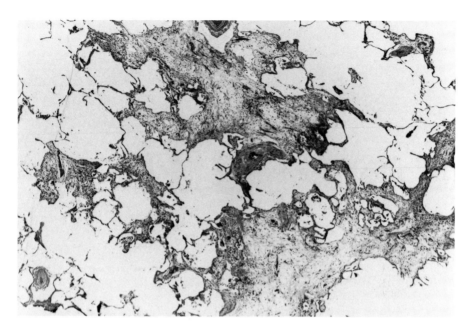

Figure 23 Chronic fibrosing interstitial pneumonia with features of UIP in mixed connective tissue disease. There is patchy scarring with relative preservation of the intervening alveolar walls.

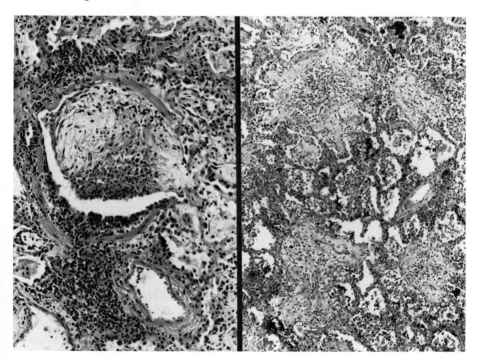

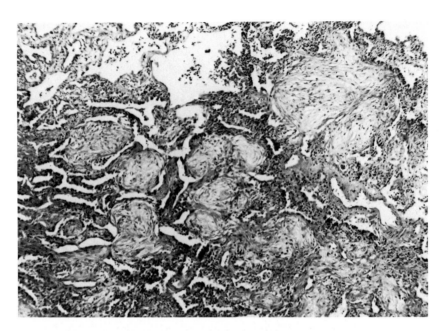

Figure 25 Bronchiolitis obliterans organizing pneumonia in polymyositis. In this case granulation extends all the way into alveolar spaces.

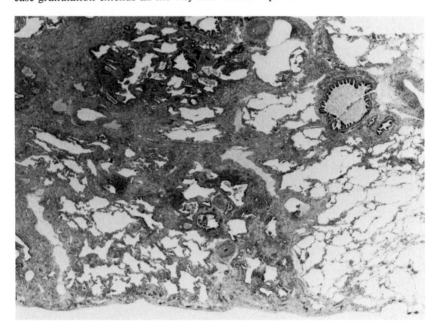

Figure 26 Chronic fibrosing interstitial pneumonia with features of usual interstitial pneumonia in polymyositis. There is a patchy fibrosing process with some preservation of pulmonary parenchyma (lower right). In other regions, there is interstitial fibrosis and microhoneycombing.

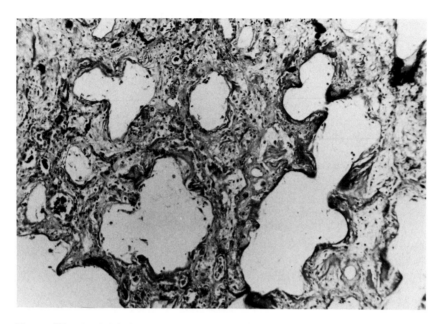

Figure 27 Fatal fulminant acute interstitial lung disease in polymyositis showing features of diffuse alveolar damage with hyaline membrane formation. No other cause was identified for the diffuse alveolar damage, which was presumed (by exclusion) to be associated with polymyositis.

irregular-size spaces with thick fibrotic walls. Nonspecific epithelial metaplasia, mucostasis, and connective tissue proliferation occur. The changes are nonspecific, and the diagnosis depends on clinical and radiographic correlation. Secondary aspergillomas occur in the abnormal airspaces.

X. Relapsing Polychondritis

In relapsing polychondritis pathologic changes occur in the cartilagenous airways, and the lung parenchyma is affected secondarily. The cartilages collapse, which causes obstruction. The acute chondritis is distinctive (Fig. 28) but only occasionally seen pathologically.

XI. Behçet's Syndrome

Patients with Behçet's syndrome may present with hemoptysis and recurrent pulmonary infiltrates; the presumed histologic correlate is vasculitis with secondary thromboses, hemorrhage, and pulmonary infarction (8,57-59).

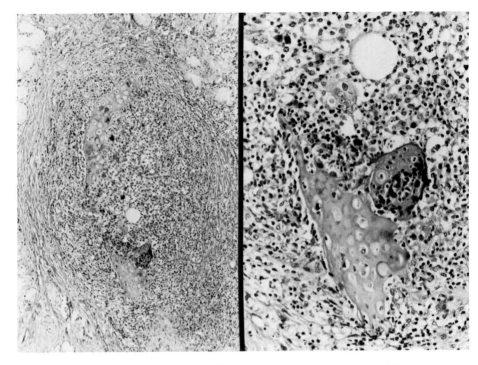

Figure 28 Autopsy examination of bronchial cartilages in a patient with relapsing polychondritis shows perichondrial fibrosis and acute inflammatory infiltrate eroding cartilagenous plates.

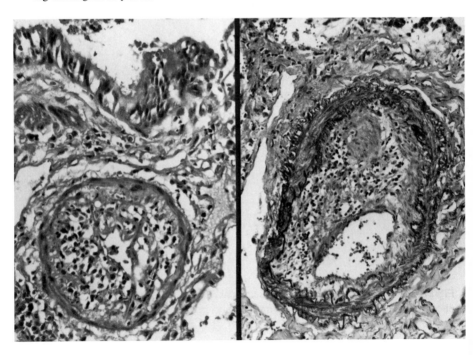

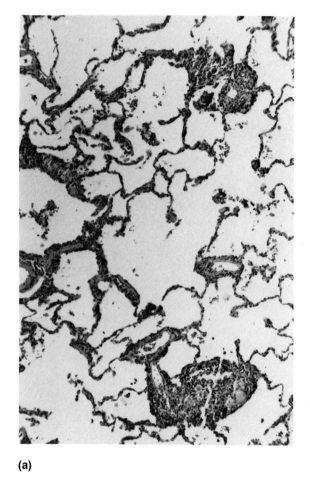

(a)

Figure 30 Chronic interstitial pneumonia with clinical evidence of mild restrictive disease in a patient with primary biliary cirrhosis. There is a nonspecific patchy inflammatory process with relative preservation of alveolar walls. Histologically, the pattern is nonspecific.

Figure 29 Pulmonary vasculitis associated with Behcet's syndrome. There is a lymphocytic vasculitis (left) associated with some endothelial thickening and fibrosis highlighted by elastic tissue (right). (Case courtesy of R. Slavin, MD, Galveston, TX.)

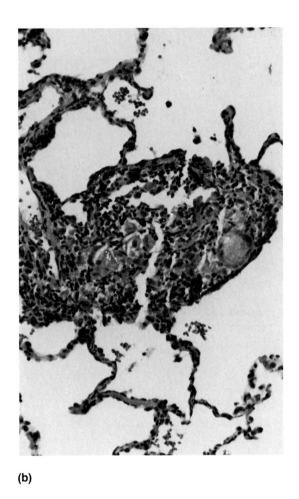

(b)

Histologically one may find acute vasculitis, lymphocytic vasculitis (Fig. 29), or scarred vessel walls, consistent with a healed vasculitis and/or thrombi depending at what stage the tissue is sampled. Circulating immune complexes are implicated in the pathogenesis (58).

XII. Primary Biliary Cirrhosis

Although a subclinical alveolitis has been described in appreciable numbers of patients with primary biliary cirrhosis (3), clinically significant pulmonary disease is unusual. A mild cellular interstitial pneumonia in a case of primary biliary cirrhosis is illustrated (Fig. 30).

XIII. Where to Biopsy?

The surgeon should select lung tissue that is abnormal but not the most abnormal, because nonspecific endstage honeycombing might be the only finding from such a biopsy. In order to avoid problems in interpretation of nonspecific changes in the tips of lobes (particularly the lingula and the right middle lobe), a biopsy size no smaller than 3 cm is recommended.

References

1. Owens, G. R., Fino, G. J., Herbert, D. L., Fino, G. J., Steen, V. D., Medsger, T. A. Jr., Pennock, B. E., Cottrell, J. J., Rodnam, G. P., and Rogers, R. M. (1983). Pulmonary function in progressive systemic sclerosis. *Chest* **84**:546-550.
2. Schneider, P. D., Wise, R. A., Hochberg, M. C., and Wigley, F. M. (1982). Serial pulmonary function in systemic sclerosis. *Am. J. Med.* **73**:385-394.
3. Wallaert, B., Bonniere, P., Prin, L., Cortet, A., Tonnel, A. B., and Voisin, C. (1986). Primary biliary cirrhosis: Subclinical inflammatory alveolitis in patients with normal chest roentgenograms. *Chest* **90**: 842-848.
4. Wallaert, B., Hatron, P. Y., Grosbois, J. M., Tonnel, A. B., Devulder, B., and Voisin, G. (1986). Subclinical pulmonary involvement in collagen-vascular diseases assessed by bronchoalveolar lavage. *Am. Rev. Respir. Dis.* **133**:574-580.
5. Churg, A. C., Franklin, W., Chan, K. W., Kopp, E., and Carrington, C. (1980). Pulmonary hemorrhage and immune-complex deposition in the lung. *Arch. Pathol. Lab. Med.* **104**:388-391.
6. Eisenberg, H., Dubois, E. L., Sherwin, R. P., and Balchum, O. J. (1973). Diffuse interstitial lung disease in systemic lupus erythematosus. *Ann. Intern. Med.* **79**:37-45.
7. Eisenberg, H. (1982). The interstitial lung disease associated with the collagen-vascular disorders. *Clin. Chest Med.* **3**:565-578.
8. Hunninghake, G. W., and Fauci, A. S. (1979). State of the art—pulmonary involvement in the collagen vascular disease. *Am. Rev. Respir. Dis.* **119**:471-503.
9. Pertschuk, L. P., Moccia, L. F., Rosen, Y., Lyons, H., Marino, E. M., Rashford, A. A., and Wellschlager, C. M. (1977). Acute pulmonary complications in systemic lupus erythematosus: Immunofluorescence and light microscopic study. *Am. J. Clin. Pathol.* **68**:553-557.
10. Rodriquez-Iturbe, B., Garcia, R., Rubio, L., and Serrano, H. (1977). Immunohistologic findings in the lung in systemic lupus erythematosus. *Arch. Pathol. Lab. Med.* **101**:342-344.

11. Turner-Warwick, M. (1974). Immunological aspects of systemic diseases of the lungs. *Proc. R. Soc. Med.* **67**:541-547.
12. Bookman, A.A.M., Urowitz, M.B., and Mitchell, R.I. (1974). Alveolar cell carcinoma in progressive systemic sclerosis. *J. Rheumatol.* **1**:466-472.
13. Anderson, N. E., and Ali, M. R. (1984). The lupus anticoagulant, pulmonary thromboembolism, and fatal pulmonary hypertension. *Ann. Rheum. Dis.* **43**:760-763.
14. Pines, A., Kaplinsky, N., Olchovsky, D., et al. (1985). Pleuropulmonary manifestations of systemic lupus erythematosis: Clinical features of its subgroups. *Chest* **88**:129-135.
15. Colby, T. V. (1988). Infiltrative lung disease. In *Pathology of the lung*. Edited by Thurlbeck, W. M.. Thieme, New York, pp. 425-518.
16. Beck, E. R., and Hoffbrand, B. I. (1966). Acute lung changes in rheumatoid arthritis. *Ann. Rheum. Dis.* **25**:459-462.
17. Burke, G. W., Carrington, C. B., and Grinnan, R. (1977). Pulmonary nodules and rheumatoid factor in the absence of arthritis. *Chest* **72**:538-540.
18. Cooney, T. P. (1981). Interrelationship of chronic eosinophilic pneumonia, bronchiolitis obliterans, and rheumatoid disease: A hypothesis. *J. Clin. Pathol.* **34**:129-137.
19. Crisp, A. J., Armstrong, R. D., Grahame, R., and Dussek, J. E. (1982). Rheumatoid lung disease, pneumothorax, and eosinophilia. *Ann. Rheum. Dis.* **41**:137-140.
20. Forman, M. B., Zwi, S., Gear, A. J., Kallenbach, J., and Wing, J. (1982). Severe airway obstruction associated with rheumatoid arthritis and Sjogren's syndrome. *S. Afr. Med. J.* **61**:674-675.
21. Geddes, D. M., Corrin, B., Brewerton, D. A., Davies, R. J., and Turner-Warwick, M. (1977). Progressive airway obliteration in adults and its association with rheumatoid disease. *Q. J. Med.* **46**:427-444.
22. Macfarlane, J. D., Dieppe, P. A., Rigden, B. G., and Clark, T. J. H. (1978). Pulmonary and pleural lesions in rheumatoid disease. *Br. J. Dis. Chest* **72**:288-300.
23. Martel, W., Abell, M. R., Mikkelsen, W. M., and Whitehouse, W. M. (1968). Pulmonary and pleural lesions in rheumatoid disease. *Radiology* **90**:641-653.
24. Yousem, S. A., Colby, T. V., and Carrington, C. B. (1985). Lung biopsy in rheumatoid arthritis. *Am. Rev. Respir. Dis.* **131**:770-777.
25. Winterbauer, R. H., Wilske, K. R., and Wheelis, R. F. (1976). Diffuse pulmonary injury associated with gold treatment. *N. Engl. J. Med.* **294**:919-921.
26. Athreya, B. H., Doughty, R. A., Bookspan, M., et al. (1980). Pulmonary manifestations of juvenile rheumatoid arthritis. *Clin. Chest Med.* **1**:361-374.

27. Romicka, A., and Maldyk, E. (1975). Pulmonary lesions in the course of rheumatoid arthritis in children. *Pol. Med. History Bull.* **18**:263-268.
28. Wagener, J. S., Taussig, L. M., DeBenedetti, C., Lemen, R. J., and Loughlin, G. M. (1981). Pulmonary function in juvenile rheumatoid arthritis. *J. Pediatr.* **99**:108-110.
29. Yousefzadeh, D. K., and Fishman, P. A. (1979). The triad of pneumonitis, pleuritis, and pericarditis in juvenile rheumatoid arthritis. *Pediatr. Radiol.* **8**:147-150.
30. Constantopoulos, S. H., Drosos, A. A., Maddison, P. J., and Moutsopoulos, H. M. (1984). Xerotrachea and interstitial lung disease in primary Sjogren's syndrome. *Respiration* **46**:310-314.
31. Constantopoulos, S. H., Papadimitriou, C. S., and Moutsopoulos, H. M. (1985). Respiratory manifestations in primary Sjogren's syndromes. *Chest* **88**:226-229.
32. Fairfax, A. J., Haslam, P. L., Pavia, D., Sheahan, N. F., Bateman, J. R. M., Agnew, J. E., Clarke, S. W., and Turner-Warwick, M. (1981). Pulmonary disorders associated with Sjogren's syndrome. *Q. J. Med.* **50**:279-295.
33. Strimlan, C. V., Rosenow, E. C., Divertie, M. B., and Harrison, E. G. (1976). Pulmonary manifestations of Sjogren's syndrome. *Chest* **70**:354-361.
34. Byrd, R. B., and Trunk, G. (1973). Systemic lupus erythematosus presenting as pulmonary hemosiderosis. *Chest* **64**:128-129.
35. Haupt, H. M., Moore, G. W., and Hutchins, G. M. (1981). The lung in systemic lupus erythematosus. *Am. J. Med.* **71**:791-798.
36. Kinney, W. W., and Angelillo, V. A. (1982). Bronchiolitis in systemic lupus erythematosus. *Chest* **82**:646-649.
37. Matthay, R. A., Schwarz, M. I., Petty, T. L., Stanford, R. E., Gupta, R. C., Sahn, S. A., and Steigerwald, J. C. (1974). Pulmonary manifestations of systemic lupus erythematosus: Review of twelve cases of acute lupus pneumonitis. *Medicine* **54**:397-409.
38. Miller, L. R., Greenberg, S. D., and McLarty, J. W. (1985). Lupus lung. *Chest* **88**:265-269.
39. Myers, J. L., and Katzenstein, A. L. A. (1986). Microangiitis in lupus-induced pulmonary hemorrhage. *Am. J. Clin. Pathol.* **85**:552-556.
40. Nadorra, R. L., and Landing, B. H. (1987). Pulmonary lesions in childhood onset systemic lupus erythematosus. *Pediatr. Pathol.* **7**:1-18.
41. Young, R. H., and Mark, G. J. (1978). Pulmonary vascular changes in scleroderma. *Am. J. Med.* **64**:998-1004.
42. D'Angelo, W. A., Fries, J. F., Masi, A. T., and Shulman, L. E. (1969). Pathologic observations in systemic sclerosis (scleroderma): A study of fifty-eight autopsy cases and fifty-eight matched controls. *Am. J. Med.* **46**:428-440.

43. Kallenbach, J., Prinsloo, I., and Zwi, S. (1977). Progressive systemic sclerosis complicated by diffuse pulmonary hemorrhage. *Thorax* **32**:767-770.
44. Salerni, R., Rodnan, G. P., Leon, D. F., and Shaver, J. A. (1977). Pulmonary hypertension in the CREST syndrome variant of progressive systemic sclerosis (scleroderma). *Ann. Intern. Med.* **86**:394-399.
45. Weaver, A. L., Divertie, M. D., and Titus, J. L. (1968). Pulmonary scleroderma. *Dis. Chest* **54**:4-12.
46. Martyn, J. B., Stein, H. B., Huang, S. H. K., Pardy, R. H., and Pare, P. D. (1985). Severe pulmonary involvement is common in mixed connective tissue disease (abstract). *Am. Rev. Respir. Dis.* **131**:A79.
47. O'Connell, D. J., and Bennett, R. M. (1977). Mixed connective tissue disease—clinical and radiological aspects of 20 cases. *Br. J. Radiol.* **50**:620-625.
48. Prakash, U. B. S., Luthra, H. S., and Divertie, M. B. (1985). Intrathoracic manifestations in mixed connective tissue disease. *Mayo Clin. Proc.* **60**:813-821.
49. Wiener-Kronish, J. P., Solinger, A. M., Warnock, M. L., Churg, A., Ordonez, M., and Golden, J. A. (1981). Severe pulmonary involvement in mixed connective tissue disease. *Am. Rev. Respir. Dis.* **124**:499-503.
50. Dickey, B. F., and Myers, A. R. (1984). Pulmonary disease in polymyositis/dermatomyositis. *Semin. Arthritis Rheum.* **14**:60-76.
51. Duncan, P. E., Griffin, J. P., Garcia, A., and Kaplan, S. B. (1974). Fibrosing alveolitis in polymyositis: A review of histologically confirmed cases. *Am. J. Med.* **57**:621-626.
52. Park, S., and Nyhan, W. L. (1974). Fatal pulmonary involvement in dermatomyositis. *Am. J. Dis. Child* **129**:723-726.
53. Salmeron, G., Greenberg, S. D., and Lidsky, M. D. (1981). Polymyositis and diffuse interstitial lung disease: A review of the pulmonary histopathologic findings. *Arch. Intern. Med.* **141**:1005-1010.
54. Schwarz, M. I., Mathay, R. A., Sahn, S. A., Stanford, R. C., Marmorstein, B. L., and Scheinhorn, D. J. (1976). Interstitial lung disease in polymyositis and dermatomyositis: Analysis of six cases and review of the literature. *Medicine* **55**:89-104.
55. Webb, D. R., and Currie, G. D. (1972). Pulmonary fibrosis masking polymyositis. *J.A.M.A.* **222**:1146-1149.
56. Rosenow, E. C., Strimlan, C. V., Muhm, J. R., and Ferguson, R. H. (1977). Pleuropulmonary manifestations of ankylosing spondylitis. *Mayo Clin. Proc.* **52**:641-649.
57. Dreisen, R. B. (1982). Pulmonary vasculitis. *Clin. Chest Med.* **3**:607-618.
58. Efthimious, J., Johnston, C., Spiro, S. G., and Turner-Warwick, M. (1986). Pulmonary diseases in Behçet's syndrome. *Q. J. Med.* (n.s.) **58**:259-280.
59. Slavin, R. E., and De Groot, W. J. (1981). Pathology of the lung in Behçet's disease. *Am. J. Surg. Pathol.* **5**:779-788.

7

Pathogenesis and Clinical Features of Pulmonary Infections

GALEN B. TOEWS and JOSEPH P. LYNCH III

University of Michigan Medical Center
Ann Arbor, Michigan

I. Introduction

The lung is an extensive epithelial interface with the external environment whose primary function is the exchange of gases at rates required by tissue metabolism. While this extensive epithelial surface allows diffusion of oxygen from the environment and elimination of carbon dioxide from the body, it also plays an essential role in the body's defenses against a potentially hostile environment. The lungs are repeatedly exposed to microorganisms from the external environment via inhalation and from the host environment via aspiration of upper airway secretions and via the circulation. A complex system of "pulmonary host defenses" have evolved to protect the structural cells that provide the architectural and functional basis for gas exchange (1-5).

II. Normal Host Defense Mechanisms

The components of the pulmonary host defense system, which are distributed throughout the respiratory tract, recognize and eliminate microorganisms before their multiplication leads to clinical disease. While defense of the lung requires many interrelated responses, they can be divided into three major parts. The resident defenses are those components that are present in healthy pulmonary parenchyma and deal with day-to-day microbial challenges. These defenses include aerodynamic filtration, the mucociliary apparatus, and alveolar macrophages. In certain circumstances, microbes overwhelm resident defenses. Fortunately, the lung possesses two additional defenses against microbes. The ability to generate an acute inflammatory response is an important factor in the clearance of most virulent bacterial pathogens. Finally, the generation and expression of immune responses in the lung are important in the defense of the lung against bacteria, mycobacteria, fungi, and certain viruses. Products of B-lymphocyte-mediated immune responses are specific antibodies that enhance phagocytosis, promote microbial killing, and neutralize toxins. Activated T lymphocytes secrete lymphokines, which are important in delayed-type hypersensitivity responses and other mediators of subacute and chronic inflammatory responses. Additionally, T-lymphocyte effectors may be cytotoxic for virally infected cells.

A. Resident Defenses

Aerodynamic defenses use inertia to remove large suspended particulates from inhaled air (3). The nose efficiently removes particules with an aerodynamic size > 10 μm. Rapid airflow, the bend in the airstream in the nose, and the bifurcating nature of the airways all favor inertial deposition of large particulates. Most particulates > 2 μm impact in the proximal airways. In contrast, particles 2 μm in diameter bypass the aerodynamic defenses and reach the alveolar surfaces (6).

The mucociliary escalator is involved in the clearance of particulates deposited in airways (2,6,7). This system consists of a ciliated epithelium with an overlying mucus layer. The mucus layer contains electrolytes, mucins, lipids, carbohydrates, nucleic acids, immunoglobulins, and enzymes that absorb gases and trap particulates. Ciliary movement (1,000-1,500 cycles/min) propels the mucus layer up the airways at progressively increasing rates. This system can clear particulates from the trachea with a half time of 30 min and from the more distal airways with a half time of several hours.

Droplets carrying infectious agents are usually < 2 μm. These particulates evade the aerodynamic and mucociliary defenses and deposit on alveolar surfaces. Physical removal of these particulates plays a relatively minor role in the defense of lung. Mechanisms that are bactericidal are quantitatively far more important (8,9). The role of mucociliary clearance in the defense of the lung against aspirated bacteria has not been studied.

Alveolar macrophages are the first line of defense against microbes that reach the alveolar surface (8-10). Alveolar macrophages ingest bacteria, fungi, and viruses. Alveolar macrophages have receptors for C3b, C3d, and the Fc portion of IgG (11-13). Optimal ingestion of microorganisms by macrophages occurs following opsonization of organisms with IgG or complement (14-15). Once phagocytosis has occurred, the phagocytic vesicles fuse with lysosomes to form phagolysosomes (16). Highly reactive toxic products of oxygen, including H_2O_2 and hydroxyl radicals (OH·), combine with hydrolytic and proteolytic enzymes from lysosomes to kill bacteria in the phagolysosomes in most instances (12,17). A 10-fold reduction in inhaled *Staphylococcus aureus* has been noted within 4 hours in absence of an inflammatory response (8-10).

B. Generation of Inflammatory Responses

While alveolar macrophages are largely responsible for the clearance of small aerosol inocula of gram-positive bacteria, effective pulmonary clearance of virulent bacteria (*Pseudomonas aeruginosa, Klebsiella pneumoniae, Haemophilus influenzae*) is dependent on the generation of an inflammatory response (18-21). In most instances, pulmonary antibacterial defenses are dependent on a dual phagocytic system that involves both alveolar macrophages and polymorphonuclear leukocytes (PMN) (20,22). The initiation of inflammation and the magnitude of the PMN response is related to bacterial species and inoculum size (23). Normal air spaces contain only small number of PMN. These cells comprise less than 2% of cells obtained by bronchoalveolar lavage. However, large numbers of PMN are sequestered in the pulmonary vasculature of normal lungs (24). This large marginating pool of PMN is available to move rapidly through the interstitium into the air space in response to inflammatory stimuli.

It is likely that chemotactic factors generated within the air spaces or the interstitium of the lung are responsible for the accumulation of PMN in alveoli (25). The C5 molecule and its fragments have been shown to be important PMN chemotaxins in murine lungs following bacterial challenges. C5-deficient mice have reduced chemotactic activity in bronchoalveolar lavage (BAL) and diminished PMN recruitment to the lung following intratracheal inoculation with *P. aeruginosa, Streptococcus pneumoniae,* and *H. influenzae* when compared to congenic C5-sufficient mice (21,26,27). The mechanism(s) responsible for the cleavage of C5 to its chemotactic fragments in the lung are unknown, but sufficient C5 is present in pulmonary secretions to provide biologically active quantities of C5 fragments (28). Bacteria are capable of activating the alternative pathway, which results in C5 cleavage, and alveolar macrophages contain proteinases capable of cleaving C5 without activation of the remainder of the complement cascade (29). Alveolar macrophages also amplify inflammation in the lung by producing noncomplement chemotactic factors for neutrophils (30-33). Macrophages also generate 5-or 11-mono-hydroxyeicosatetraenoic acids, leukotriene B$_4$, platelet activating factor (PAF), and plasminogen activator (34-37), which are known to be chemotactic substances (34-37).

Once recruited to the alveolar spaces, neutrophils ingest and destroy invading microbes. Neutrophils possess both oxygen-dependent and oxygen-independent mechanisms for killing microbes. Superoxide anion, hydroxyl radicals, and hydrogen peroxide are produced following ingestion of bacteria; all can destroy microbes (38,39). Additionally, the myeloperoxidase-H_2O_2 complex oxidizes halides to produce HOCl, chloramines, aldehydes, and singlet oxygen (40). Nonoxidative killing mechanisms included defensins and proteases (41).

C. Specific Immune Responses

Specific, local immune responses are of importance in the defense of lung against certain pathogens, particularly virulent encapsulated bacteria, intracellular organisms that survive in normal macrophages and viruses. Immune responses are generated by antigens and effected by B and T lymphocytes. The initial step in the generation of an immune response involves an antigen presenting cell which expresses class II major histocompatibility products and processes and presents the antigen to T cells (42). An effective antigen presenting cell is present in lung parenchyma, but the nature of the cell is uncertain (43,44). Alveolar macrophages are poor antigen presenting cells (45-47). While they express HLA-DR antigens, they bind resting T cells poorly (48), secrete little interleukin 1 (49), and secrete suppressive substances such as prostaglandin E_2 (50). Several studies have suggested that the antigen presenting cell is either an interstitial macrophage or a dendritic cell (43,44,51). Following antigen presentation, T-cell activation occurs, which involves T-cell production of interleukin 2 (IL-2), IL-2 receptor expression, and lymphokine secretion (52-65). T-cell activation results in the development of (a) T helper cells that are required for B-cell differentiation and antibody secretion (b) cytotoxic T cells that can lyse virally infected cells; and (c) T cells that mediate delayed type hypersensitivity and granuloma formation, which are critical to the killing of many intracellular pathogens.

The term local or pulmonary immunity can be a source of confusion. The term could refer to the intrapulmonary initiation, regulation, or expression of an immune response. It is clear that immune effector cells are present in airways and the pulmonary parenchyma under certain circumstances, but the precise site where these effector cells are generated has not been defined. Thus, the term local immunity usually refers to the functional presence of immune effectors in the lung.

Antibody-Mediated Immune Responses in the Lung

Antibodies are important in the defense of the lung against bacteria. The major role of antibody is to enhance the phagocytic and microbicidal activities of macrophages and PMN (66). Antibodies present in pulmonary parenchyma and the air spaces are derived from the circulation by transudation and produced locally by antibody forming cells in the interstitium and air spaces of the lung.

Systematic immunization clearly enhances antibacterial defenses of the lower respiratory tract. Clearance of *P. aeruginosa, Proteus mirabilis, and H. influenzae* is enhanced following systematic immunization (67-73). Both IgG (71) and IgM (69) have been proposed as the class of antibody responsible for the enhanced clearance. The intraalveolar antibodies enhance clearance by opsonizing bacteria, activating the complement cascade, and neutralizing certain exotoxins. The antibody specificities of serum and alveolar antibodies have been shown to be identical, suggesting that protective alveolar antibodies are derived in part from serum (72). Furthermore, passive immunization with specific monoclonal antibodies directed at *H. influenzae* also results in enhanced clearance of this organism (72).

Cell-Mediated Immune Responses in the Lung

The two major mechanisms by which immune T cells are involved in pulmonary host defense are lymphokine-mediated reactions and cell-mediated cytotoxic responses. Lymphokines convert resting macrophages to efficient microbicidal phagocytes, initiate delayed type hypersensitivity, and contribute to the generation of immune granulomas. Macrophage activation has been shown to largely mediate the cellular response to intracellular pathogens (74). In other instances, the interaction with antigen results in the development of cytotoxic cell effectors. Cytolytic T lymphocytes are an important defense mechanism against virally infected cells.

Lymphokine-Mediated Responses

Specific lymphokine-producing cells appear in the pulmonary parenchyma following systematic immunization and in certain disease states (74-81). Whether these cells are generated in the lung or are recruited from the circulating pool of sensitized lymphocytes is uncertain. T helper (CD4), T suppressor/cytotoxic cells (CD8), B cells, and natural killer (NK) cells can all secrete lymphokines, but CD4 cells are most proficient at the release of lymphokines. Cells producing macrophage chemotactic factor, IL-2, and gamma-interferon (γ-IFN) have been isolated from the pulmonary parenchyma (82-88).

γ-IFN is a particularly important lymphokine. Macrophage activation for enhanced antimicrobial activity has been shown to be both γ-IFN-dependent and inducible by γ-IFN only (89-92). γ-IFN treatment enhanced the ability of human monocyte-derived macrophages to kill intracellular pathogens and the ability to release H_2O_2 (89-90). γ-IFN also enhanced the in vitro antimicrobial activities of alveolar macrophages (93-95).

Although γ-IFN-stimulated macrophages are broadly activated, not all organisms are universally susceptible to activated macrophages. *Toxoplasma* gondii and *Legionella pneumophila* are killed by γ-IFN-activated human monocyte-derived macrophages (89,90,96), but certain strains of mycobacteria are resistant to the antimicrobial effect of these activated macrophages (97). However, considerable *in vitro* and *in vivo* data indicate that host defenses against mycobacteria are T-cell-dependent and likely involve γ-IFN (98-99). The role of activated macrophages in the resistance to and recovery from fungal infections is less well defined. Similarly, the efficacy of activated macrophages against extracellular pathogens such as *Pneumocystis carinii* is unknown.

Cytotoxic T Cell Responses

Specific CD8 T lymphocytes and nonspecific NK cells are present in pulmonary parenchyma (100-110). T lymphocytes that specifically kill influenza virus-infected cells *in vitro* appear in the lung parenchyma of mice 6-9 days after the induction of viral infection (101,102). Similar results have been obtained in studies of herpes simplex virus infections (100). Since cytotoxic cells do not recirculate, the possibility exists that the lung contains a subset of cytotoxic T cells that are clonally selected for by respiratory viruses. Support for this hypothesis comes from observations that cytotoxic T cells to influenza are more easily induced in the lung than in the spleen (106).

The lung also contains NK cells (107-110). There is evidence that NK cells are compartmentalized in the lung. Active NK cells are located primarily in the interstitium of the lung (110). These cells can be regulated by local lymphokines (IL-2, γ-IFN) that might be released during viral infections. Pulmonary NK cells have been shown to have a protective role in influenza infections (107). A protective role in fungal infections has also been proposed (111), but conflicting data exist. NK cells can play a role in early resistance against *C. neoformans* if the organism is delivered intravenously but did not play a role in either determining survival or resistance to infection acquired via the respiratory tract (112).

III. Host Defense Defects In Connective Tissue Disorders

A. Intrinsic Defects

Systematic Lupus Erythematosis (SLE)

Practically every aspect of the immune system has been reported to be abnormal in patients with SLE. Antibacterial activity of alveolar macrophages (AM) from both untreated and corticosteroid-treated patients with SLE is severely impaired (113). Furthermore, incubation of normal AM in SLE serum reduced phagocytosis and bactericidal activity of normal AM. Other abnormalities in macrophage function include defects in Fc receptor function and macrophage immune complex clearance (114-117). Thus, resident pulmonary host defense and systematic mononuclear-phagocyte defects are present in SLE.

Defects that could alter the generation of a protective inflammatory response have also been described. Defects include disorders of chemotaxis and phagocytic activity of both PMN and blood monocytes. Additionally, the microbicidal activity of monocytes is decreased (118-123). These defects could limit the number of inflammatory cells present in the lung following infection and adversely alter their pulmonary defense capabilities.

Both quantitative and functional abnormalities of immune cells exist. Lymphopenia is common. B cells are present in normal numbers but T lymphocytes, especially T suppressors, are decreased (124). Studies of the humoral and cellular immune responses of patients with active SLE have produced conflicting results. Serum antibody responses to immunization have been described as being normal or decreased (125,126). Primary immune responses are more deficient than secondary responses. Response to a "new" delayed type hypersensitivity antigen such as dinitrochlorobenzene is reduced, while challenges with agents such as tricophyton and *Candida* have produced variable responses (127-130).

The generation of an autologous mixed leukocyte response is also decreased (131). This reaction is believed to reflect a model system for studying normal events involved in the immunoregulation of immune response. Defects exist in the responder T-cell population and the stimulator (macrophage, dendritic cell, B cell) populations. Finally, NK cell activity is decreased in SLE, and NK cells from SLE are less responsive to the enhancing effects of interferon than normal cells (132).

Rheumatoid Arthritis (RA)

Pleuropulmonary infections occur with greater frequency in patients with RA than in those without (133-136). A twofold increase in the incidence of pneumonia was noted when RA patients were compared to those with degenerative joint disease (133). Deaths due to respiratory infection were four times greater than the expected rate for an age, sex-matched general population (134).

The factors contributing to the increased infectious complications are not clear but probably involve the use of immunosuppressive drugs. Additionally, several abnormalities in host defenses have been described. AM function in patients with RA has not been explored. Granulocyte function has been reported to be normal by some investigators (137) and impaired by others (138). Peripheral blood PMN have been reported to be deficient in their capability for both phagocytosis and response to chemoattractants (139-140).

Studies of peripheral blood lymphocytes from patients with RA have produced conflicting results. Some investigators have detected increased numbers of B lymphocytes (141), others have detected decreased numbers of B lymphocytes (142), while still others have reported no differences in B-and T-lymphocyte ratios in normal and rheumatoid patients (143). The most striking change in lymphocyte surface antigens in RA is not a fluctuation in lymphocyte subsets but an increase in Ia-positive lymphocytes. This nonspecific phenomenon is also seen after immunization with PPD and likely serves as an index of immunologic stimulation (144). Similarly, a direct correlation between disease activity and numbers of activated B lymphocytes in peripheral blood has been observed (145). Additional abnormalities that could be important in host defenses include defects in monocyte bactericidal activity, IgA deficiency, and hypogammaglobulinemia (135).

B. Drug-Induced Defects

Glucocorticoids

The history of glucocorticoid therapy and the history of collagen vascular diseases are inseparable. Unwelcome side effects frequently accompany the dramatic antiinflammatory therapeutic effect of these agents.

The effects of glucocorticoids on host defenses are exceedingly complex because glucocorticoids modify these defenses in numerous ways (146). It is not possible to identify a single mechanism of action of glucocorticoids. Glucocorticoids act by binding to a cytoplasmic receptor protein. The receptor-steroid complex then enters the nucleus, where it modifies transcription of RNA from DNA. This modification results in an alteration in the synthesis of specific proteins.

Glucocorticoid effects on host defenses include effects on leukocyte traffic, leukocyte function, and humoral factors. The effect on cellular processes is more pronounced than their effect on humoral factors. The most important effect of glucocorticoids is their ability to inhibit recruitment of neutrophils and monocytes/macrophages to the site of an infection (147).

The mechanism of the decreased accumulation of PMN is not fully understood. Glucocorticoids decrease capillary permeability, exudation of fluid, and the migration of PMN (147). Additionally, the adherence of PMN to vascular endothelium is reduced (148). The relative contributions of the vascular effect, the endothelial-PMN adherence effect, and the effect on chemotaxis to the reduction in cell accumulation at sites of infection is uncertain. Most in vitro studies have found no evidence of impaired phagocytosis or decreased bacterial killing (147).

Macrophage/monocyte traffic is also sensitive to glucocorticoids. Production of lymphokines by sensitized lymphocytes is not affected, but the ability of these mediators to recruit monocytes is decreased (149,150). The suppression of delayed hypersensitivity responses noted with glucocorticoids is probably the consequence of the decreased recruitment of macrophages necessary for this response. Steroids also antagonize the effect of migration inhibition factor and depress the bactericidal activity of monocytes (151-153). Because monocytes are critically involved in granuloma formation, the sensitivity of monocyte function to steroids may explain the increases in infections with organisms that require activated macrophages for clearance during steroid therapy.

Cyclophosphamide

Cyclophosphamide affects virtually all components of the cellular and humoral immune response (154,155). The drug acts primarily during the S phase of the cell cycle, so all rapidly dividing cells are affected. An absolute lymphocytopenia of both T and B lymphocytes occurs with early preferential depletion of B lymphocytes (156). Cyclophosphamide inhibits antibody production when given simultaneously or even after antigen exposure. Chronic therapy with cyclophosphamide leads to hypogammaglobulinemia. Suppression of *in vitro* proliferative responses of T cells to antigenic stimulation is also noted with cyclophosphamide. Delayed type hypersensitivity responses to new antigens are noted with relative sparing of established delayed type hypersensitivity (157-159).

Cyclophosphamide therapy causes suppression of all marrow elements, but neutropenia is clearly the most important consequence when host defenses are considered. Cyclophosphamide may have a cumulative effect on marrow reserves. Doses that are initially well tolerated may be associated with neutropenia with chronic administration (160).

Azathioprine

Azathioprine inhibits both humoral and cell-mediated immunity. Azathioprine causes a lymphopenia of both T and B lymphocytes (161). Immunoglobulin synthesis is suppressed, particularly secondary responses to vaccination. B lymphocyte proliferation is also suppressed (162,163). The effect of azathioprine on T lymphocytes is controversial. Little effect on mitogen-induced proliferation is noted with azathioprine therapy (164), but the induction of delayed type hypersensitivity is suppressed (163,164). Monocyte production is decreased and monocyte function is suppressed (165,166). Neutropenia occurs, and a rapid fall in PMN is noted within a week of starting therapy. Infections often occur in the face of normal granulocyte counts, suggesting that the host defense defect induced by azathioprine involves a functional impairment of immune cells involved in host defense, probably the T lymphocyte-monocyte axis.

Methotrexate

Methotrexate is a folic acid antagonist that interferes with transport of one carbon fragments required for thymidine synthesis. DNA synthesis and cellular proliferation are inhibited. Cells in the S phase are most affected.

Methotrexate exerts a profound effect on both primary and secondary antibody responses (167). Conflicting findings exist regarding its effects on T-cell function. Delayed type hypersensitivity responses are markedly reduced in animals (168), but little effect has been noted in man (167). Marrow suppression with neutropenia also occurs.

Combined Regimens

A combined regimen of cyclophosphamide and glucocorticoids is often used to treat patients with collagen vascular disease. This regimen has been shown to adversely affect pulmonary host defenses in animal models. The defect is related to both a decrease in numbers of phagocytic cells and a decrease in their function. Decreased numbers of AM and monocytes and a reduction in AM responsiveness to chemotactic stimuli have been noted. Additionally, combined therapy decreased the bactericidal capabilities of AM (169, 170).

Combined therapy also adversely affected the generation of a pulmonary inflammatory response. The chemotactic potency of AM supernatants was reduced, and the synthesis of C2 and C4 by AM was suppressed (171, 172).

IV. Infections in Connective Tissue Disorders

Infections are a frequent cause of morbidity and mortality in patients with connective tissue disorders (CTD) (173). Numerous studies have evaluated factors that correlate positively with risk of infection (174, 174a-c). These studies regarding risk factors for infection should be interpreted cautiously. None of these studies have distinguished between serious and trivial infections, nor have they analyzed the risk factors for the development of infections due to specific etiologic agents. Risk factors for opportunistic infections may differ from those for common bacterial infections. Finally, none of the studies have estimated the risk related to therapy versus underlying disease using analytical techniques that allow the relative and independent contributions of these two linked factors to be evaluated.

Several conclusions can, however, be drawn from these studies. First, SLE itself appears to be a risk factor for infection. Patients with SLE have higher rates of infection than normal adults even when infection rates are adjusted for steroid dose (174, 174a). Second, corticosteroid use and daily dose are the most consistently identified risk factors for the development of infection.

Patients on a regimen of high-dose prednisone (>40 mg/d) clearly had significantly increased (fivefold) infection rates (174b). Third, activity of disease was a risk factor in some, but not all, studies (174a,174c).

Infections are at present the commonest cause of death in SLE; 33% of patients die from infections, while 31% of patients die of active SLE (174d). If only fatal infections are considered, infections due to common bacterial organisms and those due to opportunistic organisms occur with similar frequency. Opportunistic infections were more likely to be first diagnosed at autopsy (173).

A. Bacteria

Gram-Negative Bacilli

Gram-negative bacilli (e.g., *Klebsiella pneumoniae, Escherichia coli, Pseudomonas aeruginosa*) are a frequent cause of pneumonia in patients with CTD. The high frequency of these infections is probably related to the ease with which gram-negative bacilli colonize the upper respiratory tract of patients with serious and chronic debilitating illnesses (175). These illnesses are associated with enhanced adherence of gram-negative bacteria to epithelial cells (176). These colonizing organisms reach the lower respiratory tract by aspiration of oropharyngeal secretions.

The clinical manifestations include a sudden onset of fever, chills, productive cough, and pleuritic chest pain. Leukocytosis, fever, and a new infiltrate on a chest radiograph are common clinical presentations. Consolidative lobar lesions or cavitary lesions are frequent radiographic presentations. Clinical, laboratory, and roentgenographic findings are rarely diagnostic for a specific etiologic agent in patients with CTD. Sputum should be collected for culture and staining but should be interpreted with caution because colonization is difficult to distinguish from infection. Blood cultures should be obtained.

Gram-Positive Bacteria

The incidence of pneumococcal infections in collagen vascular disease is difficult to assess accurately and may be no higher than in the general population. *S. aureus* infections, particularly *S. aureus sepsis,* are a common cause of death in patients with SLE (173). *S. aureus* pneumonia may present abruptly with high fever, chills, progressive dyspnea, and pleuritic pain or may begin insidiously with increasing fever, tachycardia, and respiratory rate as the only indication of infection. The rapid development of pleural effusions and empyema may occur.

Because a rapid definitive etiologic diagnosis is difficult to obtain in a majority of patients with CTD, early treatment is usually empiric. Any empiric therapy of a patient with CTD and suspected bacterial pneumonia should cover both *S. aureus* and gram-negative bacilli. Therapy should be instituted promptly, as pneumonia often progresses rapidly in these patients if the institution of therapy is delayed. The use of two antimicrobial agents, usually an aminoglycoside and a third-generation cephalosporin, is the preferred empiric therapy. Third-generation cephalosporins offer less nephrotoxicity and should be considered instead of aminoglycosides in patients with renal insufficiency. Aminoglycoside levels should be obtained if these agents are utilized (177-179). Vancomycin is the drug of choice if methicillin-resistant *S. aureus* infection is a significant possibility (180).

Legionella

Pneumonia due to bacteria of the family Legionellaceae occurs with increased frequency in immunocompromised patients (IPs) and patients on corticosteroid or immunosuppressive therapy (181-186), and may be fulminant (182-186). Several species and strains of Legionellaceae have been described (181,182,184,187), but over 95% of pneumonias due to *Legionella* have been due to *L. pneumophilia,* with *L. micdadei* (also known as the Pittsburgh agent, or TATLOCK bacillus) being the next most common (181,184,185). The incidence of infections due to *Legionella* species has been highly variable among different geographic regions. *Legionella* bacteria have accounted for more than 15% of pneumonias among renal transplant patients in some centers (182,183,185) but less than 3% of pneumonias in comparable patient populations in others (188). Most cases have been acquired nosocomially from environmental sources, such as contaminated water, air conditioners, or respiratory therapy equipment in hospitals (181-183,185). The clinical and radiographic features of pneumonia due to *L. pneumophilia* (legionnaire's disease), *L. micdadei,* or other *Legionella* species may be indistinguishable from other bacterial pneumonias (181,184-186,189). Extrapulmonary manifestations of headache, myalgias, confusion, and neurological and gastrointestinal symptoms are common (181,183,184), but these features do not distinguish *L. pneumophilia* from other pneumonias (189). Hyponatremia has also been a common associated laboratory finding (181,185,189). Chest radiographs typically demonstrate patchy bronchopneumonia with segmental or lobar infiltrates, which may worsen while the patient is on antibiotic therapy (181,184-186). Extensive necrosis, abscess formation, and cavitation are uncommon as initial features but may be seen in more chronic cases (181, 83,185,186). Pleural effusion occur in 10-30% of cases (181,183). Progressive hypoxemia and fatal respiratory failure may develop (181,185,186,189). Standard bacterial cultures are not helpful (181,185,186). *Legionella* bacteria stain poorly with conventional Gram stains (181-184), and alternative techniques are required to visualize the organisms. Dieterle silver impregnation stains and direct immunofluorescent stains are the most reliable means for demonstrating *Legionella* bacteria in sputum, tracheobronchial secretions, or lung tissue (181,182,184,185). Cultures for *Legionella* using specialized media are highly sensitive but may require 2-7 days (181,184,185). Indirect immunofluorescent antibody techniques detect specific antibody in sera in 75-90% of cases but may require 3-6 weeks for seroconversion so are rarely useful except in epidemiological studies (181,184).

Therapy for *Legionella* pneumonia in IPs requires prompt and aggressive reduction in the level of corticosteroid or immunosuppressive therapy in addition to antibiotics, as mortality in IPs has been as high as 30-50% even with appropriate antibiotic therapy (181,184-186). Beta-lactams and aminoglycosides are ineffective. Erythromycin has excellent activity again *Legionella* species and has been associated with the highest cure rate in clinical infections (181,185,189). Intravenous erythromycin in initial doses of 4-6 g daily is the treatment of choice (181,186). Oral therapy may be substituted after 5-7 days in patients exhibiting favorable responses to therapy. A minimum of 3 weeks of therapy is recommended (181,183,186). Rifampin has synergistic activity with erythromycin against *Legionella* in vitro, and combined therapy with erythromycin and rifampin is warranted in severely ill IPs with Legionellosis (181,184). In patients unable to tolerate erythromycin, doxycycline, a lipid-soluble tetracycline, is an acceptable alternative (181).

B. Invasive Fungal Infections

Aspergillus

Invasive infections with *Aspergillus* species *(A. fumigatus, A. flavus, A. niger)* may occur in patients with severe immune deficits and involve the lung in over 90% of cases (190-192). Host defenses against *Aspergillus* involve two distinct mechanisms. Mononuclear phagocytes (alveolar macrophages) serve as the initial barrier against *Aspergillus* and, by phagocytosing *Aspergillus* spores inhaled into the respiratory tract, may prevent tissue invasion (191,193, 194). Polymorphonuclear leukocytes have little activity against *Aspergillus* spores but are the major line of defense once the spores have germinated (191, 193,194). Patients most prone to develop invasive aspergillosis are those with severe deficits in both cellular immunity and granulocyte number or function (191,193-195). Predisposing factors for invasive aspergillosis include corticosteroid or cytotoxic therapy (190,194,196,197), recent antibiotic therapy (194,197), and severe granulocytopenia (190,191,193-195,197,198). Over 90% of cases have been reported among patients with hematological malignancies in relapse (190-192,195,197) or organ transplant recipients

(193,194,196). Although only rare cases of invasive aspergillosis complicating CTD have been described (173,192), patients on intensive corticosteroid and immunosuppressive therapy are at increased risk for *Aspergillus* infections. Invasive aspergillosis almost always begins with a bronchopulmonary infection (190-193). The most common initial finding is a new or persistent pulmonary infiltrate with fever (190-192,194,199). The sudden onset of pleuritic chest pain, hypoxemia, and hemoptysis in many patients mimics acute pulmonary embolism (191,192,194,199). The most commonly observed radiographic changes have been patchy bronchopneumonia (191,192), single or multiple nodular infiltrate (197), and cavitary lesions (191,194,199). Lobar consolidation occurs in 5-15% of cases (191-194). A diffuse miliary or interstitial pattern is less common. Progressive parenchymal necrosis may lead to cavitation and mycetoma formation (199). The propensity of *Aspergillus* to invade vessels may result in hemorrhagic infarction and massive (and sometimes fatal) hemoptysis (192,199). The clinical course of pulmonary aspergillosis is usually fulminant, with death within 2 weeks in most cases (191,194). Extrapulmonary dissemination occurs in 20-30% of cases, with a predilection for brain, gastrointestinal tract, and skin (191,192,194,197). Sinusitis, ocular invasion, and osteomyelitis have also been described (194).

Diagnosis of invasive pulmonary aspergillosis may be difficult, as sputum culture are positive in only 10-35% of cases (190,192,193,197,199,200), and blood cultures are invariably negative (192,194). The significance of positive sputum cultures remains controversial, as most positive *Aspergillus* cultures in IPs occur without evidence for invasive disease (191,194). Multiple positive sputum cultures, however, strongly suggest invasive disease (191, 194). Serological tests for *Aspergillus* antigens using immunodiffusion and CIE techniques have not been shown to be helpful (193,194). A definitive diagnosis of invasive disease requires identification of the typical septated hyphae within tissue. Fiberoptic bronchoscopy (FB) has a diagnostic yield of 40-70% for pulmonary aspergillosis and is the preferred initial invasive procedure of choice (194,199,200). Percutaneous needle aspiration (PNA) may be a superior procedure for small, localized nodular or cavitary lesions that may not be readily accessible by FB. Open lung biopsy may be necessary in cases where FB and PNA have been nondiagnostic, but even open lung biopsies may fail to substantiate the diagnosis (201,202).

Mortality from invasive pulmonary aspergillosis exceeds 80% (190-192, 194,197), but early initiation of therapy and restoration of immune function may improve survival (191,194,198,199). Amphotericin B (AmB) is the mainstay of treatment. The addition of rifampin or 5-flucytosine (5-FC) to AmB may be considered, as these drugs exhibit in vitro activity against some strains of *Aspergillus,* but there is not clear evidence that combination therapy is superior to AmB alone (193,194). The imidazole antifungal drugs miconazole and ketoconazole have minimal activity against *Aspergillus* and hav eno role in treating this disease (194). Surgical resection of *Aspergillus* mycetomas or cavities has been used as adjunctive therapy with success in some cases (190, 192,194,197), although the role of surgery remains controversial (191). The most important factors determining outcome are the status of the underlying disease and the ability to restore immune function (194,198,199). Survival has been greatest among patients in whom corticosteroid or immunosuppressive therapy has been reduced in conjunction with aggressive antifungal therapy (191,194).

Phycomycetes

Mucormycosis is a term applied to infections caused by nonseptated fungi belonging to the order Mucorales within the subclass Zygomycetes. Although infections with these nonseptated fungi are far less common than *Aspergillus* infections, Mucoraceae and *Aspergillus* share several common clinical and histological features. These fungi have a propensity to infect the lung and central nervous system (CNS) and may invade the vasculature, with resultant ischemia and hemorrhagic infarction of involved organs (193,203,204). Both types of fungi require both granulocytes and cell-mediated mechanisms for control (193). Alveolar macrophages and mononuclear phagocytes play important early roles in controlling inhaled spores, but neutrophils play the key role in killing the organism once the spores have germinated (193). High-dose corticosteroids and severe granulocytopenia are important risk factors for both *Aspergillus* and mucormycosis infections (193,203,204). Chest radiographs in pulmonary mucormycosis characteristically demonstrate patchy bronchopneumonia, consolidation, or nodular infiltrates, which may cavitate (193,203,204). Massive, fatal hemoptysis may occur, particularly in the presence of cavitary disease (193,203). The antemortem diagnosis is difficult, as blood cultures are uniformly negative and sputum cultures are rarely positive, even with invasive pulmonary disease (203,204). The diagnosis requires identification of the organism in tissue or by cultures. Fungi of the order Mucorales can be recognized by their broad, thick walls; their tendency to branch at right angles; and the lack of septations (203). Mortality with invasive pulmonary or disseminated mucormycosis has been nearly 100%, but occasionally cures with AmB have been reported when control of the underlying disease or reduction of immunosuppressive therapy can be achieved (193). Owing to the poor survival with AmB alone, we recommend combining surgical resection of localized disease (when possible) with systematic AmB, as this approach has met with the greatest success (203). The optimal dose of AmB therapy is not known, but a minimum of 2.0 g is recommended.

Histoplasma capsulatum

Histoplasmosis accounts for less than 5% of invasive fungal infections in IPs (193,205,206) but has been observed in patients with lymphopenia or impaired cellular immunity in endemic areas (205-207). Corticosteroid therapy is an important predisposing factor and has been associated with a high rate of dissemination in infected individuals (205,206). Granulocytopenia is not a major risk factor, as host defenses against *H. capsulatum* primarily involve lymphocytes and macrophages (193). Among the cases of histoplasmosis reported in immunocompromised patients (IPs), 80% have been in patients with hematological malignancies and 5-10% in organ transplant recipients, the remaining cases occurring in patients on corticosteroid or immunosuppressive therapy (205-207). Nearly 10% of published cases in IPs have been observed in patients with SLE (205,206). Chest radiographic abnormalities including diffuse or focal interstitial infiltrates, bronchopneumonia, nodular densities, or cavities are present in 60-80% of cases (206,207). Dissemination occurs in up to 70-88% of IPs with histoplasmosis (205-207). Fever and constitutional symptoms are present in virtually all patients with disseminated disease (205-207). Common sites of dissemination include bone marrow, liver, adrenals, and oropharynx (205-207). Anemia, leukopenia, and thrombocytopenia are common, reflecting bone marrow involvement (207). Cultures of bone marrow and blood have a 50-90% diagnostic yield among patients with disseminated disease (205,207). This high rate of positive blood and marrow cultures with histoplasmosis is unique to this fungus, as these sites are virtually always sterile in other invasive mycotic infections. Biopsy of oral lesions, lung, liver, or lymph nodes may also be useful. Serological or skin tests are not helpful as significant complement fixation titer rises are observed in less than 50% of cases and skin tests are negative in 85% of cases in IPs (206). Untreated, the mortality of disseminated histoplasmosis approaches 100% (206,207), but therapy with AmB may be curative in over 90% of cases if initiated early (206,207). We recommend a minimal of 1.5-2.0 g of AmB therapy, as high mortality and relapse rates have been reported in patients receiving less intensive therapy (206).

Coccidiodes immitis

Infections due to *Coccidiodes immitis* have occasionally been observed in IPs living in endemic areas but are rare (193,208). Only 13 cases of coccidiomycosis were observed in IPs seen at Stanford University over a 14-year period, despite a high prevalence of other invasive fungal infections (208). Nearly 10% of cases of coccidiomycosis in IPs have been in patients with SLE (208). Cell-mediated immune mechanisms provide the major defense against this organism, and lymphopenia and corticosteroids are common predisposing factors (208). Pulmonary manifestations usually predominate, with cough, fever, and chest radiographic abnormalities. Patchy broncho-pneumonia infiltrates have been reported most commonly, but diffuse in-terstitial or miliary infiltrates, cavities, or nodules may be observed (208,209). Fever is present in over 90% of cases. Dissemination occurs in 30-50% of IPs with coccidiomycotic infection (208). Common sites of dis-semination are lymph nodes and bone, sites rarely involved in most other mycoses. Coccidioidin skin tests are not helpful. Complement fixation tests have been positive in 65% of cases in IPs, and higher titers have been associ-ated with a higher rate of dissemination and mortality (208-210). Diagnosis requires histological or cultural confirmation. The coccidiodal spherules can be identified on cytological specimens by KOH or Papanicolaou stains. Histological stains with Gomori or methenamine silver stains will demon-strate the organism on permanent sections. Cultures may take several days (208). Sputum smears or cultures have been positive in 20-30% of cases of pulmonary coccidiomycosis (208,209). Higher yields (in the range of 40-50%) have been reported with fiberoptic bronchoscopy in the presence of cocci-diodal pneumonia but are lower when a solitary nodule is present (209). Percutaneous needle aspiration and open lung biopsy appear to have higher yields for localized nodular disease (209). Amphotericin B remains the drug of choice for coccidiomycosis (211). Most isolates are also sensitive to mico-nazole and ketoconazole. The therapeutic failure rate with AmB in IPs with miliary coccidiomycosis may approach 50% (211), most likely because of impaired host defenses. Patients failing to respond to AmB should be treated with oral ketoconazole 200-400 mg daily, as favorable responses to this agent have been achieved in 60% of patients failing on AmB (210).

Cryptococcus neoformans

IPs with defects in cellular immunity, particularly patients with Hodgkin's disease, with hematological malignancy, or receiving high-dose corticoster-oids, are prone to develop infections with *Cryptococcus neoformans* (193, 212-214). Headache, lethargy, or neurological symptoms are the most com-mon clinical manifestations, owing to a high rate of meningeal involvement (212,215,216). Pulmonary involvement may be seen as the sole or predomi-nant manifestation or in conjunction with meningeal infection (212,213). Symptoms of pulmonary cryptococcosis are often subtle, and nearly one quarter of patients are asymptomatic with incidental findings on chest ra-diograph (213). Alveolar or interstitial infiltrates are most common, but cir-cumscribed mass lesions, solitary or multiple nodules, cavities, and pleural effusions have been described (212-214). Sputum cultures are positive in ap-proximately one third of cases of cryptococcal pneumonia (213). Lung biopsy may be required to corroborate the diagnosis. Bronchoscopic yields in the range of 50% have been reported (213). Open lung biopsy may be necessary in the evaluation of solitary pulmonary nodules. The significance of positive cultures for *C. neoformans* is controversial. However, the isolation of *C. neoformans* from sputum in the IP strongly suggests infection and warrants specific antifungal therapy. Dissemination may occur in up to 80% of cases of apparent primary pulmonary cryptococcosis in IPs in the absence of therapy (213), so aggressive therapy is warranted irrespective of the status of the pulmonary process. Blood, urine, and cerebrospinal fluid (CSF) cultures are positive in most cases with disseminated disease (214).

The critical factors determining outcome are the immune status of the host, the extent of dissemination, and the presence or absence of concomitant infections (214,216). Mortality is high unless restoration of the immune status can be achieved (213-215). Of 29 patients with disseminated neoplasm and cryptococcosis treated with AmB, only nine survived 2 months (212). Higher cure rates have been achieved with aggressive antifungal therapy in conjunction with reduction in immunosuppressive therapy or control of the underlying disease (193,215). The combination of AmB and 5-FC has been associated with 60-85% survival rates even with disseminated disease (213-216). Six weeks of therapy with low-dose AmB (0.3 mg/kg/d) plus 5-FC (150 mg/kg/d in divided doses) has been shown to be more effective than conventional-dose AmB (0.4 mg/kg/d) for 10 weeks in the treatment of cryptococcal meningitis, and it has fewer side effects (215).

Nocardia asteroides

Infections due to *Nocardia asteroides* characteristically occur in IPs with severe impairment in cellular immunity or on corticosteroid therapy (217), although one third to one half of documented infections have been described in previously normal hosts (217,218). Nocardiosis may also complicate CTD, particularly SLE (219,220), and 5% of 243 cases of nocardiosis reported from 1961-72 occurred in patients with CTD (220). Although the exact prevalence of nocardial infections complicating SLE has not been clarified, nocardiosis was responsible for only 2 of 179 deaths in SLE patients in two series (173,221). As of 1980, only 13 patients with nocardiosis complicating SLE had been reported (seven of whom died of infection) (217-220). Even fewer cases have been described in other CTDs.

Prompt diagnosis is critical, as delay in initiation of therapy has resulted in high fatality rates (219) whereas cures have been achieved in over 80% of cases when therapy is initiated early (217,218). Clinical findings are often subtle, and patients may be asymptomatic in up to 30% of cases (217,222). Pulmonary involvement usually predominates, and chest radiographic abnormalities can be demonstrated in at least 70% of cases (217,218). Multiple or single nodular densities, with or without cavitation, are characteristic, but patchy bronchopneumonia or lobar consolidation have also been described (218,222,223). Dissemination to the CNS occurs in up to 20% of cases in IPs and may result in single or multiple cerebral abscesses (217,223, 224). Dissemination to soft tissue, skin, and bone with abscess formation is also common (217,218). The diagnosis of nocardiosis requires demonstration of the organism in tissue or culture. The mycelia of *Nocardia asteroides* appear as delicate, beaded, gram-positive branching filaments as well as coccobacillary forms (217). Nocardia is notoriously difficult to culture and may require 1 to 3 weeks to grow, even with specialized media (218,223). Sputum cultures have been positive in only 10-30% of cases of pulmonary nocardiosis (217,218,223). Blood cultures are invariably negative, even with disseminated disease (217,218). Invasive techniques are usually required to confirm the diagnosis of pulmonary nocardiosis (218,223). Percutaneous needle aspiration has a diagnostic yield of up to 80% and is the procedure of choice in patients with localized nodular disease (218,225). FB is a potentially useful procedure in the setting of diffuse disease or a lobar process with consolidation. Open biopsy may be diagnostic in cases where other procedures have been negative (222,226).

Treatment with sulfisoxazole 6-12 g daily has been curative in more than 80% of cases (217-219,222,223). Trimethoprim-sulfamethoxazole (TMP-SMX) is also effective (224) and may be superior to sulfisoxazole in patients with CNS involvement due to greater penetration of TMP into the cerebrospinal fluid (224) as well as synergy between TMP and SMX (217,224). Therapy should be continued for a minimum of 6-12 months (217,218).

Mycobacterial Infections

Infections with typical (*Mycobacterium tuberculosis*) and atypical mycobacteria (such as *M. kansasii* and *M. avium-intracellulare*) occur with increased frequency in IPs, although the prevalence is low compared to other opportunists (222,227-229). The incidence of mycobacterial infections complicating SLE or CTD has not been clarified. In one study, *M. tuberculosis* developed in 16 of 311 patients with SLE in Singapore (230), but this high prevalence reflects the high endemic rate of TB in that geographic area. In the United States, only sporadic cases of mycobacterial infections complicating SLE or CTD have been reported. In one autopsy series, no cases of TB were identified among 44 patients with SLE (173). In a recent study assessing infectious complications among 23 SLE patients followed for 9 years at the NIH, only one case of TB was identified (174). The actual risk of mycobacteriosis in CTD appears to be low, but it is increased in patients receiving high-dose corticosteroid or immunosuppressive therapy (174,231,227). In two large series of IPs, with *M. tuberculosis* (231,232), only one patient had received prophylactic isoniazid, suggesting that this complication may be preventable if prophylactic isoniazid therapy is administered to tuberculin-positive individuals.

Clinical signs of mycobacterial infections in IPs are nonspecific, but fever, night sweats, and fatigue are characteristic (233). Pulmonary infiltrates may be present, but in contrast to pulmonary tuberculosis in the nonimmunosuppressed individual, cavitary disease is usually absent (227,233). More common radiographic abnormalities noted include a fulminant bronchopneumonia simulating bacterial pneumonia or even adult respiratory distress syndrome (ARDS), diffuse interstitial or miliary infiltrates, or hilar adenopathy (232). Mycobacterial infections occurring in IPs are often fulminant, have a high rate of dissemination and tuberculous bronchopneumonia, and have a high mortality (227,230-233). Soft tissue or joint infections mimicking pyogenic infection are common (233). Delay in recognition and initiation of therapy appears to be the major factor responsible for the high mortality. As sputum smears and cultures are positive in only 20-50% of cases, invasive procedures are often required to establish the diagnosis (227). We believe that FB with bronchoalveolar lavage (BAL) is the preferred initial invasive procedure of choice in this setting, as diagnostic yields of 60-80% for mycobacterial pulmonary infections have been reported (234, 235). However, it should be noted that transbronchial lung biopsies are diagnostic in less than 20% of cases (234,235), and the high yields reported with FB include positive cultures, which may not be available for several weeks and may not be clinically helpful. Open lung biopsy should be considered when bronchoscopy is nondiagnostic (226,236,237).

M. tuberculosis is usually sensitive to standard antituberculous drugs, and early therapy with isoniazid and rifampin, concomitant with reduction in the level of immunosuppression, has been curative in more than 80% of cases (231,233). Cure rates for atypical mycobacterial infections in IPs are considerably lower (227). In this context, aggressive reduction of corticosteroids or immunosuppressive agents is recommended, as administration of antituberculous therapy alone in patients with persistent severe immune deficits is rarely successful (227). Aggressive chemotherapy employing five to six antituberculous drugs is recommended for atypical mycobacterial infections, but treatment failures are common (227).

Pneumocystis carinii

The prevalence of *Pneumocystis carinii* pneumonia (PCP) has increased dramatically in the past several years, owing largely to the frequency of this pathogen in patients with AIDS (238). Although less common as an opportunistic pathogen in other IPs, *P. carinii* may infect patients with severe impairment in cell-mediated immunity. Major groups at risk for PCP include organ transplant recipients (225,228,239) and patients with lymphoprolifera-tive malignancies (239,240) or on high-dose corticosteroid or immunosup-pressive therapy (239,241). In a 1974 review of 194 cases of PCP reported nationwide over a 3-year period, 65% of cases occurred in patients with leu-kemia or lymphoma, 11% in organ transplant recipients, and nine cases (4.6%) were in patients with CTD, including five patients with SLE (241). Although the overall incidence of PCP in patients with CTD is low, *P. car-inii* pneumonitis was responsible for 3 of 44 deaths in one series of SLE pa-tients (173). As therapy for *P. carinii* pneumonitis is curative in 60-80% of cases (238,239,241), early recognition and initiation of therapy are critical to optimize outcome.

In contrast to *P. carinii* in AIDS patients, which is often asymptomatic and associated with minimal radiographic abnormalities (238), most patients with *P. carinii* complicating other disorders exhibit cough, dyspnea, hypoxe-mia, and widespread diffuse interstitial or alveolar infiltrates on chest radio-graph (238,240). In one large series, over 90% of cases were hypoxemic and dyspneic, and 39% were cyanotic at the time of presentation (241). Bilateral diffuse infiltrates are found in over 95% of cases (239,241). Lobar consoli-dation or nodular or cavitary infiltrates are virtually never seen with PCP, and these suggest an alternative diagnosis (242). Duration of symptoms at the time of presentation is typically short, in the range of 5-15 days (238, 241), which contrasts with the more prolonged course observed in AIDS patients with this infection (241). Diagnosis requires histological demonstra-tion of the organism in lung tissue or BAL, as the organism has never been cultured, and sputa are rarely diagnostic. Extrapulmonary dissemination does not occur. Methenamine silver or toluidine blue stains should be done on histological material to demonstrate the *P. carinii* cysts. Fiberoptic bron-choscopy with BAL has a diagnostic yield of 70-90% of *P. carinii* (234,235) and is the preferred initial invasive diagnostic procedure. When FFB is non-diagnostic, open lung biopsy may be required to substantiate the diagnosis.

Therapy with pentamadine iesthionate 4 mg/kg/day or TMP 20 mg/kg/day with SMX 100 mg/kg/day have been associated with cure rates ranging from 40% to 80%, with higher rates observed when treatment is initiated early (238,239,241,242). Historical comparisons suggest that TMP-SMX may be superior to pentamadine in treating *P. carinii* pneumonia (239), but no controlled studies comparing these agents in adults have been done. Side effects from TMP-SMX have been reported in 10-15% of cases in the non-AIDS population in several studies (238,239,242), an incidence lower than previously observed with pentamadine (239-241). Owing to the apparent higher success rate and fewer side effects of TMP-SMX compared to penta-madine, we consider intravenous TMP-SMX to be the initial drug of choice for treatment of *P. carinii* pneumonia. Oral therapy may be substituted once response has been documented, and a 14- to 21-day course is recommended. Pentamadine has been effective in some cases failing on TMP-SMX (241, 242).

D. Viral Infections

Infections with DNA viruses (cytomegalovirus, herpes simplex, and herpes varicella-zoster) are more common in patients with profound and sustained defects in cellular immunity (243,244). Groups at highest risk for these infections are organ transplant recipients (245-247) and patients with AIDS (248) or hematological malignancy (245), but severe viral infections in patients with CTD on intensive corticosteroid or immunosuppressive therapy have been described. Predisposing factors for DNA-viral infections among transplant recipients include pretransplant seropositivity of the recipient, receipt of blood products or organs from a seropositive donor, and the intensity of immunosuppression (245). As patients with CTD rarely receive as intense immunosuppressive therapy as transplant recipients and are not exposed to virus from donor blood or organ products, CMV or herpetic viral infections complicating CTD are rare.

Cytomegalovirus

Cytomegalovirus (CMV) is the most important cause of serious viral infections in IPs. Disseminated visceral infection and pneumonia, uncommon manifestations of viruses of the herpes simplex-varicella-zoster group, complicate 10-40% of symptomatic CMV infections and may be lethal (249-252). Cytomegalovirus may cause a wide spectrum of disease in the IP, ranging from asymptomatic viral shedding to a fulminant lethal pneumonia and disseminated disease (245,258). Prolonged fever, anemia, leukopenia, abnormal liver function tests, and an atypical mononucleosislike syndrome are the most common manifestations of overt CMV infection in IPs (252,254). Pneumonitis may occur in up to 10-20% of infected patients (245). Virtually all patients with CMV pneumonitis are febrile (245,252). Diffuse interstitial or alveolar infiltrates on chest radiograph are characteristic (252,253). Large nodular mass densities or cavities are never seen; these would suggest an alternative diagnosis. Hypoxemia may antedate the development of pulmonary infiltrates by several days (252). A miliary pattern on chest radiograph, often with fulminant respiratory failure and alveolar hemorrhage, usually reflects hematogenous seeding from viremia and disseminated infection (253). Patients with an interstitial pattern tend to have a more insidious onset, and blood cultures are less frequently positive in this setting (253). Infection with CMV has been shown to interfere with cell-mediated immunity and may predispose to serious superinfections with bacteria, fungi, and protozoan opportunists that may contribute to death (252,254).

The diagnosis of CMV pneumonitis can be established by demonstrating the characteristic large cells containing intranuclear inclusions and multiple smaller cytoplasmic inclusions in lung tissue or cytological specimens (245,255). Basophilic intranuclear inclusions (Cowdry type A) with an owl's eye appearance can best be demonstrated on hematoxylin and eosin stains of infected tissue or on Papanicolaou stains of cytological material (245, 255). Wright's Giemsa-stained touch imprints of infected lung tissue may provide a rapid diagnosis prior to permanent sections and are superior to hematoxylin and eosin in demonstrating the intracytoplasmic inclusions (255). Cultures ae highly sensitive, with a diagnostic accuracy of 80-90% of cases (249,250,256) but may require 2-6 weeks to grow. Immunofluorescent (IF) studies using monoclonal antibodies against CMV antigens have enabled a rapid (within 3-4 h) diagnosis of CMV-infected cells in BAL fluid or tissue, with a diagnostic accuracy comparable to or exceeding conventional cytological and cultural techniques (250,256,257). Additional techniques using in situ hybridization with specific cDNA probes against CMV-viral DNA appear to have comparable accuracy to the IF techniques (250,257) but are complex procedures to perform and require 2-3 days to complete.

Results of antiviral therapy for CMV pneumonia have been disappointing to date. Treatment with adenine arabinoside (vidarabine), alpha-interferon (α-IFN), or a combination of vidarabine and α-IFN have had no significant benefit in human CMV infections, and significant toxicity has been noted with these agents (245,252,258). Acyclovir, a guanosine analog that selectively inhibits herpes viral DNA polymerase and inhibits herpes and CMV virus replication (259), has been tried in the treatment of CMV pneumonitis, but the results have been unimpressive (247,249,260). Despite anecdotal reports of cures of CMV infections with parenteral acyclovir (246), acyclovir has not been shown to improve survival in patients with established CMV pneumonitis. A newer guanosine analog similar to acyclovir, 9-(1,3-dihydroxy-2-propoxymethyl) guanine, also known as DHPG or gancyclovir, exhibits 10- to 100-fold more potent activity against CMV than acyclovir and has some promise (248,261). DHPG has resulted in virologic and clinical improvement in patients with CMV retinitis (248) and may suppress excretion of CMV from respiratory secretions (262), but it has not been shown to prolong survival in patients with CMV pneumonia. An additional antiviral agent, trisodium phosphonoformate (foscarnet), is a potent inhibitor of herpesvirus DNA polymerases and has modest activity against CMV (263,264). Foscarnet has been used in Europe to treat CMV pneumonitis in organ transplant recipients, with favorable clinical and virological responses in 50% of cases (263,264), but it is not yet available in this country. Despite the discouraging results to date, the advent of more rapid diagnostic techniques to diagnose CMV infections earlier (250,256) and the recognition of the importance of reducing the level of immunosuppressive agents suggest that new antiviral agents may have a role in selected patient populations.

Herpes Simplex

Severe or disseminated herpes simplex (HSV) or varicella-zoster (VZ) infections may occur in IPs (244,254). Individuals at highest risk are organ transplant recipients and children with acute leukemia, where the incidence may approach 30-40% (243,244,265). Severe herpetic infections complicating CTD are rare, but the importance of cellular immunity in controlling the extent and recovery from herpesvirus infections (265) suggests that patients on intensive immunosuppressive therapy for CTD are at increased risk for disseminated or visceral infections. Humoral antibodies play a role in modulating herpetic infections but are of lesser importance than cell immune mechanisms (244,265).

Pneumonia due to HSV in IPs may occur from extension from esophageal or oropharyngeal disease, or from hematogenous seeding. Herpetic lesions involving the lip or oropharynx preceding or occurring simultaneously with the pulmonary lesion have been described in 80-90% of cases (266,267). HSV is far less common than CMV pneumonitis, and as of 1982 only 41 cases of lower respiratory tract infection due to HSV had been reported, most of which were diagnosed at necropsy (266). As more cases of HSV tracheobronchial infection or pneumonia have become recognized, its protean clinical features have become apparent. Cough, dyspnea, and hypoxemia are typical. In the mildest form, herpetic infection may present as a mild extension of oropharyngitis (244,266), but a more generalized diffuse tracheobronchitis extending into bronchioles and a diffuse hemorrhagic pneumonia may occur (266). Extensive involvement of trachea and bronchi with gross punctate mucosal ulcerations, edema, and thick tracheobronchial membranes may be observed (266,267). The additional finding that open lung biopsies have often been negative even in necropsy-proven HSV pneumonia supports the concept that HSV respiratory tract infection most often arises intrabronchially (266,267). Patients with fulminating HSV pneumonia often have widespread pulmonary edema due to diffuse lung injury, with massive pulmonary hemorrhage as a terminal event (244). Both focal pneumonia with consolidation and diffuse interstitial infiltrates on chest radiograph have been described (267). Cavitation does not occur. It is likely that the focal pneumonic infiltrates represent direct extension from oropharyngeal herpetic infection, while the diffuse radiographic pattern reflects hematogenous spread (267). Bacterial or fungal superinfection supervenes in 50% or more of cases and is an important contributory cause of death (244,266,267).

HSV may be identified by cytologies or cultures from lung, bronchial tissue, or BAL fluid (254,266). Eosinophilic intranuclear inclusions and multinucleated (syncytial) giant cells may be detected in infected tissue, although identical cytological changes may be found in VZ infections (266). More recently, diagnostic techniques using immunofluorescence and monoclonal antibodies and in situ DNA hybridization have promise (244,267). Mortality from HSV pneumonia exceeds 80%. Acyclovir has been efficacious in limiting herpetic mucocutaneous (268) and visceral infections in IPs (258) and is effective prophylaxis against HSV infections in bone marrow transplant recipients (244,258). Although data confirming its efficacy in HSV pneumonitis are lacking, we recommend IV acyclovir 250 mg/mm^2 q8h for a 7-to-10-day course. It is likely that the outcome depends more on the immune status of the host and the presence or absence of complicating superinfections than on the influence of antiviral therapy.

Varicella-Zoster

As with HZV, VZ has the potential to cause a rapidly progressive hemorrhagic pneumonia in susceptible hosts (244,254). However, life-threatening VZ infections are rare and pulmonary lesions are infrequent even with disseminated zoster (244,254). The cutaneous exanthem of zoster, with grouped vesicles on an erythematous base, usually precedes the onset of pneumonia by 1-7 days (254). With VZ pneumonia cough, dyspnea, and fever are usually present (244,254). Chest radiographs demonstrate patchy or diffuse interstitial and alveolar infiltrates, with a peribronchiolar distribution, but lobar pneumonia, mimicking a bacterial process, has been described (243). Histological and cytological features of VZ pneumonia are identical to HSV pneumonia (244), and cultural identification is required for differentiation. Spontaneous resolution of VZ infections is characteristic, even in IPs, but acyclovir, α-IFN, and vidarabine have been shown to reduce viral shedding and accelerate healing in IPs with VZ (254,269). Intravenous acyclovir is superior to vidarabine as therapy of localized cutaneous zoster in IPs (254) and is the treatment of choice of VZ pneumonia. Untreated, the mortality of VZ pneumonia in IPs has been 15-35%, but acyclovir has reduced mortality to approximately 10% (244,254). Simply reducing the level of immunosuppressive therapy may hasten the resolution of the lesions and prevent dissemination (244,254).

E. Invasive Diagnostic Techniques

The approach to the patient with CTD and pulmonary infiltrates should be thorough and immediate. Appropriate serologies should be done to exclude flare of the underlying disease. A careful drug history is important, as certain agents such as methotrexate, gold, and cytotoxic agents are known to be capable of causing lung injury. Sputum smears and cultures for bacteria, viruses, AFB, fungi, and *Legionella* should be done to exclude infection.

Papincolaou smears of sputum by be useful to identify fungi, virocytes, or *P. carinii.* Lumbar puncture to include India ink prep, cryptococcal antigen, and cultures is indicated in any patient with neurological signs or symptoms. Aspiration, biopsy, or culture of any extrapulmonary lesions should be done. In many cases, however, invasive techniques are required to establish a specific etiological diagnosis. The decision to proceed with invasive procedures depends on multiple factors, including the severity and acuteness of illness, the pattern on chest radiograph, and the potential morbidity of biopsy. In patients with a clinical course compatible with bacterial illness, empirical broad-spectrum parenteral antibiotics should be initiated immediately. Examination of sputum Gram stain may guide therapy if a predominant organism is visualized, but it is rarely definitive and may be misleading. Accordingly, aggressive initial coverage combining a beta-lactam and an aminoglycoside is recommended until results of sputum and blood cultures have become available.

Patients failing to respond to antibiotics may require a more aggressive evaluation, possibly including FB. Findings on chest radiograph may be a clue to the likely etiology. For example, a lobar infiltrate with air bronchograms is far more likely to represent a bacterial or mycotic process, whereas diffuse interstitial or miliary infiltrates are rarely due to bacteria and strongly suggest opportunistic infection (270,271). In this context, biopsy should be performed promptly, as noninvasive techniques are rarely diagnostic. Open lung biopsy provides the highest yield (237,272), but the need for general anesthesia and the potential for serious complications make this unsuitable as the initial invasive diagnostic procedure in most cases.

In our opinion, FB is the preferred initial invasive procedure in the diagnostic evaluation of pulmonary infiltrates in IPs. By combining BAL, bronchial brushings, and transbronchial biopsy (TBB), specific etiological diagnoses can be established in 50-90% of cases in this patient population (234, 235,270,273,274). For *P. carinii* pneumonitis, BAL and TBB have comparable yields, in the range of 85-90% (234,235). BAL is superior to TBB in the detection of other opportunists such as fungi, AFB, and viruses, with 50-80% yields (234,235). The higher yield of BAL compared to TBB for certain opportunists probably reflects the large alveolar surface area covered by BAL and the small sample size of TBB. It should be noted, however, that these high yields from BAL also include positive culture results which may not be available for several days or weeks and may be of no clinical value. BAL is least useful in nonspecific interstitial pneumonitis and malignancy, although negative results of BAL in such cases make the diagnosis of a specific treatable infection less likely (273). False-positive results have not been a major problem, but fungal organisms demonstrated on BAL may occasionally represent colonization rather than invasive infection. Unless concurrent TBBs demonstrate fungal hyphae invading lung parenchyma, one cannot reliably distinguish colonization from invasion. Combining both TBB and BAL increases the yield slightly compared to either procedure alone as well as the specificity (234,275) and is recommended in patients in whom no contraindications to biopsy exist. As TBB has a greater potential for complications including pneumothorax or hemorrhage, BAL alone is reasonable in patients who are thrombocytopenic or in respiratory failure. FB is of limited value in the diagnostic evaluation of bacterial pneumonia, but bronchial brushings and cultures utilizing a sheathed catheter to eliminate oropharyngeal contamination may permit more precise identification of bacterial pathogens (276). Nonspecific inflammatory changes (NSC) or fibrosis may be seen in up to 30-50% of TBBs in IPs (275,277). The significance of such changes is controversial. Some investigators have concluded that NSC are infrequently associated with a specific treatable disorder and that more aggressive diagnostic procedures are rarely warranted (273,277). Others have noted that NSC should not be considered definitive, as open lung biopsy may establish a specific and treatable etiology diagnosis in some cases (201,272,275). The decision to proceed with an open lung biopsy needs to be individualized. If FB is nondiagnostic and the patient is not responding to therapy, open lung biopsy should be considered.

References

1. Newhouse, M., Sanchis, J., and Bienenstock, J. (1976). Lung defense mechanisms. *N. Engl. J. Med.* **295**:990-998; 1045-1052.
2. Green, G. M., Jakab, G. J., Low, R. B., and Davis, G. S. (1977). Defense mechanisms of the respiratory membrane. *Am. Rev. Respir. Dis.* **115**:479-514.
3. Brain, J. D., Proctor, D. F., and Reid, L. M. (eds) (1977). *Respiratory Defense Mechanisms*, parts I and II. Marcel Dekker, New York.
4. Toews, G. B. (1983). Pulmonary clearance of infectious agents. In *Respiratory Infections: Diagnosis and Management*. Edited by Pennington, J. E. Raven Press, New York, pp. 31-39.
5. Toews, G. B. (1986). Determinants of bacterial clearance from the lower respiratory tract. *Semin. Respir. Infect.* **1**:68-78.
6. Proctor, D. F. (1977). The upper airway. I. Nasal physiology and defense of the lung. II. The larynx and trachea. *Am. Rev. Respir. Dis.* **115**:97-129; 315-342.
7. Wanner, A. (1977). Clinical aspects of mucociliary clearance. *Am. Rev. Respir. Dis.* **116**:73-125.
8. Laurenzi, G. A., Berman, L., First, M., and Kass, E. H. (1965). A quantitative study of the deposition and clearance of bacteria in the murine lung. *J. Clin. Invest.* **43**:759-768.

9. Green, G. M., and Kass, E. H. (1964). The role of the alveolar macrophage in the clearance of bacteria from the lung. *J. Exp. Med.* **119**:167-176.

10. Goldstein, E., Lippert, W., and Warshauer, D. (1974). Pulmonary alveolar macrophage. Defender against bacterial infection in the lung. *J. Clin. Invest.* **54**:519-528.

11. Hocking, W. G., and Golde, D. W. (1979). The pulmonary-alveolar macrophage. *N. Engl. J. Med.* **301**:580-587.

12. Nathan, C. F., Murray, H. W., and Cohn, Z. A. (1980). The macrophage as an effector cell. *N. Engl. J. Med.* **303**:622-626.

13. Reynolds, H. Y., Atkinson, J. P., Newball, H. H., and Frank, M. M. (1975). Receptors for immunoglobulin and complement on human alveolar macrophages. *J. Immunol.* **114**:1813-1819.

14. Reynolds, H. Y., and Thompson, R. E. (1973). Pulmonary host defenses. I. Analysis of protein and lipids in bronchial secretions and antibody responses after vaccination with *Pseudomonas aeruginosa*. *J. Immunol.* **11**:358-368.

15. Reynolds, H. Y., and Newball, H. H. (1976). Fluid and cellular milieu of the human respiratory tract. In *Immunologic and Infectious Reactions in the Lung*. Edited by Kirkpatrick, C. H., and H. Y. Reynolds. Marcel Dekker, New York, pp. 3-27.

16. Stossel, T. P. (1974). Phagocytosis. *N. Engl. J. Med.* **290**:717-724; 833-839.

17. Babior, B. M. (1978). Oxygen-dependent microbial killing by phagocytes. *N. Engl. J. Med.* **298**:659-668; 721-725.

18. Southern, P. M., Mayes, B. B., Pierce, A. K., and Sanford, J. P. (1970). Pulmonary clearance of *Pseudomonas aeruginosa*. *J. Lab. Clin. Med.* **76**:548-559.

19. Pierce, A. K., Reynolds, R. C., and Harris, G. D. (1977). Leukocytic response to inhaled bacteria. *Am. Rev. Respir. Dis.* **116**:679-684.

20. Toews, G. B., Gross, G. N., and Pierce, A. K. (1979). The relationship of inoculum size to lung bacterial clearance and phagocytic cell response in mice. *Am. Rev. Respir. Dis.* **120**:559-566.

21. Toews, G. B., Vial, W. C., and Hansen, E. J. (1985). Role of C5 and recruited neutrophils in early clearance of nontypable *Haemophilus influenzae* from murine lungs. *Infect. Immun.* **50**:207-212.

22. Rehm, S. R., Gross, G. N., and Pierce, A. K. (1980). Early bacterial clearance from murine lungs: Species-dependent phagocyte response. *J. Clin. Invest.* **66**:194-199.

23. Onofrio, J. M., Toews, G. B., Lipscomb, M. F., and Pierce, A. K. (1983). Granulocyte-alveolar macrophage interaction in the pulmonary clearance of *Staphylococcus aureus*. *Am. Rev. Respir. Dis.* **127**:335-341.

24. Cohen, A., Batra, G., Petersen, R., Podany, J., and Nguyen, D. (1979). Size of the pool of alveolar neutrophils in normal rabbit lungs. *J. Appl. Physiol.* **47**:440-444.
25. Vial, W. C., Toews, G. B., and Pierce, A. K. (1984). Early pulmonary granulocyte recruitment in response to *Streptococcus pneumonia*. *Am. Rev. Respir. Dis.* **129**:87-91.
26. Larsen, G. L., Mitchel, B. C., Harper, T. B., and Henson, P. M. (1982). The pulmonary response of C5 sufficient and deficient mice to *Pseudomonas aeruginosa*. *Am. Rev. Respir. Dis.* **126**:306-311.
27. Toews, G. B., and Vial, W. C. (1984). The role of C5 in polymorphonuclear leukocyte recruitment in response to *Streptococcus pneumoniae*. *Am. Rev. Respir. Dis.* **129**:82-86.
28. Kolb, W. B., Kolb, L. M., Wetsel, R. A., Rogers, R. W., and Shaw, J. O. (1981). Quantitation and stability of the fifth component of complement (C5) in bronchoalveolar lavage fluid obtained from nonhuman primates. *Am. Rev. Respir. Dis.* **123**:226-231.
29. Snyderman, R., Skin, H. S., and Dannenberg, A. M. (1977). Macrophage proteinase and inflammation: The production of chemotactic activity from the fifth component of complement by macrophage proteinase. *J. Immunol.* **109**:896-898.
30. Kazmierowski, J. A., Gallin, J. I., and Reynolds, H. Y. (1977). Mechanisms for the inflammatory response in primate lungs: Demonstration and partial characterization of an alveolar macrophage-derived chemotactic factor with preferential activity for polymorphonuclear leukocytes. *J. Clin. Invest.* **59**:273-281.
31. Hunninghake, G. W., Gallin, J. I., and Fauci, A. S. (1978). Immunologic reactivity of the lung. The in vitro generation of a neutrophil chemotactic factor by alveolar macrophages. *Am. Rev. Respir. Dis.* **117**:15-23.
32. Hunninghake, G. W., Gadek, J. E., Fales, H. M., and Crystal, R. G. (1980). Human alveolar macrophage-derived chemotactic factor for neutrophils, stimuli and partial characterization. *J. Clin. Invest.* **66**:473-483.
33. Merrill, W. W., Naegel, G. P., Matthay, R. A., and Reynolds, H. Y. (1980). Alveolar macrophage-derived chemotactic factor, kinetics of in vitro production and partial characterization. *J. Clin. Invest.* **65**:268-276.
34. Ford-Hutchinson, S. W., Bray, M. A., Doinong, M. U., Shipley, M. E., and Smith, M. J. (1980). Leukotriene B, a potent chemokinetic and aggregating substance released from polymorphonuclear leukocytes. *Nature* **286**:264-265.
35. Valone, F. H., Franklin, M., Sun, F. F., and Goetzl, E. J. (1980). Alveolar macrophage lipoxygenase products of arachidonic acid: Isolation and recognition as the predominant constituents of the neutrophil chemotactic activity elaborated by alveolar macrophages. *Cell Immunol.* **54**:390-401.

36. Arnoux, B. A., Duval, D., and Benveniste, J. (1980). Release of platelet activating factor from alveolar macrophages by the calcium ionophore A23187 and phagocytosis. *Eur. J. Clin. Invest.* **10**:437-441.
37. Fel, A. O. S., and Cohn, Z. A. (1986). The alveolar macrophage. *J. Appl. Physiol.* **60**:353-369.
38. Badwey, J. A., and Karnovsky, M. L. (1980). Active oxygen species and the functions of phagocytic leukocytes. *Annu. Rev. Biochem.* **49**:695-726.
39. Babior, B. M. (1984). The respiratory burst of phagocytes. *J. Clin. Invest.* **73**:599-601.
40. Rosen, H., and Klebanoff, S. J. (1979). Bactericidal activity of a superoxide anion-generation system. A model for the polymorphonuclear leukocyte. *J. Exp. Med.* **149**:27-39.
41. Zeya, H. I., and Spitznagel, J. K. (1968). Arginine-rich proteins of polymorphonuclear leukocyte lysosomes. Antimicrobial specificity and biochemical heterogeneity. *J. Exp. Med.* **12**:927-941.
42. Unanue, E. R., Beller, D. I., Lu, C. Y., and Allen, P. M. (1984). Antigen presentation: Comments on its regulation and mechanism. *J. Immunol.* **132**:1-5.
43. Weissler, J. C., Lyons, C. R., Lipscomb, M. F., and Toews, G. B. (1986). Human pulmonary macrophages. Functional comparison of cells obtained from whole lung and by bronchoalveolar lavage. *Am. Rev. Respir. Dis.* **133**:473-477.
44. Nicod, L. P., Lipscomb, M. F., Weissler, J. C., Lyons, C. R., Albertson, J., and Toews, G. B. (1987). Mononuclear cells in human lung parenchyma: Characterization of a potent accessory cell not obtained by bronchoalveolar lavage. *Am. Rev. Respir. Dis.* **136**:818-823.
45. Toews, G. B., Vial, W. C., Dunn, M. M., et al. (1984). The accessory cell function of human alveolar macrophages in specific T cell proliferation. *J. Immunol.* **132**:181-186.
46. Mayernik, D. G., Ul-Hag, A., and Rinehart, J. J. (1983). Differentiation-associated alteration in human monocyte-macrophage accessory function. *J. Immunol.* **130**:2156-2160.
47. Ettensohn, D. B., and Robert, N. J. Jr. (1983). Human alveolar macrophage support of lymphocyte responses to mitogens and antigens. *Am. Rev. Respir. Dis.* **128**:516-522.
48. Lyons, C. R., Ball, E. J., Toews, G. B., Weissler, J. C., Stastny, P., and Lipscomb, M. F. (1986). Inability of human alveolar macrophages to stimulate resting T cells correlates with decreased anitgen specific T cell-macrophage binding. *J. Immunol.* **137**:1173-1180.
49. Wewers, M. D., Rennard, S. I., Hance, A. J., Bitterman, P. B., and Crystal, R. G. (1984). Normal human alveolar macrophages obtained

by bronchoalveolar lavage have a limited capacity to release interleukin-1. *J. Clin. Invest.* **74**:2208-2218.

50. McCombs, C. C., Michalski, J. P., Westerfield, B. T., and Light, R. W. (1982). Human alveolar macrophages suppress the proliferative response of peripheral blood lymphocytes. *Chest* **82**:266-271.

51. Sertl, K., Takemura, T., Tschachler, E., Ferrans, V. J., Kaliner, M. A., and Shevack, E. M. (1986). Dendritic cells with antigen presenting capability resideon airway epithelium, lung parenchyma and visceral pleura. *J. Exp. Med.* **163**:436-451.

52. Robb, R. J., Munck, A., and Smith, K. (1981). T cell growth factor receptors and quantitation, specificity and biological relevance. *J. Exp. Med.* **154**:1455-1474.

53. Uchiyama, T., Broder, S., and Waldmann, T. A. (1981). A monoclonal antibody (anti-Tac) reactive with activated and functionally mature human T cells. I. Production of anti-Tac monoclonal antibody and distribution of Tac (+) cells. *J. Immunol.* **126**:1393-1397.

54. Meuer, S. C., Hussey, R. E., Cantrell, D. A., et al. (1984). Triggering of the T_3-T_1 antigen-receptor complex results in clonal T-cell proliferation through an interleukin 2-dependent autocrine pathway. *Proc. Natl. Acad. Sci. USA* **81**:1509-1513.

55. Milestone, L. M., and Waksman, B. H. (1970). Release of virus inhibitor from tuberculin-sensitized peritoneal cells stimulated by antigen. *J. Immunol.* **105**:1068-1071.

56. Croll, A. D., and Morris, A. G. (1986). The regulation of gamma-interferon production by interleukins 1 and 2. *Cell Immunol.* **102**:33-42.

57. Mizel, S. B. (1982). Interleukin-1 and T cell activation. *Immunol. Rev.* **63**:51-72.

58. Kirchner, H., Bauer, A., Moritz, T., and Herbst, F. (1986). Lymphocyte activation and induction of interferon gamma in human leukocyte cultures by the mitogen in *Mycoplasma arthritidis* supernatant (MAS). *Scand. J. Immunol.* **24**:609-613.

59. Le, J., Lin, J. X., Henriksen-DeStefano, D., and Vilcek, J. (1986). Bacterial lipopolysaccharide-induced interferon-γproduction: Roles of interleukin 1 and interleukin 2. *J. Immunol.* **135**:4525-4530.

60. Murray, H. W., Welte, K., Jacobs, J. L., Rubin, B. Y., Mertelsmann, R., and Roberts. R. B. (1985). Production of an in vitro response to interleukin 2 in the acquired immunodeficiency syndrome. *J. Clin. Invest.* **76**:1959-1964.

61. Pearlstein, K. T., Palladino, M. A., Welte, K., and Vilcek, J. (1983). Purified human interleukin-2 enhances induction of immune interferon. *Cell Immunol.* **80**:1-9.

62. Reem, G. H., and Yeh, N. H. (1984). Interleukin 2 regulates expression of its receptor and synthesis of gamma interferon by human T lymphocytes. *Science* **255**:429-430.
63. Vilcek, J., Henriksen-DeStefano, J., Siegel, D. D., Klion, A., Robb, R. J., and Le, J. (1985). Regulation of IFN-γ induction in human peripheral blood cells by exogenous and endogenously produced interleukin 2. *J. Immunol.* **135**:1851-1856.
64. Palacios, R. (1984). Production of lymphokines by circulating human T lymphocytes that express or lack receptors for interleukin 2. *J. Immunol.* **132**:1833-1836.
65. Croll, A. D., Wilkinson, M. F., and Morris, A. G. (1985). Interleukin 2 receptor blockade by anti-Tac antibody inhibits IFN-γ induction. *Cell Immunol.* **92**:182-189.
66. Reynolds, H. Y., and Thompson, R. E. (1973). Pulmonary host defenses II. Interaction of respiratory antibodies with *Pseudomonas aeruginosa* and alveolar macrophages. *J. Immunol.* **111**:369-380.
67. Jakab, G. J. (1976). Factors influencing the immune enhancement of intrapulmonary bactericidal mechanisms. *Infect. Immun.* **14**:389-398.
68. Pennington, J. E. (1979). Lipopolysaccharide *Pseudomonas* vaccine: Efficacy against pulmonary infection with *Pseudomonas aeruginosa*. *J. Infect. Dis.* **140**:73-80.
69. Pennington, J. E., and Kuchmy, D. (1980). Mechanisms for pulmonary protection by lipopolysaccharide *Pseudomonas* vaccine. *J. Infect. Dis.* **142**:191-198.
70. Pennington, J. E., Hickey, W. F., Blackwood, L. L., and Arnaut, M. A. (1981). Active immunization with lipopolysaccharide *Pseudomonas* antigen for chronic *Pseudomonas* bronchopneumonia in guinea pigs. *J. Clin. Invest.* **68**:1140-1148.
71. Dunn, M. M., Toews, G. B., Hart, D., and Pierce, A. K. (1985). The effects of systematic immunization on pulmonary clearance of *Pseudomonas aeruginosa*. *Am. Rev. Respir. Dis.* **131**:426-431.
72. Toews, G. B., Hart, D. A., and Hansen, E. J. (1985). Effect of systematic immunication on pulmonary clearance of *Haemophilus influenzae* type b. *Infect. Immun.* **48**:343-349.
73. Hansen, E. J., Hart, D. A., McGehee, J. L., and Toews, G. B. (1988). Immune enhancement of pulmonary clearance of nontypable *Haemophilus influenzae*. *Infect. Immun.* **56**:182-190.
74. McLeod, R. E., Wing, J., and Remington, J. S. (1985). Lymphocytes and macrophages in cell-mediated immunity. In *Principles and Practice of Infectious Diseases*. Edited by Mandell, G. L., Douglas, R. G. Jr., and Bennet, J. E. John Wiley, New York, pp. 72-93.

75. Galindo, B., and Myrvik, Q. N., (1970). Migratory response of granulomatous alveolar cells from BCG-sensitized rabbits. *J. Immunol.* **105**:227-237.
76. Waldman, R. H., and Henney, C. S. (1971). Cell-mediated immunity and antibody response in the respiratory tract after local and systematic immunization. *J. Exp. Med.* **134**:482-494.
77. Waldman, R. H., Spencer, C. S., and Johnson, J. E. (1972). Respiratory and systematic cellular and humoral immune responses to influenza virus vaccine administered parenterally or by nose drops. *Cell Immunol.* **3**:294-300.
78. Jurgensen, P. F., Olsen, G. N., Johnson, J. E. III, et al. (1973). Immune response of the human respiratory tract. II. Cell-mediated immunity in the lower respiratory tract to tuberculin, mumps, and influenza viruses. *J. Infect. Dis.* **128**:730-735.
79. Nash, D. R., and Holle, B. (1973). Local and systematic cellular immune responses in guinea pigs given antigen parenterally or directly into the lower respiratory tract. *Clin. Exp. Immunol.* **13**:573-583.
80. Reynolds, H. Y., Thompson, R. E., and Devlin, H. B. (1974). Development of cellular and humoral immunity in the respiratory tract of rabbits to *Pseudomonas* lipopolysaccharide. *J. Clin. Invest.* **53**:1351-1358.
81. Burell, R., and Hill, J. O. (1975). The effect of respiratory immunization on cell-mediated immune effector cells in the lung. *Clin. Exp. Immunol.* **24**:116-124.
82. Nugent, K. M., Glazier, J., Monick, M. M., and Hunninghake, G. W. (1985). Stimulated human alveolar macrophages secrete interferon. *Am. Rev. Respir. Dis.* **131**:714-718.
83. Robinson, B. W., McLemore, T. L., and Crystal, R. G. (1985). Gamma interferon is spontaneously released by alveolar macrophages and lung T lymphocytes in patients with pulmonary sarcoidosis. *J. Clin. Invest.* **75**:1488-1495.
84. Moseley, P. L., Hemken, C., Monick, W., Nugent, K. M., and Hunninghake, G. W. (1986). Interferon and growth factor for human lung fibroblasts. Release from bronchoalveolar cells from patients with active sarcoidosis. *Chest* **89**:657-662.
85. Hancock, W. W., Kobzik, L., Colby, A. J., O'Hara, C. J., Cooper, A. G., and Godleski, J. J. (1986). Detection of lymphokines and lymphokine receptors in pulmonary sarcoidosis: Immunohistologic evidence that inflammatory macrophages express IL-2 receptors. *Am. J. Pathol.* **123**:1-8.
86. Hunninghake, G. W., Gadek, J. E., Young, R. C. Jr., Kawanami, O., Fenans, V. J., and Crystal, R. G. (1980). Maintenance of granuloma

formation in pulmonary sarcoidosis by T lymphocytes within the lung. *N. Engl. J. Med.* **302**:594-598.

87. Pinkston, P., Bitterman, P. B., and Crystal, R. G. (1983). Spontaneous release of interleukin-2 by lung T-lymphocytes in active pulmonary sarcoidosis. *N. Engl. J. Med.* **308**:793-800.

88. Hunninghake, G. W., Bedell, G. N., Zavala, D. C., Monick, M., and Brady, M. (1983). Role of interleukin-2 release by lung T cells in active pulmonary sarcoidosis. *Am. Rev. Respir. Dis.* **128**:634-638.

89. Nathan, C. F., Murray, H. W., Wiebe, M. E., and Rubin, B. Y. (1983). Identification of interferon-γ as the lymphokine that activates human macrophage oxidative metabolism and antimicrobial activity. *J. Exp. Med.* **158**:670-689.

90. Murray, H. W., Rubin, B. Y., and Rothermel, C. D. (1983). Killing of intracellular *Leishmania donovani* by lymphokine-stimulated mononuclear phagocytes. Evidence that interferon-γ is the activating lymphokine. *J. Clin. Invest.* **72**:1506-1510.

91. Rothermel, C. D., Rubin, B. Y., and Murray, H. W. (1983). γ-interferon is the factor in lymphokine that activates human macrophages to inhibit intracellular *Chlamydia psittaci* replication. *J. Immunol.* **131**:2542-2544.

92. Rubin, B. Y., Bartal, A. H., Anderson, S. L. Millet, S. K., Hirshaut, Y., and Feit, C. (1983). The anticellular and protein-inducing activities of human gamma interferon preparations are mediated by interferon. *J. Immunol.* **130**:1019-1020.

93. Murray, H. W., Gellene, R. A., Libby, D. M., Rothermel, C. D., and Rubin, B. Y. (1985). Activation of tissue macrophages from AIDS patients: In vitro response of AIDS alveolar macrophages to lymphokines and gamma-interferon. *J. Immunol.* **135**:2374-2377.

94. Black, C. M., Catterall, J. R., and Remington, J. S. (1987). In vivo and in vitro activation of alveolar macrophages by recombinant interferon-γ. *J. Immunol.* **138**:491-495.

95. Jensen, W. A., Rose, R. M., Wasserman, A. S., Kalb, T. H., Anton, K., and Remold, H. G. (1987). In vitro activation of the antibacterial activity of human pulmonary macrophages by recombinant gamma interferon. *J. Infect. Dis.* **155**:574-577.

96. Bhardwaj, N., Nash, T. W., and Horwitz, M. A. (1986). Interferon-γ-activated human monocytes inhibit the intracellular replication of *Legionella pneumophilia*. *J. Immunol.* **137**:2662-2669.

97. Douvas, G. S., Looker, D. L., Vatter, A. E., and Crowle, A. J. (1985). Gamma interferon activates human macrophages to become tumoricidal and leishmanicidal but enhances replication of macrophage-associated mycobacteria. *Infect. Immun.* **80**:1-8.

98. Chaparas, S. D. (1982). The immunology of mycobacterial infections. *CRC Crit. Rev. Microbiol.* **9:**139-197.
99. Edwards, C. K. III, Hedegaard, H. B., Zlotnik, A., Gangadharam, P. R.. Johnston, R. B. Jr., and Pabst, M. J. (1986). Chronic infection due to *Mycobacterium intracellulare* in mice: Association with macrophage release of prostaglandin and reversal by injection of indomethacin, muramyl dipeptide, or interferon-gamma. *J. Immunol.* **136:**1820-1827.
100. Clancy, R., Rawls, W. E., and Jagannath, S. (1977). Appearance of cytotoxic cells within the bronchus after local infection with herpes simplex virus. *J. Immunol.* **119:**1102-1105.
101. Wyde, P. R., and Cate, T. R. (1978). Cellular changes in lungs of mice infected with influenza virus: characterization of the cytotoxic responses. *Infect. Immun.* **22:**423-429.
102. Yap, K. L., Ada, G. L., and McKenzie, I. F. (1978). Transfer of specific cytotoxic T lymphocytes protects mice inoculated with influenza virus. *Nature* **273:**238-239.
103. Caldwell, J. L., and Kaltreider, H. B. (1980). Cytolytic activity of pulmonary and systematic lymphoid cells from C57B1/6 mice following intrapulmonary or intraperitoneal immunization with allogeneic tumor cells. *Exp. Lung Res.* **1:**99-110.
104. Emeson, E. E., Norin, A. J., and Veith, F. J. (1982). Antigen-induced recruitment of circulating lymphocytes to the lungs and hilar lymph nodes of mice challenged intratracheally with alloantigens. *Am. Rev. Respir. Dis.* **125:**453-459.
105. Liu, M. D., Ishizaka, K., and Plaut, J. J. (1982). T lymphocyte-responses of murine lung: Immunization with alloantigen induces accumulation of cytotoxic and other T lymphocytes in the lung. *J. Immunol.* **129:**2653-2661.
106. Stein-Streilein, J., Witte, P., Streilein, J. W., and Guffee, J. (1985). Local cellular defenses in influenza infected lungs. *Cell Immunol.* **95:**234-246.
107. Mann, D., Sonnenfield, G., and Stein-Streilein, J. (1985). Pulmonary compartmentalization of interferon and natural killer cell activity. *Proc. Soc. Exp. Biol. Med.* **180:**224-230.
108. Stein-Streilein, J., and Guffee, J. (1986). In vivo treatment of mice and hamsters with antibodies to Asialo GM1 increases morbidity and mortality to pulmonary influenza infection. *J. Immunol.* **136:**1475-1441.
109. Robinson, B. W. S., Pinkston, B., and Crystal, R. G. (1984). Natural killer cells are present in the normal lung but are functionally impotent. *J. Clin. Invest.* **74:**942-950.

110. Weissler, J. C., Nicod, L. P., Lipscomb, M. F., and Toews, G. B. (1987). Natural killer cell function in human lung is compartmentalized. *Am. Rev. Respir. Dis.* **135**:942-949.

111. Murphy, J. W., and McDaniel, D. O. (1982). In vitro activity of natural killer (NK) cells against *Cryptococcus neoformans. J. Immunol.* **128**:1577-1583.

112. Lipscomb, M. F., Alvarellos, T., Toews, G. B., et al. (1987). Role of natural killer cells in resistance to *Cryptococcus neoformans* infections in mice. *Am. J. Path.* **128**:354-361.

113. Wallaert, B., Aerts, C., Bort, F., et al. (1987). Alveolar macrophage dysfunction in systematic lupus erythematosis. *Am. Rev. Respir. Dis.* **136**:293-297.

114. Frank, M. M., Hamburger, P. I., Lawley, T. J., Kimberley, R. P., and Plotz, P. H. (1979). Defective reticuloendothelial system Fc receptor function in systematic lupus erythematosis. *N. Engl. J. Med.* **300**:518-523.

115. Katayama, S., Chia, D., Knutson, D. W., and Barnett, E. V. (1983). Decreased Fc receptor avidity and degradative function of monocytes from patients with systematic lupus erythematosis. *J. Immunol.* **131**:217-222.

116. Parris, T. M., Kimberly, R. P., Inman, R. D., McDougal, J. S., Gibofsky, A., and Christian, C. L. (1982). Defective Fc-mediated function of the mononuclear phagocyte system in lupus nephritis. *Ann. Intern. Med.* **97**:526-532.

117. Salmon, J. E., Kimberley, R. P., Gibofsky, A., and Fotino, M. (1984). Defective mononuclear phagocyte function in systematic lupus erythematosus: Dissociation of Fc receptor-ligand binding and internalization. *J. Immunol.* **133**:2525-2531.

118. Brandt, L., and Hedberg, H. (1969). Impaired phagocytosis by peripheral blood granulocytes in systematic lupus erythematosus. *Scand. J. Haematol.* **6**:348-353.

119. Clark, R. A., Kimball, H. R., and Decker, J. L. (1974). Neutrophil chemotaxis in systematic lupus erythematosus. *Ann. Rheum. Dis.* **33**:167-172.

120. Alvarez, I., Vazquez, J. J., Fontan, G., Gil, A., Barbado, J., and Ojeda, J. A. (1978). Neutrophil chemotaxis and serum chemotaxis activity in systematic lupus erythematosus. *Scand. J. Rheumatol.* **7**:69-74.

121. Al-Dadithy, H., Insenberg, D. A., Addison, I. E., Goldstone, A. H., and Snaith, M. L. (1982). *Ann. Rheum. Dis.* **41**:33-38.

122. Svensson, B., and Bedberg, H. (1973). Impaired phagocytosis by macrophages in SLE. *Scand. J. Rheumatol.* **2**:78-80.

123. Philips, R., Lomnitzer, R., Wadee, A. A., and Rabson, A. R. (1985). Defective monocyte function in patients with systematic lupus erythematosus. *Clin. Immunol. Immunopathol.* **34**:69-76.

124. Steinberg, A. D., Klassen, L. W., Budman, D. R., and Williams, G. W. (1979). Immunofluorescence studies of anti-T cell antibodies and T cells in systematic lupus erythematosis: Selective loss of brightly staining T cells in active disease. *Arthritis Rheum.* **22**:114-122.

125. Louie, J. S., Nies, K. M., Shoji, K. T., et al. (1978). Clinical and antibody responses after influenza immunization in systematic lupus erythematosis. *Ann. Intern. Med.* **88**:790-792.

126. Ristow, S. C., Douglas, R. C. Jr., and Condemi, J. J. (1978). Influenza vaccination of patients with systematic lupus erythematosus. *Ann. Intern. Med.* **88**:786-789.

127. Hahn, B. H., Bagby, M. K., and Osterland, C. K. (1973). Abnormalities of delayed hypersensitivity in systematic lupus erythematosus. *Am. J. Med.* **55**:25-31.

128. Rosenthal, C. J., and Franklin, E. C. (1975). Depression of cellular-mediated immunity in systematic lupus erythematosus. *Arthritis Rheum.* **18**:207-217.

129. Abe, T., and Homma, M. (1971). Immunological reactivity in patients with systematic lupus erythematosus. *Acta Rheum. Scand.* **17**:35-46.

130. Horwitz, D. A. (1972). Impaired delayed hypersensitivity in systematic lupus erythematosus. *Arthritis Rheum.* **15**:353-359.

131. Sakane, T., Steinberg, A. D., and Green, I. (1978). Failure of autologous mixed lymphocyte reactions between T and non-T cells in patients with systematic lupus erythematosus. *Proc. Natl. Acad. Sci. USA* **75**:3464-3468.

132. Strannegard, O., Hermodsson, S., and Westberg, G. (1982). Interferon and natural killer cells in systematic lupus erythematosus. *Clin. Exp. Immunol.* **50**:246-252.

133. Walker, W. C. (1967). Pulmonary infections and rheumatoid arthritis. *Q. J. Med.* **36**:239-251.

134. Monson, R. R., and Hall, A. P. (1976). Mortality among arthritics. **29**:459-467.

135. Bamji, A., and Cooke, N. (1985). Rheumatoid arthritis and chronic bronchial suppuration. *Scand. J. Rheumatol.* **14**:15-21.

136. Mitchell, D. M., Spitz, P. W., Young, D. Y., Bloch, D. A., McShane, D. J., and Fries, J. F. (1986). Survival, prognosis, and causes of death in rheumatoid arthritis. *Arthritis Rheum.* **29**:706-714.

137. Hallgren, R., Hukansson, L., and Venge, P. (1978). Kinetic studies of phagocytosis. I. The serum independent particle uptake by PMN from patients with rheumatoid arthritis and SLE. *Arthritis Rheum.* **21**:107-113.

138. Corberand, J., Amigues, H., deLarrard, B., and Pradere, J. (1977). Neutrophil functions in rheumatoid arthritis. *Scand. J. Rheumatol.* **6**:49-52.
139. Mowat, A. G., and Baum, J. (1971). Chemotaxis of polymorphonuclear leukocytes from patients with rheumatoid arthritis. *J. Clin. Invest.* **50**:2541-2549.
140. Turner, R. A., Schumacher, H. R., and Myers, A. R. (1973). Phagocytic function of polymorphonuclear leukocytes in rheumatic diseases. *J. Clin. Invest.* **52**:1632-1635.
141. Mellbye, O. J., Messner, R. P., DeBord, J. R., and Williams, R. C. (1972). Immunoglobulin and receptors for C3 on lymphocytes from patients with rheumatoid arthritis. *Arthritis Rheum.* **15**:371-380.
142. Papamichael, M., Brown, J. C., and Holborow, E. J. (1971). Immunoglobulins on the surface of human lymphocytes. *Lancet* **2**:850-852.
143. Micheli, A., and Bron, J. (1974). Studies on blood T and B lymphocytes in rheumatoid arthritis. *Ann. Rheum. Dis.* **33**:435-436.
144. Yu, D. T., Winchester, R. J., Fu, S. M., Gibofsky, A., Ko, H. S., and Kunkel, H. G. (1980). Peripheral blood Ia-positive T cells, increases in certain diseases and after immunization. *J. Exp. Med.* **151**:91-100.
145. Carter, S. D., Bacon, P. A., and Hall, N. D. (1981). Characterization of activated lymphocytes in the peripheral blood of patients with rheumatoid arthritis. *Ann. Rheum. Dis.* **40**:293-298.
146. Cupps, T. R., and Fauci, A. S. (1982). Corticosteroid-mediated immunoregulation in man. *Immunol. Rev.* **65**:133-155.
147. Parrillo, J. E., and Fauci, A. S. (1979). Mechanisms of glucocorticoid action on immune processes. *Ann. Rev. Pharmacol. Toxicol.* **19**:179-201.
148. MacGregor, R. R. (1977). Granulocyte adherence changes induced by hemodialysis, endotoxin, epinephrine, and glucocorticoids. *Ann. Intern. Med.* **86**:35-39.
149. Cummings, M. M., and Hudgins, P. C. (1952). The influence of cortisone on the passive transfer of tuberculin hypersensitivity in the guinea pig. *J. Immunol.* **69**:331-335.
150. Weston, W. L., Mandel, M. J., Yeckley, J. A., Krueger, G. G., and Claman, H. N. (1973). Mechanism of cortisol inhibition of adoptive transfer of tuberculin sensitivity. *J. Lab. Clin. Med.* **82**:366-371.
151. Balow, J. E., and Rosenthal, A. S. (1973). Glucocorticoid suppression of macrophage migration inhibitory factor. *J. Exp. Med.* **137**:1031-1041.
152. Rinehart, J. J., Balcerzak, S. P., Sagone, A. L., and LoBuglio, A. F. (1974). Effects of corticosteroids on human monocyte function. *J. Clin. Invest.* **54**:1337-1343.

153. Rinehart, J. J., Sagone, A. L., Balcerzak, S. P., Ackerman, G. A., and LoBuglio, A. F. (1975). Effects of corticosteroid therapy on human monocyte function. *N. Engl. J. Med.* **292**:236-241.
154. Makinodan, T., Santos, G. W., and Quinn, R. P. (1970). Immunosuppressive durgs. *Pharmacol. Rev.* **22**:189-247.
155. Shand, F. L. (1979). The immunopharmacology of cyclophosphamide. *Int. J. Pharmacol.* **1**:165-171.
156. Cupps, T. R., Edgar, L. C., and Fauci, A. S. (1982). Suppression of human B lymphocyte function by cyclophosphamide. *J. Immunol.* **128**:2453-2457.
157. Berenbaum, M. C., and Brown, I. N. (1964). Dose-response relationships for agents inhibiting the immune response. *Immunology* **7**:65-71.
158. Askenase, P. W., Hayden, B. J., and Gershon, R. K. (1975). Augmentation of delayed type hypersensitivity of doses of cyclophosphamide which do not effect antibody responses. *J. Exp. Med.* **141**:697-702.
159. Sy, M. S., Miller, S. D., and Claman, H. N. (1977). Immune suppression with supraoptimal doses of antigen in contact sensitivity. I. Demonstration of suppressor cells and their sensitivity to cyclophosphamide. *J. Immunol.* **119**:240-244.
160. Schein, P. S., and Winokur, S. T. (1975). Immunosuppressive and cytotoxic chemotherapy: Long-term complications. *Ann. Intern. Med.* **82**:84-95.
161. Yu, D. T., Clements, P. J., Peter, J. B., Levy, J., Paulus, H. E., and Barnett, E. V. (1974). Lymphocyte characteristics in rheumatic patients and the effect of azathioprine therapy. *Arthritis Rheum.* **17**:37-45.
162. Levy, J., Barnett, E. V., MacDonald, N. S., Klinenberg, J. R., and Pearson, C. M. (1972). The effect of azathioprine on gammaglobulin synthesis in man. *J. Clin. Invest.* **51**:2233-2238.
163. Maibach, H. I., and Epstein, W. L. (1965). Immunologic responses of healthy volunteers receiving azathioprine (Imuran). *Int. Arch. Allergy* **27**:102-109.
164. Sharbaugh, R. J., Ainsworth, S. K., and Fitts, C. T. (1976). Lack of effect of azathioprine on phytohemagglutinin-induced lymphocyte transformation and established delayed cutaneous hypersensitivity. *Int. Arch. Allergy Appl. Immunol.* **51**:681-686.
165. Gassman, A. E., and Van Furth, R. (1975). The effect of azathioprine (Imuran) on the kinetics of monocytes and macrophages during the normal steady state and an acute inflammatory reaction. *Blood* **46**: 51-64.
166. Phillips, S. M., and Zweiman, B. (1973). Mechanisms in the suppression of delayed hypersensitivity in the guinea pig by 6-mercaptopurine. *J. Exp. Med.* **137**:1494-1510.

167. Mitchell, M. S., Wade, M. E., DeConti, R. C., Bertino, J. R., and
      Calabresi, P. (1969). Immunosuppressive effects of cytosine arabin-
      oside and methotrexate in man. *Ann. Intern. Med.* **70**:535-547.
168. Gabrielsen, A. E., and Good, R. A. (1967). Chemical suppression of
      adaptive immunity. *Adv. Immunol.* **6**:91-229.
169. Pennington, J. E. (1977). Bronchoalveolar cell response to bacterial chal-
      lenge in the immunosuppressed lung. *Am. Rev. Respir. Dis.* **116**:885-893.
170. Pennington, J. E. (1977). Quantitative effects of immunosuppres-
      sion on bronchoalveolar cells. *J. Infect. Dis.* **136**:127-131.
171. Pennington, J. E., and Harris, E. A. (1981). Influence of immuno-
      suppression on alveolar macrophage chemotactic activities in guinea
      pigs. *Am. Rev. Respir. Dis.* **123**:299-304.
172. Pennington, J. E., Matthews, W. J. Jr., Marino, J. T., and Colten,
      H. R. (1979). Cyclophosphamide and cortisone acetate inhibit com-
      plement biosynthesis by guinea pig bronchoalveolar macrophages. *J.
      Immunol.* **123**:1318-1321.
173. Hellman, D. B., Petri, M., and Whiting-O'Keefe, Q. (1987). Fatal
      infections in systemic lupus erythematosis: The role of opportunis-
      tic organisms. *Medicine* **66**:341-348.
174. Staples, P., Gerding, D., Decker, J., and Gordon, R. Jr. (1974). In-
      cidence of infection in systemic lupus erythematosus. *Arthritis Rheum.*
      17:1-10.
174a. Nived, O., Sturfelt, G., and Wollheim, F. (1985). Systematic lupus
      erythematosus and infection: A controlled and prospective study in-
      cluding an epidemiological group. *Q. J. Med.* **55**:271-287.
174b. Ginzler, E., Diamond, H., Kaplan, D., Weiner, M., Schlesinger,
      M., and Seleznick, M. (1978). Computer analysis of factors influenc-
      ing frequency of infection in systemic lupus erythematosus. *Arthritis
      Rheum.* **21**:37-44.
174c. Perez, H., Andron, R., and Goldstein, I. (1979). Infections in pa-
      tients with systemic lupus erythematosus. *Arthritis Rheum.* **22**:1326-
      1333.
174d. Rosner, S., Ginzler, E., Diamond, H., et al. (1982). A multicenter
      study of outcome in systemic lupus erythematosus. II. Causes of death.
      Arthritis Rheum. **25**:612-617.
175. Johanson, W. G., Pierce, A. K., and Sanford, J. P. (1969). Chang-
      ing pharyngeal bacterial flora of hospitalized patients. *N. Engl. J.
      Med.* **281**:137-140.
176. Woods, D. E., Straus, D. C., Johanson, W. G., and Bass, J. A. (1983).
      Factors influencing the adherence of *Pseudomonas aeruginosa* to
      mammalian buccal epithelial cells. *Rev. Infect. Dis.* **5**(Suppl.):846-851.

177. Toews, G. B. (1987). Nosocomial pneumonia. *Clin. Chest Med.* **8:** 467-479.
178. Pennington, J. E. (1986). Gram negative bacterial pneumonia in the immunocompromised host. *Semin. Respir. Infect.* **1(3):**145-150.
179. Valdivieso, M., Gil-Extremera, B., Zornoza, J., Rodriguez, V., and Bodees, G. P. (1977). Gram negative bacillary pneumonia in the compromised host. *Medicine* **56:**241-254.
180. Musher, D. M., and McKenzie, S. O. (1977). Infections due to *Staphylococcus aureus*. *Medicine* **56:**383-409.
181. Davis, G. S., and Winn, W. C. (1987). Legionnaire's disease: Respiratory infections caused by *Legionella* bacteria. *Clin. Chest Med.* **8:**419-439.
182. Dowling, J. N., Pasculle, A. W., Frola, F. N., Zaphyr, M. K., and Yee, R. B. (1983). Infection caused by *Legionella micdadei* and *Legionella pneumophilia* among renal transplant recipients. *J. Infect. Dis.* **149:**703-713.
183. Marshall, W., Foster, R. S., and Winn, W. (1981). Legionnaire's disease in renal transplant patients. *Am. J. Med.* **141:**423-427.
184. Gump, D. W., and Keegan, M. (1986). Pulmonary infections due to *Legionella* in immunocompromised patients. *Semin. Respir. Infect.* **1(3):**151-159.
185. Muder, R. R., Yu, V. L., and Zuravleff, J. J. (1983). Pneumonia due to the Pittsburgh pneumonia agent: New clinical perspective with a review of the literature. *Medicine* **62:**120-128.
186. Saravolatz, L. D., Burch, K. H., Fisher, E., et al. (1979). The compromised host and legionnaire's disease. *Ann. Intern. Med.* **90:**533-537.
187. Fang, G., Yu, V. L., and Vickers, R. M. (1987). Infections caused by the Pittsburgh pneumonia agent. *Semin. Respir. Infect.* **2(4):**262-266.
188. Goldstein, J. D., Keller, J. L., Winn, W. C. Jr., and Myerowitz, R. L. (1982). Sporadic Legionellaceae pneumonia in renal transplant recipients. *Arch. Pathol. Lab. Med.* **106:**108-111.
189. Yu, V. L., Kroboth, F. J., Shonnard, J., Brown, A., McDearman, S., and Magnussen, M. (1982). Legionnare's disease: New clinical perspective from a prospective pneumonia study. *Am. J. Med.* **73:**357-361.
190. Fisher, B. D., Armstrong, D., Yu, B., and Gold, J. W. (1981). Invasive aspergillosis: Progress in early diagnosis and treatment. *Am. J. Med.* **71:**571-577.
191. Pennington, J. E. (1980). Aspergillus lung disease. *Med. Clin. North Am.* **64:**475-488.
192. Young, R. C., Bennett, J. E., Vogel, C. L., Carbone, P. P., and Devita, V. T. (1970). Aspergillosis: The spectrum of disease in 98 patients. *Medicine* **49:**147-173.

193. Cairns, M. R., and Durack, D. T. (1986). Fungal pneumonia in the immunocompromised host. *Semin. Respir. Infect.* **1(3)**:166-185.
194. Rinaldi, M. G. (1983). Invasive aspergillosis. *Rev. Infect. Dis.* **5**:1061-1077.
195. Gerson, S. L., Talbot, G. H., Hurwitz, S., Strong, B. L., Lusk, E. J., and Cassileth, P. A. (1984). Prolonged granulocytopenia: The major risk factor for invasive pulmonary aspergillosis in patients with leukemia. *Ann. Intern. Med.* **100**:345-351.
196. Gustafson, T., Schaffner, W., Lavely, G. B., Stratton, C. W., Johnson, H. K., and Hutcheson, R. H. Jr. (1983). Invasive aspergillosis in renal transplant recipients: Correlation with corticosteroid therapy. *J. Infect. Dis.* **148**:230-238.
197. Meyer, R. D., Young, L. S., Armstrong, D., and Yu, B. (1973). Aspergillosis complicating neoplastic disease. *Am. J. Med.* **54**:6-15.
198. Aisner, J., Schimpff, S. C., and Wiernik, P. H. (1977). Treatment of invasive aspergillosis: Relation of early diagnosis and treatment to response. *Ann. Intern. Med.* **86**:539-543.
199. Sinclair, A. J., Rossof, A. H., and Coltman, C. A. Jr. (1978). Recognition and successful management in pulmonary aspergillosis in leukemia. *Cancer* **42**:2019-2024.
200. Albelda, S. M., Talbot, G. H., Gerson, S. L., Miller, W. T., and Cassileth, P. A. (1984). Role of fiberoptic bronchoscopy in the diagnosis of invasive pulmonary aspergillosis in patients with acute leukemia. *Am. J. Med.* **76**:1027-1034.
201. Hiatt, J. R., Gong. H., Mulder, D. G., and Ramming, K. P. (1982). The value of open lung biopsy in the immunocompromised patient. *Surgery* **92**:285-291.
202. McCabe, R. E., Brooks, R. G., Mark, J. B., and Remington, J. S. (1985). Open lung biopsy in patients with acute leukemia. *Am. J. Med.* **78**:609-616.
203. Lehrer, R. I. (1980). Mucormycosis. *Ann. Intern. Med.* **93**:93-108.
204. Meyer, R. D., Rosen, P., and Armstrong, D. (1972). Phycomycosis complicating leukemia and lymphoma. *Ann. Intern. Med.* **77**:871-879.
205. Dismukes, W. E., Royal, S. A., and Tynes, B. S. (1978). Disseminated histoplasmosis in corticosteroid-treated patients. Report of five cases. *J.A.M.A.* **240**:1495-1498.
206. Kauffman, C. A., Israel, K. S., Smith, J. W., White, A. C., Schwarz, J., and Brooks, G. F. (1978). Histoplasmosis in immunosuppressed patients. *Am. J. Med.* **64**:923-932.
207. Davies, S. F., Sarosi, G. A., Peterson, P. K., et al. (1979). Disseminated histoplasmosis in renal transplant recipients. *Am. J. Surg.* **137**:686-691.

208. Deresinski, S. C., and Stevens, D. A. (1974). Coccidiomycosis in compromised hosts. *Medicine* **54**:377-395.
209. Wallace, J. M., Catanzaro, A., Moser, K. M., and Harrell, J. H. (1981). Flexible fiberoptic bronchoscopy for diagnosing pulmonary coccidioidomycosis. *Am. Rev. Respir. Dis.* **123**:286-290.
210. Brass, C., Galgiani, J. N., Campbell, S. C., and Stevens, D. A. (1980). Therapy of disseminated or pulmonary coccidioidomycosis with ketoconazole. *Rev. Infect. Dis.* **2(4)**:656-660.
211. Bayer, A. S. (1981). Fungal pneumonias: Pulmonary coccidioidal syndromes. *Chest* **79**:686-691.
212. Kaplan, M. H., Rosen, P. P., and Armstrong, D. (1977). Cryptococcosis in a cancer hospital. *Cancer* **39**:2265-2274.
213. Kerkering, T. M., Duma, R. J., and Shadomy, S. (1981). The evolution of pulmonary cryptococcosis. *Ann. Intern. Med.* **94**:611-616.
214. Perfect, J. R., Durack, D. T., and Gallis, H. A. (1983). Cryptococcemia. *Medicine* **62**:98-109.
215. Bennett, J. E., Dismukes, W. E., Duma, R. J., et al. (1979). A comparison of amphotericin B alone and combined with flucytosine in the treatment of cryptococcal meningitis. *N. Engl. J. Med.* **301**:126-131.
216. Dismukes, W. E., Cloud, G., Gallis, H. A., et al. (1987). Treatment of cryptococcal meningitis with combination amphotericin B and flucytosine for four as compared with six weeks. *N. Engl. J. Med.* **317**: 334-341.
217. Palmer, D. L., Harvey, R. L., and Wheeler, J. D. (1974). Diagnostic and therapeutic considerations in *Nocardia asteroides* infection. *Medicine* **53**:391-401.
218. Simpson, G. L., Stinson, E. G., Egger, M. J., and Remington, J. S. (1981). Nocardial infections in the immunocompromised host: A detailed study in a defined population. *Rev. Infect. Dis.* **3**:492-507.
219. Gorevic, P. D., Katler, E. I., and Agus, B. (1980). Pulmonary nocardiosis: Occurrence in men with systemic lupus erythematosus. *Arch. Intern. Med.* **140**:361-363.
220. Santen, R. J., and Wright, I. S. (1967). Systemic lupus erythematosis associated with pulmonary nocardiosis. *Arch. Intern. Med.* **119**:202-205.
221. Dubois, E. L. (1974). *Lupus Erythematosus: A Review of the Current Status of Discoid and Systemic Lupus Erythematosus*, 2d ed. University of Southern California Press, Los Angeles.
222. Ramsey, P. G., Rubin, R. H., Tolkoff-Rubin, N. E., Cosimi, A. B., Russell, P. S., and Greene, R. (1980). The renal transplant patient with fever and pulmonary infiltrates: Etiology, clinical manifestations, and management. *Medicine* **59**:206-222.

223. Young, L. S., Armstrong, D., Blevins, A., and Lieberman, P. (1971). *Nocardia asteroides* infection complicating neoplastic disease. *Am. J. Med.* **50**:357-367.

224. Maderazo, E. G., and Quintiliani, R. (1974). Treatment of nocardial infection with trimethoprim and sulfamethoxazole. *Am. J. Med.* **57**: 671-675.

225. Mammana, R. B., Petersen, E. A., Fuller, J. K., Siroky, K., and Copeland, J. G. (1983). Pulmonary infections in cardiac transplant patients: Modes of diagnosis, complications, and effectiveness of therapy. *Ann. Thorac. Surg.* **36**:700-705.

226. Cheson, B. D., Samlowski, W. E., Tang, T., and Spruance, S. L. (1985). Value of open lung biopsy in 87 immunocompromised patients with pulmonary infiltrates. *Cancer* **55**:453-459.

227. Gold, J. W. M. (1986). Mycobacterial infection in immunosuppressed patients. *Semin. Respir. Infect.* **1(3)**:160-165.

228. Dummer, J. S., Hardy, A., Poorsattar, A., and Ho, M. (1983). Early infections in kidney, heart, and liver transplant recipients on cyclosporin. *Transplantation* **36**:259-267.

229. Peterson, P. K., Ferguson, R., Fryd, D. S., Balfour, H. H. Jr., Rynasiewicz, J., and Simmons, R. L. (1982). Infectious diseases in hospitalized renal transplant recipients: A prospective study of a complex and evolving problem. *Medicine* **61**:360-372.

230. Feng, P., and Tan, T. (1982). Tuberculosis in patients with systemic lupus erythematosus. *Ann. Rheum. Dis.* **41**:11-14.

231. Sahn, S. A., and Lakshminarayan, S. (1976). Tuberculosis after corticosteroid therapy. *Br. J. Chest Dis.* **70**:195-205.

232. Kaplan, M. H., Armstrong, D., and Rosen, P. (1974). Tuberculosis complicating neoplastic disease. *Cancer* **33**:850-858.

233. Lloveras, J., Peterson, P. K., Simmons, R. L., and Najarian, J. S. (1982). Mycobacterial infections in renal transplant recipients. *Arch. Intern. Med.* **142**:888-892.

234. Stover, D. E., Zaman, M. B., Hajdu, S. I., Lange, M., Gold, J., and Armstrong, D. (1984). Bronchoalveolar lavage in the diagnosis of diffuse pulmonary infiltrates in the immunosuppressed host. *Ann. Intern. Med.* **101**:1-7.

235. Stover, D. E., White, D. A., Romano, P. A., and Gellene, R. A. (1985). Diagnosis of pulmonary disease in acquired immune deficiency syndrome (AIDS). Role of bronchoscopy and bronchoalveolar lavage. *Am. Rev. Respir. Dis.* **130**:659-662.

236. Cockerill, F. R. III, Wilson, W. R., Carpenter, H. A., Smith, T. F., and Rosenow, E. C. III (1985). Open lung biopsy in immunocompromised patients. *Arch. Intern. Med.* **145**:1398-1404.

237. Rossiter, S. J., Miller, D. C., Churg, A. M., Carrington, C. B., and Mark, J. B. (1979). Open lung biopsy in the immunosuppressed patient. Is it really beneficial? *J. Thorac. Cardiovasc. Surg.* **77**:338-345.
238. Kovacs, J. A., Hiemenz, J. W., Macher, A. M., et al. (1984). *Pneumocystis carinii* pneumonia: A comparison between patients with the acquired immunodeficiency syndrome and patients with other immunodeficiencies. *Ann. Intern. Med.* **100**:663-671.
239. Young, L. S. (1982). Treatment of *Pneumocystis carinii* pneumonia in adults with trimethoprim/sulfamethoxazole. *Rev. Infect. Dis.* **4**:608-613.
240. Rosen, P., Armstrong, D., and Ramos, C. (1972). *Pneumocystis carinii* pneumonia. A clinicopathologic study of twenty patients with neoplastic diseases. *Am. J. Med.* **53**:428-436.
241. Walzer, P. D., Perl, D. P., Krogstad, D. J., Rawson, P. G., and Schultz, M. G. (1974). *Pneumocystis carinii* pneumonia in the United States: Epidemiologic, clinical and diagnostic features. *Ann. Intern. Med.* **80**:83-93.
242. Young, L. S. (1986). Protozoal infections in the lungs of immunosuppressed patients. *Semin. Respir. Infect.* **1(3)**:186-192.
243. Shanley, J. D., and Jordan, M. C. (1986). Viral pneumonia in the immunocompromised patient. *Semin. Respir. Infect.* **1(3)**:193-201.
244. Feldman, S., and Stokes, D. C. (1987). Varicella zoster and herpes simplex virus pneumonias. *Semin. Respir. Infect.* **2(2)**:84-94.
245. Klotman, M. E., and Hamilton, J. D. (1987). Cytomegalovirus pneumonia. *Semin. Respir. Infect.* **2(2)**:95-103.
246. Nunan, T. O., King, M., Bull, P., Banatvala, J. E., Jones, N. F., and Hilton, P. J. (1984). Parenteral acyclovir therapy for cytomegalovirus infection after renal transplantation. *Clin. Nephrol.* **22**:28-31.
247. Wade, J. C., McGuffin, R. W., Springmeyer, S. C., Newton, B., Singer, J. W., and Meyers, J. D. (1983). Treatment of cytomegaloviral pneumonia with high dose acyclovir and human leukocyte interferon. *J. Infect. Dis.* **148**:557-562.
248. Masur, H., Lane, H. C., Palestine, A., et al. (1986). Effect of 9-(2-hydroxy-2-propoxymethyl) guanine on serious cytomegalovirus disease in eight immunosuppressed homosexual men. *Ann. Intern. Med.* **104**:41-44.
249. Dummer, J. S., White, L. T., Ho, M., Griffith, B. P., Hardesty, R. L., and Bahnson, H. T. (1985). Morbidity of cytomegalovirus infection in recipients of heart or heart-lung transplants who received cyclosporine. *J. Infect. Dis.* **152**:1182-1191.
250. Hackman, R. C., Myerson, D., Meyers, J. D., et al. (1985). Rapid diagnosis of cytomegaloviral pneumonia by tissue immunofluorescence with a murine monoclonal antibody. *J. Infect. Dis.* **151**:325-329.

251. Meyers, J. D., Reed, E. C., Shepp, D. H., et al. (1988). Acyclovir for prevention of cytomegalovirus infection and disease after allogenic marrow transplantation. *N. Engl. J. Med.* **318**:70-75.
252. Peterson, P. K., Balfour, H. H. Jr., Marker, S. C., Fryd, D. S., Howard, R. J., and Simmons, R. L. (1980). Cytomegalovirus disease in renal allograft recipients: A prospective study of the clinical features, risk factors, and impact on renal transplantation. *Medicine* **59**:283-300.
253. Beschorner, W. E., Hutchins, G. M., Burns, W. H., Saral, R., Tutschka, P. J., and Santos, G. W. (1980). Cytomegalovirus pneumonia in bone marrow transplant recipients: Miliary and diffuse patterns. *Am. Rev. Respir. Dis.* **122**:107-114.
254. Straus, S. E., Ostrove, J. M., Inschauspe, G., et al. (1988). Varicella-zoster virus infections. Biology, natural history, treatment, and prevention. *Ann. Intern. Med.* **108**:221-237.
255. Shulman, H. M., Hackman, R. C., Sale, G. E., and Meyers, J. D. (1982). Rapid cytologic diagnosis of cytomegalovirus interstitial pneumonia on touch imprints from open-lung biopsy. *Am. J. Clin. Pathol.* **77**:90-94.
256. Emanuel, D., Peppard, J., Stover, D., Gold, J., Armstrong, D., and Hammerling, U. (1986). Rapid immunodiagnosis of cytomegalovirus pneumonia by bronchoalveolar lavage using human and murine monoclonal antibodies. *Ann. Intern. Med.* **104**:476-481.
257. Myerson, D., Hackman, R. C., and Meyers, J. D. (1984). Diagnosis of cytomegaloviral pneumonia by in situ hybridization. *J. Infect. Dis.* **150**:272-277.
258. Hirsch, M. S., and Schooley, R. T. (1983). Treatment of herpes virus infections. *N. Engl. J. Med.* **309**:1033-1039.
259. Dorsky, D. I., and Crumpacker, C. S. (1987). Drug five years later: Acyclovir. *Ann. Intern. Med.* **107**:859-874.
260. Wade, J. C., Hintz, M., McGuffin, R. W., Springmeyer, S. C., Connor, J. D., and Meyers, J. D. (1982). Treatment of cytomegalovirus pneumonia with high dose acyclovir. *Am. J. Med.* **73**(Suppl. 1a):249-256.
261. Whitley, R. (1988). Ganclicovir—Have we established clinical value in the treatment of cytomegalovirus infections? *Ann. Intern. Med.* **108**: 452-454.
262. Shepp, D. H., Dandliker, P. S., de Miranda, P., et al. (1985). Activity of 9-(2-hydroxy-1-(hydroxymethyl)-ethoxymethyl) guanine in the treatment of cytomegalovirus pneumonia. *Ann. Intern. Med.* **103**:368-373.

263. Jacobson, M. A., and Mills, J. (1988). Serious cytomegalovirus disease in the acquired immunodeficiency syndrome (AIDS). Clinical findings, diagnosis, and treatment. *Ann. Intern. Med.* **108**:585-594.
264. Ringden, O., Lonnquist, B., Paulin, T., et al. (1986). Normal metabolism, safety and preliminary clinical experiences using foscarnet in the treatment of cytomegalovirus infections in bone marrow and renal transplant recipients. *Antimicrob. Chemother.* **17**:373-387.
265. Rand, K. H., Rasmussen, L. E., Pollard, R. B., Arvin, M., and Merigan, T. C. (1977). Cellular immunity and herpes virus infections in cardiac-transplant patients. *N. Engl. J. Med.* **296**:1372-1377.
266. Graham, B. S., and Snell, J. D. (1983). Herpes simplex virus infection of the adult lower respiratory tract. *Medicine* **62**:384-393.
267. Ramsey, P. G., Fife, K. H., Hackman, R. C., Meyers, J. D., and Corey, L. (1982). Herpes simplex virus pneumonia. Clinical virologic, and pathologic features in 20 patients. *Ann. Intern. Med.* **97**:813-820.
268. Mitchell, C. D., Bean, B., Gentry, S. R., Grothe, K. E., Boen, J. R., and Balfour, H. H. Jr. (1981). Acyclovir therapy for mucocutaneous Herpes simplex infections in immunocompromised patients. *Lancet* **1**:1389-1392.
269. Balfour, H. H. Jr., Bean, B., Laskin, O. L., et al. (1983). Acyclovir halts progression of herpes zoster in immunocompromised patients. *N. Engl. J. Med.* **308**:1448-1453.
270. Springmeyer, S. C., Silvestri, R. C., Sale, G. E., et al. (1982). The role of transbronchial biopsy for the diagnosis of diffuse pneumonias in immunocompromised marrow transplant recipients. *Am. Rev. Respir. Dis.* **126**:763-765.
271. Tenholder, M. F., and Hooper, R. G. (1980). Pulmonary infiltrates in leukemia. *Chest* **78**:468-473.
272. Toledo-Pereyra, L. H., DeMeester, T. R., Kinealey, L., MacMahon, H., Churg, A., and Golomb, H. (1980). The benefits of open lung biopsy in patients with previously non-diagnostic transbronchial lung biopsy. *Chest* **77**:647-650.
273. Cordonnier, C., Bernaudin, J., Fleury, J., et al. (1985). Diagnostic yield of bronchoalveolar lavage in pneumonitis occurring after allogeneic bone marrow transplantation. *Am. Rev. Respir. Dis.* **132**:1118-1123.
274. Young, J. A., Hopkin, J. M., and Cuthbertson, W. R. (1984). Pulmonary infiltrates in immunocompromised patients: Diagnosis by cytological examination of bronchoalveolar lavage fluid. *J. Clin. Pathol.* **37**:390-397.
275. Nishio, J. N., and Lynch, J. P. III (1980). Fiberoptic bronchoscopy in the immunocompromised host: Significance of a nonspecific transbronchial biopsy. *Am. Rev. Respir. Dis.* **121**:307-312.

276. Wimberley, N., Foling, L. J., and Bartlett, J. (1979). A fiberoptic bronchoscopy technique to obtain uncontaminated lower airway secretions for bacterial culture. *Am. Rev. Respir. Dis.* **119**:337-343.
277. Poe, R. H., Utell, M. J., Israel, R. H., Hall, W. J., and Eshleman, J. D. (1979). Sensitivity and specificity of the nonspecific transbronchial lung biopsy. *Am. Rev. Respir. Dis.* **119**:25-31.

Part III

**PULMONARY INVOLVEMENT WITH
RHEUMATIC DISEASES**

8

Rheumatoid Arthritis

DUNCAN A. GORDON

University of Toronto and
Toronto Western Hospital
Toronto, Ontario, Canada

ROBERT H. HYLAND

University of Toronto and
Wellesley Hospital
Toronto, Ontario, Canada

IRVIN BRODER

University of Toronto
Gage Research Institute and
Toronto Western Hospital
Toronto, Ontario, Canada

I. Introduction

Pulmonary involvement in rheumatoid arthritis (RA) was first recognized by Ellman and Ball in 1948 (1). As the systemic nature of RA was further explored, lung disorders were recognized as a characteristic and common component of this disease. The pulmonary manifestations in RA include pleuritis, pleural effusion, nodules, pneumonitis, interstitial fibrosis, airway obstruction, and vasculitis (2-5) (Table 1). These abnormalities will be referred to as primary pulmonary manifestations of RA because they are felt to be the result of the systemic inflammation of RA and to be inherent to the disease. Our present understanding of the pathophysiology for the development of parenchymal lung and pleural manifestations is presented in Chapters 1 and 2, respectively. In this chapter, the different clinical components of the primary pulmonary manifestations of RA are discussed, the potential risk factors for these complications are reviewed, and the clinical evaluation of pulmonary disease in the RA patient is outlined.

In addition to the primary pulmonary manifestations of RA, environmental exposures, infectious agents, and antirheumatic drug reactions may

Table 1 Pulmonary Manifestations of Rheumatoid Arthritis

Primary disorders
  Pleuritis
  Pleural effusion
  Nodules
  Pneumonitis/interstitial fibrosis
  Airway obstruction
  Vasculitis
Secondary disorders
  Rheumatoid pneumoconiosis (Caplan's syndrome)
  Pulmonary reactions to antirheumatic drugs
  Pulmonary infection

be associated with the development of pulmonary disease in RA patients (2, 6-12). These complications will be referred to as secondary pulmonary diseases (Table 1). An association of coal dust exposure and the development of pulmonary nodules in coal miners affected by RA has long been recognized as Caplan's syndrome (13). Rheumatoid pneumoconiosis (Caplan's syndrome) is the only secondary pulmonary manifestation discussed in this chapter. The effects of rheumatic disorders on host defense mechanisms that resist contagious disease and the infectious agents that require particular attention in RA patients are reviewed in Chapter 7. The pulmonary complications of antirheumatic drug therapy are reviewed in Chapter 14.

II. Clinical Manifestations of Pulmonary Disease in Rheumatoid Arthritis

A. Pleuritis and Pleural Effusion

Pleural involvement may be the most common pulmonary manifestation in RA patients, although the exact incidence is unknown. The variation in reported frequency of pleural disease is in part the result of differences in the diagnostic (clinical, radiographic, or pathologic) criteria used in these studies. Studies of clinical pleuritic symptoms have given variable results. In one controlled series, 21% of 516 patients had pleurisy sometime during their disease, whereas only 12% of a control group of 301 patients with degenerative joint disease showed pleurisy (14). Moreover, in our series pleuritic symptoms were reported in 11% of 155 RA patients, which was no different from our control population (5). A changing severity of extraarticular disease in RA patients with time (15) has been suggested as an explanation for the changing prevalence of pleural disease in RA patients reported in these temporally separated studies. Radiographic studies have noted pleural effusions in 5% of patients (16,17). Autopsy series have noted pleural abnormalities in 38-73% patients with RA (18,19). These data demonstrate that pleural disease is common in patients with RA but suggest that the pathologic evidence of pleural involvement in RA may be more common than the clinical and radiographic manifestations of this complication.

The clinical manifestations of pleural involvement are pleuritis, pleural friction rub, and effusion on chest radiographs, although it should be recognized that many patients with pleural disease will have normal X-rays. Although a diagnosis of RA is established in most patients before the onset of pleuritis, pleuritic chest pain may herald the onset of RA (16). A fever may be seen with the acute onset of pleurisy in RA patients (20). The radiographic manifestations of pleuritis and pleural effusions are described in Chapter 4. The effusions may be unilateral or bilateral and commonly loculated (2,21-23). Patients with pleuritis will rarely have underlying parenchymal lung disease on X-ray (23).

Pleural effusions in RA patients are most frequently exudates and in some instances may have characteristics mimicking an empyema (24). The characteristics and suspected pathophysiology of these effusions are fully described in Chapter 2. The fluid is usually cloudy in appearance. A milky appearance may be seen in long-standing pleural effusions because of cholesterol crystals (16) or because of true chylous effusions (25). White cell count is generally below $5,000/mm^3$ with predominantly mononuclear cells and occasionally eosinophils (21). A distinctive cytological pattern has also been reported as characteristic of rheumatoid pleuritis (26). Biochemical analysis will generally show elevated protein (3-7 g/dl), elevated lactate dehydrogenase (LDH), low glucose (frequently less than 30 g/dl), and low pH (17,27). Serologic analysis of pleural effusions has demonstrated the presence of rheumatoid factor and immune complexes (28,29). Rheumatoid factors may be produced locally (30). Depletion of complement is also reported (31). Because many of the features of pleural effusions in RA patients are similar to those seen with infection, pleural fluid should always be cultured to exclude the possibility of infection. Particular attention should be taken to culture for infectious agents, including anaerobes, in RA patients with effusion who have fever, pleural fluid white cell count of greater than $50,000/mm^3$, and/or a history of treatment with corticosteroids (32,33).

The pleural pathology in RA is fully described in Chapter 6. Typically, the pleura has a granular appearance on the parietal surface with focal involvement (34). Thus, a blind pleural biopsy may not detect an abnormality because of sampling error (16,17,21), and pleuroscopy may be required (34). Management of pleural disease must be integrated with the total therapeutic plans for all components of the patient's RA. In most cases, the adequate control of the articular symptoms with an appropriate medical program will suppress the clinical pleuritic symptoms. Frequently pleural effusion will resolve spontaneously within a few months. In refractory cases, systemic corticosteroids may be required, although the response is variable (16). The local injection of corticosteroids has been successfully used in the treatment of refractory rheumatoid pericardial effusions (35), but there is limited experience with this procedure in the management of rheumatoid pleural effusions (36). We have found intrapleural injection of tetracycline effective in controlling symptomatic pleural effusions. Surgical decortication has been successfully employed in rare cases with pleural thickening and fibrotic lung entrapment (37).

B. Pulmonary Nodules

Lung nodules are rare in RA. In Walker and Wright's series only two examples were found among 516 patients with RA (16,22). In most cases, pulmonary nodules are asymptomatic and discovered as an incidental finding on chest radiographs (38). Symptomatic presentations for pulmonary nodules are rare and include hemoptysis after cavitation of the nodule (16,21) (Fig. 1A) and pneumothorax if erosion into the pleural space occurs (Fig. 1B).

Radiographic features of pulmonary nodules are discussed in Chapter 4. The nodules are usually located subpleurally in the upper lung fields (23, 39) and may vary in size from a few millimeters to several centimeters. Single, multiple, unilateral, and bilateral distributions are reported. Atypical radiographic presentations may resemble fibrocavitary lesions such as that seen with tuberculosis or ankylosing spondylitis (40). Histologic features of pulmonary nodules are described in Chapter 6. Characteristically these nodules resemble peripheral subcutaneous rheumatoid nodules with central necrosis, palisading epithelioid cells, infiltrating mononuclear cells, and obliterative vasculitis (21).

When a pulmonary nodule is discovered in a patient with RA, other potential causes must be excluded. Appropriate tests must be taken to rule out malignancy or infection. Comparison to previous chest X-rays, sputum cytology, transbronchial biopsy (21,41), and potentially open lung biopsy should be employed as indicated, depending on clinical judgment and other associated signs, symptoms, and risk factors. In rare situations, pulmonary nodules may precede the development of arthritis (38,39) or resolve spontaneously (23).

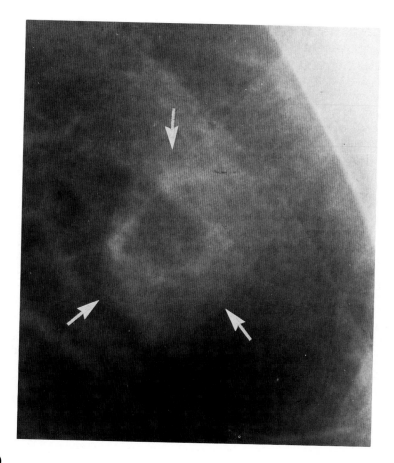

(A)

Figure 1   (A) Chest X-ray showing in the left lower lobe a solitary rheumatoid lung nodule (biopsy proven) with cavitation (arrows) in a 60-year-old man with seropositive, nodular, erosive RA of 20 years' duration. (B) Subsequent chest X-ray from the same patient taken 1 year later showing left pyopneumothorax after sudden hemoptysis and formation of a bronchopleural fistula attributed to rupture of the necrotic nodule shown in Figure 1A. Surgical drainage was complicated by persistent empyema and formation of a skin fistula requiring thoracoplasty 4 years later. Courtesy Dr. M. L. Russell (2).

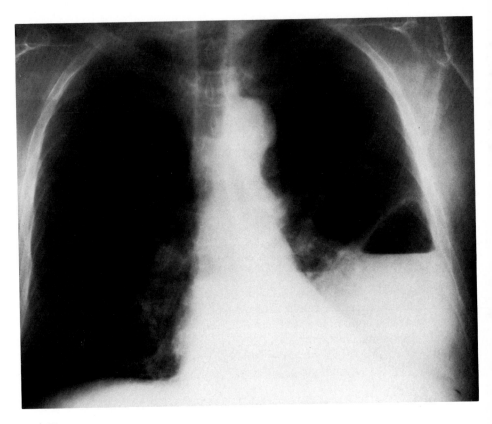

(B)

Figure 1 (continued)

C. Rheumatoid Pneumoconiosis (Caplan's Syndrome)

Caplan's syndrome is the combination of multiple pulmonary nodules and mining dust exposure in patients with RA. In 1953, Caplan described the development of multiple peripheral lung nodules in Welsh coal miners who developed RA (13). In 1969, Scadding broadened the concept of Caplan's syndrome to include exposure to other dusts, such as silica and asbestos (38). Occupations at risk for these dust exposures include carbon electrode occupations, boiler scalers, asbestos workers, gold miners, tile makers, chalk workers, foundry workers, grinders, and those exposed to rubber dusts (3). This syndrome appears to be rare in the United States, although exposure to tuberculosis and silica has been reported to cause a granulomatous lung reaction in American miners with RA (42). Although the pathophysiology of this process remains undefined, the epidemiologic data suggest an enhancement of the development of pulmonary disease in RA patients with pneumoconiosis.

The majority of patients with Caplan's syndrome are rheumatoid factor positive (43). Radiographic findings of Caplan's syndrome are discussed in Chapter 4. These radiographic findings in Caplan's syndrome include nodule cavitation, nodule calcification, pleural effusions, and, rarely, pneumothorax. The lung nodules in Caplan's syndrome show histologic lesions similar to those described above except for the presence of a peripheral pigmented ring of dust surrounding the lesion (38). Rheumatoid factor has been detected within the lung nodules (44).

The understanding of the natural history of Caplan's syndrome requires a comparison of RA patients with pneumoconiosis and the pneumoconiosis that develops in normal subjects after similar mining dust exposures. After 5-10 years, depending on the intensity of the mineral dust exposure, several pulmonary complications may develop in normal individuals (43,45). In more than 50% of asymptomatic coal miners without RA, the chest radiograph will show a simple pneumoconiosis. About 20% of miners will slowly develop cough, exertional dyspnea, and radiologic signs of central conglomerate lesions known as progressive massive fibrosis (PMF). This pneumoconiosis is associated with progressive chronic airway obstruction and pathologic focal emphysema. Tuberculosis has also been implicated in the pathogenesis of this syndrome. Most PMF develops in patients without RA. Although 14% of PMF cases are rheumatoid factor positive, these individuals do not have clinical RA (43,46).

Miners with RA show an increased risk for the development of PMF and Caplan's syndrome. PMF may develop in 50% of miners with RA, although these RA subjects only represent 3% of total PMF cases in all miners (47). Twenty-five percent of all miners who develop RA show simple pneumoconiosis without progression, but another 25% may rapidly develop Caplan's syndrome with the onset of their RA (47). Caplan's syndrome may appear within weeks of the polyarthritis as asymptomatic crops of peripheral lung nodules 1-2 cm in diameter. The nodules may progress to cavitation or calcification with pleural effusions or, rarely, pneumothorax (47). Ordinarily, lung disability is not associated with these lesions, but pulmonary function tests show signs of mild airway obstruction, unlike the progressive respiratory failure seen in PMF (48).

The radiographic features of Caplan's syndrome may appear with or after the onset of RA in about half the cases (47). However, 50% of miners with the radiographic features of multiple pulmonary nodules resembling Caplan's syndrome will not have RA (47). Rheumatoid factor is positive in 50% of these patients with radiographic findings similar to Caplan's syndrome, but who do not have clinical RA (30,47).

D. Pneumonitis/Pulmonary Fibrosis

Interstitial inflammatory lung disease in RA patients appears to run a continuum from mild pneumonitis to severe pulmonary fibrosis and restrictive lung disease. These inflammatory pulmonary disorders represent the most common abnormality affecting the pulmonary parenchyma in RA (49). Understandably, the variable frequency of its detection in RA has depended on the case selection and type of investigative methods used. For example, Walker and Wright reported an incidence of 1.6% based on abnormal chest radiographs (16,22), whereas Frank et al. reported an incidence of 41% when pulmonary function tests were used (50). Unfortunately, interpretation of the results of pulmonary function tests such as diffusing capacity may be confounded by the patient's previous occupation, smoking habits, medications, or hemoglobin concentration.

Nonproductive cough and progressive dyspnea are the most common symptoms. Chest crackles were detected in 10% of unselected patients with RA, and their presence correlated strongly with chest radiographic changes and a decrease in some pulmonary function variables (5). Clubbing and hypertrophic pulmonary osteoarthropathy may be seen in patients with RA and pulmonary fibrosis (51). Polyarthritis usually precedes the onset of pulmonary fibrosis, although lung involvement and RA may appear together, or sometimes the lung disease may precede the articular symptoms of RA (16).

The usual radiographic changes are initially an increased reticulation with a fluffy pattern early in the course, characteristic of an exudative inflammatory alveolar reaction, but with progression later to fibrosis with a fine nodularity and honeycomb pattern (23) (Fig. 2). The lower lobes are typically most affected, with the apices rarely affected (40). Radiographic findings in interstitial pulmonary fibrosis are described fully in Chapter 4. Gallium scan uptake may detect active inflammation, but its utility in assessing the activity of alveolitis in RA patients has not been clearly established, as discussed in Chapter 5.

The identification of alveolitis and even fibrosis in RA patients may often precede the appearance of pulmonary symptoms if sensitive methods to detect abnormalities of pulmonary function are used. Abnormal pulmonary function tests are frequently found in the presence of normal chest films (50-56).

Many of these studies, however, were uncontrolled (50,51,57) or failed to take smoking history fully into account (50-57). When pulmonary function abnormalities are present, pulmonary restriction with decreased compliance and defects in gas transfer are the most common abnormalities. Pulmonary function testing in RA patients is fully described in Chapter 3.

Open lung biopsy is the definitive procedure for proving the diagnosis of pulmonary fibrosis, particularly if impaired gas exchange is the only abnormality (58). However, open biopsy is now being complemented or replaced

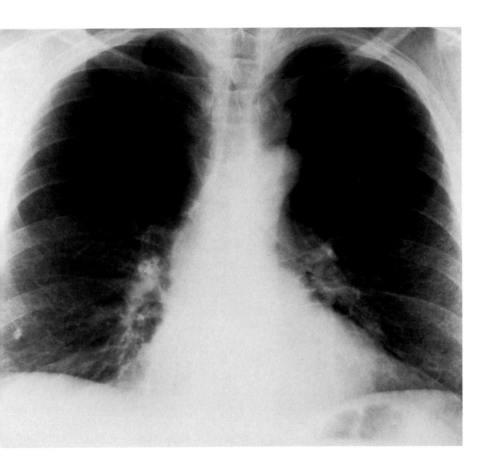

Figure 2A Chest X-ray showing diffuse pulmonary fibrosis affecting both lower lung fields in a 50-year-old man with nodular, seropositive, erosive polyarthritis of 8 years' duration. After 4 years of polyarthritis, nodules appeared with skin vasculitis, peripheral neuropathy, nonproductive cough, exertional dyspnea, and bilateral basal crackles. Rheumatoid factor was 1:1,280; ANA 1:30; cryoglobulins and circulating immune complexes were detected, and typing for protease inhibitors was normal. Pulmonary function tests showed evidence of obstruction and restriction. For over 8 years he has taken corticosteroids, a single daily dose of prednisone 15-20 mg, without worsening of his symptoms, pulmonary function, or appearance of the chest film.

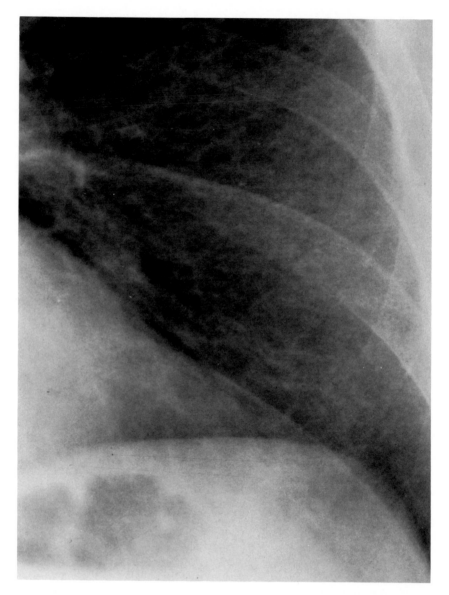

Figure 2B Characteristic radiographic fine nodular reticular pattern affecting the left lower lung field in the patient described in Figure 2A. Courtesy Dr. D. A. Gordon (2).

by fiberoptic bronchoscopy and bronchoalveolar lavage (BAL) (59). BAL may show a neutrophilic (60) and/or eosinophilic (61) cellular response with increased IgG, suggesting active inflammatory disease. The use of BAL is fully described in Chapter 5. As described in Chapter 6, lung pathology can show a variety of diseases. The different histologic patterns include cellular interstitial infiltrates without significant fibrosis, interstitial fibrosing pneumonia resembling usual interstitial pneumonia (UIP) with pulmonary fibrosis, desquamative interstitial pneumonia, and lymphocytic interstitial pneumonia.

The exact pathogenesis of interstitial lung disease in RA patients is unknown. The development of interstitial lung disease correlates with increased manifestations of autoimmunity. Tomasi et al. (62) and Lawrence et al. (63) showed an association of radiographic evidence of pulmonary fibrosis and production of rheumatoid factor in RA, and a number of investigators showed correlations of abnormal pulmonary function tests with either rheumatoid factor, antinuclear antibodies (ANA), immune complexes, or cryoglobulinemia in patients with RA (54,57,64). Immunofluorescent studies from biopsy material obtained from patients with RA have shown deposition of IgG and complement in pulmonary capillaries (54,65,66). As described below in the section on risk factors, there may be a genetic predisposition to the development of pulmonary diseases.

Corticosteroids, azathioprine, and cyclophosphamide have been employed in the treatment of interstitial lung disease in RA patients. The success of therapy probably depends on the relative amounts of reversible active inflammation and irreversible fibrosis that are present when treatment is initiated. Once the fibrotic phase develops, the prognosis is poor, and the interstitial lung disease is resistant to treatment. The detection of active inflammation by BAL (60,67,68) or gallium scanning (67) may aid in the identification of patients with the highest potential for response to treatment. The presence of increased lymphocytes on BAL correlated with a good response to corticosteroid and a good prognosis in one study (68). However, the presence of increased numbers of eosinophils in BAL fluid is associated with progressive lung disease and a poor prognosis despite the use of corticosteroids (61). The precise role of BAL in the evaluation and management of the rheumatoid lung awaits more definitive study.

E. Airway Obstruction

Upper Airway Obstruction

Upper airway obstructions may evolve from synovitis of the cricoarytenoid joint (69), a rheumatoid nodule of the vocal cord (70), or arteritis of the vasa nervorum of the recurrent laryngeal and vagus nerves (71).

Cricoarytenoid arthritis is commonly asymptomatic. It may be associated only with hoarseness, or it may progress to cause upper airway obstruction (69). With acute laryngeal obstruction, the patient presents with dysphagia, dysphonia, and throat pain. Occasionally deep esophageal ulcers may develop at the level of the larynx in association with this involvement (72). The cricothyroid joints may also be affected. Systemic or inhaled corticosteroids have been used in this condition. Acute stridor with progressive upper airway obstruction may lead to suffocation unless tracheostomy is performed. The treatment of acute upper airway obstruction may be helped by use of helium oxygen mixtures (73).

Chronic forms of cricoarytenoid synovitis may cause exertional dyspnea and stridor that is slowly progressive or episodic. Hoarseness and fullness of the throat radiating to the ipsilateral meatus of the ear are frequently overlooked symptoms. Chronic involvement may cause cricoarytenoid joint ankylosis and risk of further episodes of laryngeal obstruction. Evaluation should include direct fiberoptic laryngoscopy and high-resolution computerized tomography (74). Pulmonary function tests, particularly respiratory flow-volume loops, are important in monitoring the patient's progress after treatment (73). A superimposed viral infection may change an asymptomatic condition into an acute laryngeal obstruction.

Laryngeal dysfunction associated with arteritis or vasculitis of the vasa nervorum of the recurrent laryngeal and vagus nerve may occur (71). Corticosteroids and immunosuppressive treatment have been effective in controlling this problem.

Awareness of cricoarytenoid involvement or vocal cord fixation is important in the patient with RA requiring general anesthesia. Preoperative attention is required if tracheostomy is to be avoided. The fiberoptic laryngoscope allows transnasal intubation under direct vision. Postoperative vigilance should be maintained to detect postextubation obstruction.

Lower Airway Obstruction

Obstruction of the lower respiratory tract airways in patients with RA has only recently gained attention. Peribronchiolar fibrosis and inflammation may be associated with diffuse pulmonary fibrosis (75), but patients with RA without pulmonary fibrosis or emphysema may develop an acute progressive bronchiolitis obliterans associated with hyperinflated lungs (76). Chronic slowly progressive obstruction of the small airways associated with a normal chest radiograph has also been reported in patients with RA (77,78). These chronic changes seem aggravated or induced by cigarette smoking (5), the presence of alpha-1-antitrypsin deficiency (79), or certain antirheumatic medication (8,80). A chronic obstructive picture may also affect a subset of nonsmokers with Sjogren's syndrome (81,82).

F. Acute Obliterative Bronchiolitis

Bronchiolitis obliterans is a rare pulmonary complication of RA. In 1977, a rapidly progressive airway obliteration resembling childhood viral bronchiolitis was reported in five women (76). At least 15 additional cases have subsequently been described (8-10). Affected patients had nonproductive cough, progressive dyspnea, and diffuse crackles with characteristic midexpiratory squeak. The chest X-ray either was normal or showed distended lungs (Fig. 3).

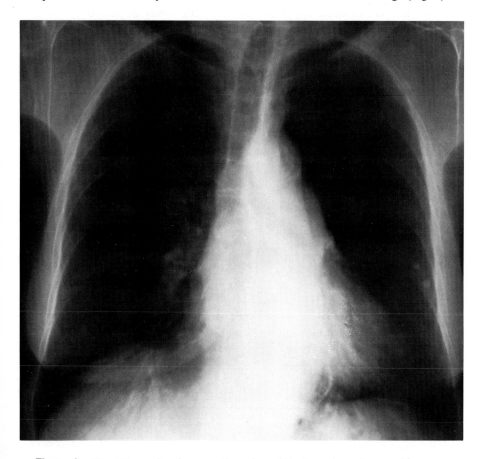

Figure 3 Chest X-ray showing overdistension of the lungs in a 69-year old woman in acute respiratory failure. The patient, a nonsmoker, had a 30-year history of seropositive, erosive RA. Two years earlier she developed exertional dyspnea that worsened 18 months later. Penicillamine was administered for a few weeks. The penicillamine was switched to azathioprine, but she became more incapacitated by shortness of breath. Pulmonary function tests showed increasing small airways obstruction in keeping with acute obliterative bronchiolitis. Courtesy Drs. M. A. Hutcheon and P. Lee (2).

Table 2 Characteristics of 155 Patients with Rheumatoid Arthritis and 95 Control Subjects by Smoking Category

	Nonsmokers			Ex-smokers			Current smokers		
	Rheumatoid	Control	P Value[a]	Rheumatoid	Control	P Value[a]	Rheumatoid	Control	P Value[a]
No. of subjects	64	40		46	31		45	24	
Age	55 ± 12	59 ± 15		57 ± 15	59 ± 11˙		57 ± 12	55 ± 14	
Female	78%	85%		39%	48%		42%	63%	
Pack-years	0	0		21 ± 17	22 ± 24		32 ± 17	33 ± 22	
Years of arthritis	12 ± 10	10 ± 9		10 ± 7	9 ± 10		7 ± 7	9 ± 7	
Oral corticosteroids ever	38	5%	.0002	48%	10%	.0005	27%	13%	
Gold salts ever	60%	3%	.0001	68%	0%	.0002	64%	4%	.0001
Penicillamine ever	16%	0%	.01	24%	0%	.003	20%	0%	.02
Cough	3%	8%		9%	13%		20%	17%	
Shortness of breath	8%	8%		24%	10%		18%	13%	
Rhonchi	0%	0%		9%	0%		18%	13%	
Crackles	11%	5%		22%	3%		22%	8%	

		P[a]			P[a]			P[a]
Lansbury index	37 ± 38	2 ± 10	.001	39 ± 49	0%	.001	34 ± 45	0%	.0002
Subcutaneous nodules	13%	0%	.02	15%	0%	.03	42%	0%	.05
Chest X-ray abnormal	15%	6%		22%	10%		30%	5%	.03
FVC[b]	107 ± 18	110 ± 19		103 ± 20	109 ± 20		101 ± 17	101 ± 22	.05
TLC	101 ± 16	102 ± 11		100 ± 15	102 ± 18		99 ± 13	104 ± 15	
RV	87 ± 25	92 ± 24		96 ± 30	87 ± 28		95 ± 26	97 ± 21	
TGV	112 ± 18	113 ± 25		114 ± 31	110 ± 27		109 ± 18	123 ± 21	
FEV_1	115 ± 19	117 ± 21		105 ± 23	112 ± 22		98 ± 22	110 ± 24	.05
V_{max} 50% VC[c]	105 ± 34	101 ± 31		83 ± 40	99 ± 45		76 ± 32	83 ± 35	.05
V_{max} 25% VC[d]	69 ± 42	66 ± 33		50 ± 28	55 ± 23		43 ± 28	47 ± 34	
$DLCO_{sb}$	78 ± 13	78 ± 12		74 ± 20	77 ± 20		71 ± 13	63 ± 14	

[a]Chi-square or t-tests. A blank indicates a P value □ .05.
[b]Pulmonary function results are expressed as percentage of normal predicted values.
[c]V_{max} 50% VC = maximum expired flow at 50% vital capacity.
[d]V_{max} 25% VC = maximum expired flow at 25% vital capacity.
Abbreviations: FVC, forced vital capacity; TLC, total lung capacity; RV, residual volume; $DLCO_{sb}$, single-breath diffusion capacity carbon monoxide.
Source: Hyland et al. (5).

The patients were mostly seropositive for rheumatoid factor. Pulmonary function tests showed a reduction in helium dilution lung volumes with severe air flow obstruction. When lung volumes were measured by body plethysmography, hyperinflation was present, confirming that the low lung volumes measured by helium dilution were artifactual owing to poor gas mixing (76). Postmortem examinations showed only obliterative bronchiolitis without mucous gland hypertrophy or significant emphysema. The prognosis for this condition is poor. Five of the first six cases died within 18 months of disease onset despite corticosteroid treatment.

The pathophysiology of this condition is unknown. Although bronchiolitis obliterans has been reported in patients with RA taking D-penicillamine and other antirheumatic drugs (10), it has also been reported in RA patients not receiving these agents (76). The potential relationship of antirheumatic drug therapy to the development of bronchiolitis obliterans is discussed in Chapter 14. The development of bronchiolitis obliterans has only been reported in patients with RA receiving D-penicillamine and not in patients receiving D-penicillamine for a nonrheumatic disease such as Wilson's disease. These data would imply that bronchiolitis obliterans is a potential complication of RA, with an associated increased risk of developing this form of airway obstruction in patients receiving D-penicillamine or other antirheumatic drugs.

G. Chronic Obstructive Airways Disease

The evaluation of chronic obstructive airways disease in RA patients has produced conflicting and confusing results. Part of this confusion may have resulted from failure to consider the effects of smoking, restrictive lung disease, and impairment secondary to respiratory muscle weakness (81).

Collins et al. (77) and Geddes et al. (78) reported the presence of chronic airway obstruction in 61% and 32% of patients with RA, respectively, independent of their smoking status. The Collins study consisted mainly of men with RA who were current smokers and included only 15 control subjects (77). Although Geddes et al. separated their patients into smokers and non-smokers, this division was based on the smoking status at the time of evaluation. The study did not consider the possibility of pulmonary damage in patients who had previously smoked (78). In this study the pulmonary function changes attributed to obstructive lung disease could also have been explained by a restrictive ventilatory defect or respiratory muscle weakness (81).

In our prospective study of 155 patients with RA and 95 control subjects, the smoking status was defined in all individuals (Table 2). Participants were classified as nonsmokers, ex-smokers, or current smokers. There were no significant differences in pulmonary function tests in RA patients and controls in the nonsmoker and ex-smoker groups (Table 2) (5). RA patients who were currently smoking had a significantly lower FEV_1 than control subjects who were current smoking. However, the FEV_1/FVC ratio and flow rates were similar in the two groups. These data suggest that the difference in FEV_1 in these patients was a result of more severe restrictive lung disease in RA patients rather than more obstructive lung disease in RA patients.

Begin et al. reported a subset of patients with well-established seropositive nodular erosive RA who had never smoked yet showed progressive chronic airways obstruction (81,82). None of these six patients had bronchitis, bronchiectasis, or asthma. All patients had sicca syndrome with histopathologic evidence of Sjogren's autoimmune exocrinopathy. Lung biopsies in four cases showed peribronchiolar lymphoplasmacytic infiltration. The airway obstruction in these patients progressed much more rapidly than that seen in smokers with chronic lung disease. Gold and D-penicillamine were not implicated. HLA-DR4 was more frequent in RA patients with this airways disease (82). The pulmonary abnormalities associated with Sjogren's disease (59) are discussed in full in Chapter 13.

In summary, studies evaluating chronic obstructive airways disease in RA patients are confusing and incomplete. Observations to date would suggest that this problem is relatively uncommon if it occurs at all. Pulmonary function tests evaluating this disorder are difficult to interpret in view of the possible confounding effects of smoking, concurrent restrictive disease, and ventilatory muscle weakness.

H. Vasculitis

Pulmonary vascular abnormalities can include arteritis, vasculitis associated with rheumatoid nodules, and pulmonary hypertension. In some patients with RA, systemic polyarteritis may emerge and affect the lungs. Although this complication has been documented in seropositive nodular RA (16), it is important to differentiate these patients from subjects with polyarteritis nodosa. Vasculitis is an inherent feature of the rheumatoid nodule and other extraarticular features of RA. Moreover, immunofluorescence studies of lung biopsies have shown immunoglobulin deposition in pulmonary arterioles (65). Pulmonary hypertension from necrotizing pulmonary panarteritis without parenchymal disease or systemic vasculitis has been reported (80). Immunofluorescence studies in these patients did not demonstrate deposition of immunoglobulins or complement (80).

III. Risk Factors

Certain risk factors may be associated with pulmonary abnormalities in RA. The first risk factor recognized was the association of rheumatoid pneumoconiosis (Caplan's syndrome) in miners who developed RA. Although most

risk factors cannot be altered to reduce the probability of developing pulmonary complications of RA, an understanding of these risk factors may
assist us in understanding the pathogenesis of these lesions.

A. Age and Sex

Pulmonary data on elderly patients with RA have not been reported. Although the role of age as a risk factor for pulmonary complications is unknown, the patient's sex may influence the frequency of lung involvement.
Seropositive men with RA have more extra-articular features including pulmonary abnormalities than women (83,84). In our series, we found more
males showed extra-articular features, however, pulmonary restriction in
smokers or non-smokers was not greater in men than in women (5).

B. Duration, Severity, and Course of RA

While patients with extraarticular features of RA, including pulmonary abnormalities (83), have more severe disease, these manifestations of RA are
not merely a reflection of the duration of disease. Sometimes pulmonary
abnormalities such as effusion, nodules, and diffuse fibrosis may actually
herald the onset of polyarthritis (20,38,39). Although the view has been held
that in the presence of extraarticular features, joint disease is more likely
quiescent, this has not been our experience (83) and was not the case in a
series of 34 cases of Felty's syndrome seen in our center (85). We found that
a decrease in lung volume measurement was associated with an increased
number of joint effusions, high sedimentation rate, and circulating immune
complexes (5) (Table 3). Sjogren's syndrome, another expression of disease
severity, may be associated with bronchiolar obstruction (81,82), as discussed
in Chapter 13. These data would all suggest that pulmonary involvement is
more common in patients with more severe RA.

C. Genetic Factors

Genetic predisposition has been implicated in the pathogenesis of RA and
diffuse pulmonary fibrosis (6,86,87). There are also HLA-DR immunogenetic correlations with Sjogren's syndrome in RA patients with airways obstruction (82) and correlations with susceptibility to nephrotoxicity after
gold or D-penicillamine (87). Pleural effusions appear more commonly in
male RA patients with HLA-B8 and HLA-DR3 (88). A significant increase
in the frequency of the heterozygous alpha-1-antitrypsin Pi-type MZ was
found among patients with diffuse pulmonary fibrosis with and without RA
when compared to a healthy control population (6). The relation of HLA-DR
and alpha-1-antitrypsin deficiency is unknown. These data would suggest

Table 3 Association of Pulmonary Abnormalities in Patients with Rheumatoid Arthritis (n = 155)

Clinical variables and pulmonary abnormalities	Clinical variable absent or below median	Clinical variable present or above median	P Value[a]
Gold salts now (no vs. yes)	90	65	
Chest X-ray abnormal	13%	33%	0.005
TGV[b]	117 ± 23	105 ± 19	0.02
Gold salts previously (no vs. yes)	57	33	
Chest X-ray abnormal	10%	9%	
TGV	117 ± 21	118 ± 28	
Joint effusions (2 vs. > 2)	108	47	
FVC	106 ± 19	99 ± 17	0.04
TLC	102 ± 14	96 ± 15	0.05
Sedimentation rate (mm/h)	39 ± 29	53 ± 29	0.006
Clq binding units	26 ± 21	32 ± 23	
Sedimentation rate (<37 vs. > 37)	78	76	
Joint effusions	1.9 ± 3.0	3.6 ± 5	0.02
FVC	108 ± 17	100 ± 20	0.02
TLC	102 ± 13	98 ± 16	
Clq binding units	23 ± 18	33 ± 24	0.004

[a]Chi-square or t-tests. A blank indicates a P value □ 0.05.
[b]Pulmonary function results are expressed as percentage of normal predicted values.
Source: Hyland et al. (5).

that genetic factors may play a role in predisposing a patient toward the development of pulmonary complications of RA, but they certainly do not explain the majority of cases.

D. Occupational Considerations

The clinical features of rheumatoid pneumoconiosis (Caplan's syndrome) are discussed earlier in this chapter. Although patients with hypersensitivity pneumonitis from exposure to mold may develop rheumatoid factors (89), the effects of hypersensitivity pneumonitis in RA patients are unknown except as described in Chapter 14 for drug-induced pulmonary reactions. The effect of chemical irritants and organic dusts have not been reported in patients with RA.

E. Cigarette Smoking

Smoking clearly causes lung damage in RA patients; however, it is unclear if the damage in RA patients is more severe than that seen in normal controls. The effects of cigarette smoking on the development of rheumatoid pneumoconiosis and pulmonary fibrosis, severity of chronic obstructive pulmonary disease, and limitation of diffusing capacity have been examined.

Patients who smoke and then develop RA may be at increased risk for the development of pulmonary abnormalities analogous to the Caplan's syndrome in miners (5). The additive effects of smoking and pneumoconiosis in RA patients are unknown. Pulmonary fibrosis may develop more frequently in RA patients who are heavy smokers (16,90).

An earlier section of this chapter reviews the effects of smoking on the development of chronic obstructive pulmonary disease in RA patients. Obstructive pulmonary disease may occur in RA patients who smoke, but it is debated whether the severity or prevalence of this problem is increased in RA patients who smoke. In our comparison of 155 RA patients and 95 control subjects who were separated into groups by smoking history, RA patients who smoked had reduced FEV_1 when compared to control subjects who smoked. There were no significant differences between RA patients who had never smoked or ceased smoking and matched control subjects. This finding was explained by lung volume restriction rather than airways obstruction.

Interpretations of the effects of RA on gas transfer are controversial. In our study, RA patients did not differ significantly from the controls in their diffusing capacity (Table 2). The single-breath diffusing capacity of carbon monoxide (DLCOsb) tended to decrease in direct relation to smoking status. Again, no difference was found in another study using steady-state method (91). One study reported an abnormal DLCOsb in 41% of RA patients (50). In males, this correlated with smoking history and airway obstruction, while in females, the low DLCOsb did not appear to correlate with smoking but was related to mild restriction. In another series, an abnormal DLCOsb was found in 24% of patients with RA and correlated strongly with smoking history (53). In these last two studies, the patients with RA and control subjects were not tested in the same laboratory but were classified as normal or abnormal based on expected values obtained from prediction formulae. Other studies have found low DLCO in RA patients but provided inadequate smoking data to interpret the results (50,52,64,92). Thus, when smoking history is taken into account, the collected findings on the diffusing capacity do not support the presence of a gas transfer defect in RA independent of the effects of cigarette smoking. Limitations of this approach are significant, as discussed in Chapter 3.

Another factor that can influence diffusing capacity in the RA patient is hemoglobin concentration. Since patients with advanced RA are commonly anemic, a decrease in diffusing capacity might be expected. Our study and others have seldom taken this factor into account even though we found no change in diffusing capacity not explained by smoking status of patients.

IV. Clinical Evaluation of Pulmonary Disease in the RA Patient

A systematic approach to a RA patient with pulmonary complaints is required to confirm a correct diagnosis and establish an appropriate management plan. Although many patients' symptoms will be a manifestation of underlying RA, it is important to exclude other causes of lung complaints. Special attention should be taken to rule out the possibility of infection.

A. Review of Underlying Rheumatic Diagnosis

When a patient carrying a diagnosis of RA develops pulmonary symptoms, pleural effusions, or interstitial fibrosis, other rheumatic diseases should be considered despite the original diagnosis. Several diffuse connective tissue diseases may resemble RA at presentation, and additional manifestations may develop later. These diseases include systemic lupus erythematosus, polymyositis, dermatomyositis, polyarteritis nodosa, Wegener's granulomatosis, ankylosing spondylitis (40), and hypertrophic pulmonary osteoarthropathy (93). A complete review of the total clinical status of the patient is important in addition to attention to the new pulmonary complaints. In some cases this evaluation will detect significant changes in the status of other organ involvement and influence the clinical diagnosis and management.

B. Differential Diagnosis of Pulmonary Syndromes Unrelated to RA

The presence of RA does not protect the patient from the development of other new pulmonary diseases or complications. The evaluation of any RA patient with pulmonary symptoms requires an open mind to detect abnormalities associated with the underlying disease and/or unrelated independent pulmonary diseases. Unrelated explanations of pleuritis, pleural effusions, pulmonary nodules, and parenchymal lung disease are reported in RA patients.

Rib fractures may mimic symptoms of pleurisy. Patients with osteoporosis secondary to RA or corticosteroid therapy may experience vertebral collapse or rib fractures after minor trauma or coughing. Rib fractures may also lead to hemothorax or bronchopneumonia. Rib fractures in RA patients should not be confused with the erosive superior rib margin defects associated with severe shoulder disease (94). Corticosteroid therapy can also lead to an abnormal chest X-ray secondary to mediastinal widening from fatty infiltration.

Pleural effusions may be secondary to congestive heart failure, pulmonary infarction, hypothyroidism with polyserositis, idiopathic or infectious granulomatous disease, malignancies, pancreatitis, or carcinomatosis (95-97). Evaluation of all clinical features of the patient with thoracentesis and pleural fluid analysis will assist in the differential diagnosis.

Multiple or single pulmonary nodules in RA patients present difficult diagnostic challenges. Multiple pulmonary nodules may represent malignancy (95) or septic emboli. Solitary rheumatoid nodules may be confused with tuberculosis (98) or carcinoma (97). In many cases, excision of the nodule and pathologic examination are required to establish a diagnosis (97).

Parenchymal lung involvement may represent a myriad of unrelated pulmonary diseases. Alveolar cell carcinoma may arise in well-established diffuse pulmonary fibrosis and should be suspected when a patient with pulmonary fibrosis deteriorates rapidly. Leukemic infiltrates and lymphangitic carcinoma (Fig. 4) may mimic the picture of diffuse pulmonary fibrosis in a patient with RA. Confusion may arise in recognizing pulmonary edema when superimposed on diffuse pulmonary fibrosis. Aspiration pneumonitis, sarcoidosis and Loeffler's syndrome, or bronchocentric granulomatosis may present diagnostic difficulties (99,100). BAL may help in establishing the diagnosis without having to resort to lung biopsy.

C. Pulmonary Infections

A variety of pulmonary infections may arise in RA patients with or without underlying pulmonary parenchymal disease (14,101). The detection of infection in RA patients is often difficult because with severe RA the patients may be asymptomatic without fever of leukocytosis. Bronchitis, pneumonia, and tuberculosis have been reported commonly in men with RA (14). In a controlled study, 43 of 230 women with RA had a history of bronchitis and bronchiectasis that actually preceded RA in 28 of the 43 (102). Infectious pneumonia and pleurisy seen in 20 patients preceded RA in 17. In one series of 516 patients with RA, almost twice as many pulmonary infections were seen in RA patients, particularly males, as in controls (14). The association of bronchiectasis in RA should not be overlooked (16,22,102). The obliterative bronchiolitis described in some patients with RA may be the result of

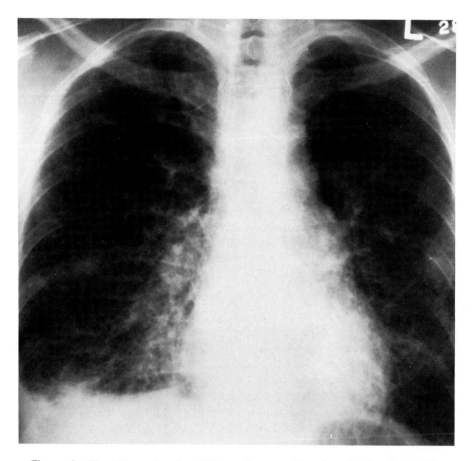

Figure 4 Chest X-ray showing diffuse pulmonary fibrosis and right pleural effusion in a 40-year-old woman with a 3-year history of seropositive, nodular RA. Two years earlier her polyarthritis had responded to gold injections, but she then developed progressive dyspnea, nonproductive cough, and medium basal crackles. Pleural fluid glucose was normal, but a transbronchial lung biopsy showed adenocarcinoma in keeping with lymphangitic spread. Courtesy Dr. E. C. Keystone (2).

viral infection or disturbed immunoregulation by corticosteroids, immunosuppressives, or D-penicillamine.

The frequency and morbidity of pulmonary infections in RA patients have been debated. A higher prevalence of respiratory infections in RA patients has not been confirmed by ourselves and others (5,103); however, we observed that intercurrent infections were associated with general debility and contributed to death in patients with RA (83). Autopsy studies of patients with RA have shown an increased frequency of bronchitis and bronchiectasis compared with matched controls (2). In one large series 1,035 patients with RA were compared with 617 persons with osteoarthritis (104). Deaths from all causes were increased by 86% in RA patients, commonly due to respiratory infection. In the RA group respiratory deaths were observed 57, expected 13, whereas in the osteoarthritis group results were observed 20, expected 13 (104). Patients with RA may be predisposed to infections because of impaired cellular immunity or neutropenia associated with the disease itself (105). Chapter 7 further reviews the pulmonary infections and changes in host defense mechanisms in patients with rheumatic diseases. Although additional information will be needed to reach a final conclusion on the significance of pulmonary infections in patients with RA, these data suggest that RA patients do not have an increased incidence of pulmonary infections but that they may experience an increased morbidity and mortality when infectious events occur.

V. Summary

The pulmonary manifestations in RA include pleuritis, pleural effusion, nodules, rheumatoid pneumoconiosis, pneumonitis, interstitial fibrosis, airway obstruction, and vasculitis. In addition to these diseases, which are specifically seen in RA, these individuals may experience pulmonary ailments as the result of antirheumatic drugs, infectious agents, or a multitude of unrelated pulmonary conditions. When a patient with RA presents with new pulmonary complaints, the diagnosis should be reviewed and non-RA-related etiologies excluded. This evaluation should particularly rule out infectious causes.

References

1. Ellman, P., and Ball, R. E. (1948). "Rheumatoid disease" with joint and pulmonary manifestations. *Br. Med. J.* **2**:816.
2. Gordon, D. A., Hyland, R. H., and Broder, I. (1985). Clinical presentation and differential diagnosis of pulmonary abnormalities. In *Rheumatoid Arthritis—Etiology, Diagnosis, Management.* Edited by Utsinger, P. D., N. J. Zvaifler, and G. E. Ehrlich. Lippincott, Philadelphia, pp. 441-463.
3. Hurd, E. R. (1979). Extraarticular manifestations of rheumatoid arthritis. *Semin. Arthritis Rheum.* **8**:151-176.
4. Turner, R., Collins, R., and Nomeir, A. M. (1979). Extraarticular manifestations of rheumatoid arthritis. *Bull. Rheum. Dis.* **29**:986-990.

5. Hyland, R. H., Gordon, D. A., Broder, I., et al. (1983). A systematic controlled study of pulmonary abnormalities in rheumatoid arthritis. *J. Rheumatol.* **10**:395-405.

6. Geddes, D. M., Webley, M., Brewerton, D. A., et al. (1977). Alpha-1-antitrypsin phenotypes in fibrosing alveolitis and rheumatoid arthritis. *Lancet* **2**:1049-1051.

7. Gould, P. W., McCormack, P. L., and Palmer, D. G. (1977). Pulmonary damage associated with sodium aurothiomalate therapy. *J. Rheumatol.* **4**:252-260.

8. Penny, W. J., Knight, R. K., Rees, A. M., Thomas, A. L., and Smith, A. P. (1982). Obliterative bronchiolitis in rheumatoid arthritis. *Ann. Rheum. Dis.* **41**:469-472.

9. Lyle, W. H. (1988). D-penicillamine and fatal obliterative bronchiolitis. (Letter.) *Br. Med. J.* **1**:105.

10. Wolfe, F., Schurle, D. R., Lin, J. J., et al. (1983). Upper and lower airway disease in penicillimine treated patients with rheumatoid arthritis. *J. Rheumatol.* **10**:406-410.

11. Sternlieb, I., Bennett, B., and Scheinberg, I. H. (1975). D-penicillamine induced Goodpasture's syndrome in Wilson's disease. *Ann. Intern. Med.* **82**:673-676.

12. Lang, A. E., Humphrey, J. G., and Gordon, D. A. (1981). Plasma exchange therapy for severe pencillamine induced myasthenia gravis. *J. Rheumatol.* **8**:303-307.

13. Caplan, A. (1953). Certain unusual radiological appearances in the chest of coal-miners suffering from rheumatoid arthritis. *Thorax* **8**:29-37.

14. Walker, W. C., and Wright, V. (1967). Rheumatoid pleuritis. *Ann. Rheum. Dis.* **26**:467-474.

15. Fleming, A., Dodman, S., Crown, J. M., et al. (1976). Extraarticular features in early rheumatoid disease. *Br. Med. J.* **1**:1241-1243.

16. Walker, W. C., and Wright, V. (1968). Pulmonary lesions and rheumatoid arthritis. *Medicine* **47**:501-520.

17. Lillington, G. A., Carr, D. T., and Mayne, J. G. (1971). Rheumatoid pleurisy with effusion. *Arch. Intern. Med.* **128**:764-768.

18. Baggenstoss, A. H., and Rosenberg, E. F. (1943). Visceral lesions associated with chronic infectious (rheumatoid) arthritis. *Arch. Pathol.* **35**: 503-516.

19. Fingerman, D. L., and Andrus, F. C. (1943). Visceral lesions associated with rheumatoid arthritis. *Ann. Rheum. Dis.* **3**:168-181.

20. MacFarlane, J. D., Dieppe, P. A., Rigden, B. G., and Clark, T. J. (1978). Pulmonary pleural lesions in rheumatoid disease. *Br. J. Dis. Chest* **72**: 288-300.

21. Turner-Warick, M., and Courtney, E. R. (1977). Pulmonary manifestations of rheumatoid disease. *Clin. Rheum. Dis.* **3**:549-564.

22. Walker, W. C., and Wright, V. (1967). Rheumatoid pleuritis. *Q. J. Med.* **36**:239-251.
23. Martel, W., Abell, M. R., Mikkelsen, W. M., and Whitehouse, W. M. (1968). Pulmonary and pleural lesion in rheumatoid disease. *Radiology* **90**:641-653.
24. Maude, M. A. J., Watson, J. I., Henderson, J. A. M., and Wang, N. (1969). Pleural fluid in rheumatoid pleuritis. *Arch. Intern. Med.* **124**: 373-376.
25. Baim, S., Samuelson, C. O., and Ward, J. R. (1979). Rheumatoid arthritis, amyloidosis, and chylous effusions. *Arthritis Rheum.* **22**:182-185.
26. Shinto, R., and Prete, P. (1988). Characteristic cytology in rheumatoid pleural effusion. *Am. J. Med.* **85**:587.
27. Sahn, S. A., Kaplan, R. L., Maulitz, R. M., and Good, J. T. Jr. (1980). Rheumatoid pleurisy, observations on the development of low pleural fluid pH and glucose level. *Arch. Intern. Med.* **140**:1237-1238.
28. Halla, J. T., Schrohenloher, R. E., and Volanakis, J. E. (1980). Immune complexes and other laboratory features of pleural effusions: A comparison of rheumatoid arthritis, systemic lupus erythematosus and other diseases. *Ann. Intern. Med.* **92**:748-752.
29. Halla, J. T., Schrohenloher, R. E., and Volanakis, J. E. (1980). Observations on some properties of immune complexes in a rheumatoid arthritis patient presenting with simultaneous synovitis and pleurisy. *Arthritis Rheum.* **23**:1318-1320.
30. Halla, J. T., Koopman, W. J., Schrohenloher, R. E., Darby, W. L., and Heck, L. W. (1983). Local synthesis of IgM and IgM rheumatoid factor in rheumatoid pleuritis. *J. Rheumatol.* **10**:204-209.
31. Hunder, G. G., McDuffie, F. C., and Hepper, G. G. (1972). Pleural fluid complement in systemic lupus erythematosus and rheumatoid arthritis. *Ann. Intern. Med.* **76**:357-363.
32. Storey, D. D., Dines, D. E., and Coles, D. T. (1976). Pleural effusion. A diagnostic dilemma. *J.A.M.A.* **236**:2183-2186.
33. Dieppe, P. A. (1975). Empyema in rheumatoid arthritis. *Ann. Rheum. Dis.* **34**:181-185.
34. Faurschou, P., Francis, D., and Faarup, P. (1985). Thoracoscopic, histological, and clinical findings in nine cases of rheumatoid pleural effusion. *Thorax* **40**:371-375.
35. Gordon, D. A., Richards, A. J., Koehler, B. E., and Broder, I. (1978). Intrapericardial steroids in rheumatoid disease. (Letter.) *Arthritis Rheum.* **21**:280.
36. Russell, M. L., Gladman, D. D., and Mintz, S. (1986). Rheumatoid pleural effusion: Lack of response to intrapleural corticosteroid. *J. Rheumatol.* **13**:412-415.

37. Yarbrough, J. W., Sealy, W. C., and Miller, J. A. (1975). Thoracic surgical problems associated with rheumatoid arthritis. *J. Thorac. Cardiovasc. Surg.* **69**:347-354.

38. Scadding, J. G. (1969). The lungs in rheumatoid arthritis. *Proc. R. Soc. Med.* **62**:227-238.

39. Eraut, D., Evans, J., and Caplin, M. (1978). Pulmonar necrobiotic nodules without rheumatoid arthritis. *Br. J. Dis. Chest* **72**:301-306.

40. Yue, C. C., Park, C. H., and Kushner, I. (1986). Apical fibrocavitary lesions of the lung in rheumatoid arthritis. Report of two cases and review of the literature. *Am. J. Med.* **81**:741-746.

41. Tishler, M., Grief, J., Fireman, E., Yaron, M., and Topilsky, M. (1986). Bronchoalveolar lavage—a sensitive tool for early diagnosis of pulmonary involvement in rheumatoid arthritis. *J. Rheumatol.* **13**:547-550.

42. Benedek, T. G. (1973). Rheumatoid pneumoconiosis: Documentation of onset and pathogenic considerations. *Am. J. Med.* **55**:515-524.

43. Caplan, A., Payne, R. R. B., and Withey, J. L. (1962). A broader concept of Caplan's syndrome related to rheumatoid factors. *Thorax* **17**:205-212.

44. Wagner, J. C., and McCormick, J. N. (1967). Immunological investigations of coal workers' disease. *J. R. Coll. Physicians* **2**:49-56.

45. Wagner, J. C. (1977). Pulmonary fibrosis and mineral dusts. *Ann. Rheum. Dis. (Suppl.)* **36**:42.

46. Miall, W. E. (1955). Rheumatoid arthritis in males: An epidemiological study of a Welsh mining community. *Ann. Rheum. Dis.* **14**:150-158.

47. Miall, W. E., Caplan, A., Cochrane, A. L., et al. (1953). An epidemiological study of rheumatoid arthritis associated with characteristic chest x-ray appearances in coal-workers. *Br. Med. J.* **2**:1231-1236.

48. Constanindis, K., Musk, A. W., Jenkins, J. P. R., and Berry, G. (1978). Pulmonary function in coal workers with Caplan's syndrome and nonrheumatoid complicated pneumonconiosis. *Thorax* **33**:764-768.

49. Roschmann, R. A., and Rothenberg, R. J. (1987). Pulmonary fibrosis in rheumatoid arthritis: A review of clinical features and therapy. *Semin. Arthritis Rheum.* **16**:174-185.

50. Frank, S. T., Weg, J. G., Harkeroad, L. E., et al. (1973). Pulmonary dysfunction in rheumatoid disease. *Chest* **63**:27-34.

51. Huang, C. T., and Lyons, H. A. (1966). Comparison of pulmonary function in patients with systemic lupus erythematosus, scleroderma and rheumatoid arthritis. *Am. Rev. Respir. Dis.* **93**:865-875.

52. Whorwell, P. J., Wojtulewski, J. A., and Lacey, B. W. (1975). Respiratory function in rheumatoid disease. *Br. Med. J.* **2**:175.

53. Davidson, C., Brooks, A. G. F., and Bacon, P. A. (1974). Lung function in rheumatoid arthritis. A clinical survey. *Ann. Rheum. Dis.* **33**:293-297.

54. Cervantes-Perez, P., Toro-Perez, A. H., and Rodriguez-Jurado, P. (1980). Pulmonary involvement in rheumatoid arthritis. *J.A.M.A.* **243**: 1715-1719.
55. Popper, M. S., Bogdonoff, M. L., and Hughes, R. L. (1972). Interstitial rheumatoid lung disease. A reassessment and review of the literature. *Chest* **62**:243-250.
56. Sievers, K., Aho, K., Hurri, I., et al. (1964). Studies of rheumatoid pulmonary disease. A comparison of roetgenological findings among patients with high rheumatoid factor titers and with completely negative reactions. *Acta Tuberc. Scand.* **35**:21-34.
57. Erhardt, C. C., Mumford, P., and Maini, R. N. (1979). The association of cryoglobulinaemia with nodules, vasculitis and fibrosing alveolitis in rheumatoid arthritis and their relationship to serum C1q binding activity and rheumatoid factor. *Clin. Exp. Immunol.* **38**:405-413.
58. Yousem, S. A., Colby, T. V., and Carrington, C. B. (1985). Lung biopsy in rheumatoid arthritis. *Am. Rev. Respir. Dis.* **131**:770-777.
59. Hatron, P. Y., Wallaert, B., Gosset, D., et al. (1987). Subclinical lung inflammation in primary Sjogren's syndrome. Relationship between bronchoalveolar lavage cellular analysis findings and characteristics of the disease. *Arthritis Rheum.* **30**:1226-1231.
60. Garcia, J. G. N., James, H. L., Zinkgraf, S., Perlman, M. B., and Deogh, B. A. (1987). Lower respiratory tract abnormalities in rheumatoid interstitial lung disease—potential role of neutrophils in lung injury. *Am. Rev. Respir. Dis.* **136**:811-817.
61. Peterson, M. W., Monick, M., and Hunningshake, G. W. (1987). Prognostic role of eosinophils in pulmonary fibrosis. *Chest* **92**:51-56.
62. Tomasi, T. B. Jr., Fudenberg, H. H., and Finby, M. (1962). Possible relationship of rheumatoid factors and pulmonary disease. *Am. J. Med.* **33**:243-248.
63. Lawrence, J. D., Locke, G. B., and Ball, J. (1971). Rheumatoid serum factor in populations in the U.K. 1. Lung disease and rheumatoid serum factor. *Clin. Exp. Immunol.* **8**:723.
64. Schernthaner, G., Scherak, O., Kolarz, G., and Kummer, F. (1976). Seropositive rheumatoid arthritis associated with decreased diffusion capacity of the lung. *Ann. Rheum. Dis.* **35**:258-262.
65. DeHoratius, R. J., Abruzzo, J. L., and Williams, R. C. (1972). Immunofluorescent and immunologic studies of rheumatoid lung. *Arch. Intern. Med.* **129**:441-446.
66. Turner-Warwick, M. (1967). Autoallergy in lung disease. *J. R. Coll. Physicians* **2**:57-66.
67. Greene, N. B., Solinger, A. M., and Baughman, R. P. (1987). Patients with collagen vascular disease—the value of gallium scanning and bron-

chioalveolar lavage in predicting response to steroid therapy and clinical outcome. *Chest* **91**:698-703.

68. Raghu, G. (1987). Idiopathic pulmonary fibrosis. A rational approach. *Chest* **92**:148-154.
69. Geterud, A., Ejnell, H., Mansson, I., Sandberg, N., Bake, B., and Bjelle, A. (1986). Severe airway obstruction caused by laryngeal rheumatoid arthritis. *J. Rheumatol.* **13**:948-951.
70. Friedman, B. A., and Rice, D. H. (1975). Rheumatoid nodules of the larynx. *Arch. Otolaryngol.* **101**:361-363.
71. Lovoy, M. R., and Hughes, G. R. V. (1980). Laryngeal dysfunction and rheumatoid arthritis. A case report. (Letter.) *J. Rheumatol.* **7**:759-760.
72. Montgomery, W. W., and Goodman, M. L. (1980). Rheumatoid cricoarytenoid arthritis complicated by upper esophageal ulcerations. *Ann. Otol. Rhinol. Laryngol.* **89**:6-8.
73. Skrinskas, G. J., Hyland, R. H., and Hutcheon, M. A. (1983). Using helium-oxygen mixtures in the management of acute upper airway obstruction. *Can. Med. Assoc. J.* **128**:555-558.
74. Brazeau-Lamontagne, L., Charlin, B., Levesque, R. Y., and Lussier, A. (1986). Cricoarytenoiditis: CT assessment in rheumatoid arthritis. *Radiology* **158**:463-466.
75. Fulmer, J. D., Roberts, W. C., Von Gal, E. R., and Crystal, R. G. (1979). Morphologic-physiologic correlates of the severity of fibrosis and degree of cellularity in idiopathic pulmonary fibrosis. *J. Clin. Invest.* **63**:665-676.
76. Geddes, D. M., Corrin, B., Brewerton, D. A., et al. (1977). Progressive airway obliteration in adults and its association with rheumatoid disease. *Q. J. Med.* **46**:427-444.
77. Collins, R. L., Turner, R. A., Johnson, M., Whitley, N. O., and McLean, R. L. (1976). Obstructive pulmonary disease in rheumatoid arthritis. *Arthritis Rheum.* **19**:623-628.
78. Geddes, D. M., Webley, W., and Emerson, P. A. (1979). Airways obstruction in rheumatoid arthritis. *Ann. Rheum. Dis.* **38**:222-225.
79. Cox, D. W., and Huber, O. (1980). Association of severe rheumatoid arthritis with heterozygosity for alpha-1-antitrypsin deficiency. *Clin. Genet.* **17**:153-160.
80. Baydur, A., Mongan, E. S., and Slager, U. T. (1979). Acute respiratory failure and pulmonary arteritis without parenchymal involvement: Demonstration in a patient with rheumatoid arthritis. *Chest* **75**:518-520.
81. Begin, R., Masse, S., Cantin, A., Menard, H. A., and Bureau, M. A. (1982). Airway disease in a subset of nonsmoking rheumatoid patients. Characterization of the disease and evidence for an autoimmune pathogenesis. *Am. J. Med.* **72**:743-750.

82. Radoux, V., Menard, H. A., Begin, R., Decary, F., and Koopman, W. J. (1987). Airways disease in rheumatoid arthritis patients. One element of a general exocrine dysfunction. *Arthritis Rheum.* **30**:249-256.

83. Gordon, D. A., Stein, J. L., and Broder, I. (1973). The extra-articular features of rheumatoid arthritis. A systematic analysis of RA. *Am. J. Med.* **54**:445-452.

84. Gordon, D. A., Koehler, B. E., and Russell, M. L. (1975). The clinical significance of immune complexes in rheumatoid disease. *Ann. N.Y. Acad. Sci.* **256**:338.

85. Sienknecht, C. W., Urowitz, M. B., Pruzanski, W., and Stein, H. B. (1977). Felty's syndrome. Clinical and serological analysis of 34 cases. *Ann. Rheum. Dis.* **36**:500-507.

86. Hilton, R. D., and Pitkeathly, D. A. (1974). Familial association of rheumatoid arthritis and fibrosing alveolitis. *Ann. Rheum. Dis.* **33**:191-195.

87. Wooley, P. H., Griffin, J., Panayi, G. S., Batchelor, J. R., Welsh, K. I., and Gibson, T. J. (1980). HLA-DR antigens and toxic reactions to sodium aurothiomalate and D-penicillamine in patients with rheumatoid arthritis. *N. Engl. J. Med.* **303**:300-302.

88. Hakala, M., Tiilikainen, A., Hameenkorpi, R., et al. (1986). Rheumatoid arthritis with pleural effusion includes a subgroup with autoimmune features and HLA-B8, Dw3 association. *Scand. J. Rheumatol.* **15**:290-296.

89. Banaszak, E. F., Theide, W. H., and Find, J. N. (1970). Hypersensitivity pneumonitis due to contamination of an air conditioner. *N. Engl. J. Med.* **283**:271-276.

90. Walker, W. C., and Wright, V. (1969). Diffuse interstitial pulmonary fibrosis and rheumatoid arthritis. *Ann. Rheum. Dis.* **28**:252-259.

91. Hills, E. A., Davies, S., and Geary, M. (1979). Frequency dependence of dynamic compliance in patients with rheumatoid arthritis. *Thorax* **34**:755-761.

92. Laitinen, O., Salorinne, Y., and Poppius, H. (1973). Respiratory function in systemic lupus erythematosus, scleroderma, and rheumatoid arthritis. *Ann. Rheum. Dis.* **32**:531-535.

93. Schechter, S. L., and Bole, G. G. (1976). Hypertrophic osteoarthropathy and rheumatoid arthritis. *Arthritis Rheum.* **19**:639-643.

94. McKendry, R. J. R., and Hogan, D. B. (1981). Superior margin rib defects in rheumatoid arthritis. *J. Rheumatol.* **8**:673-678.

95. Sahn, S. A., and Neff, T. A. (1976). Cavitary pulmonary lymphosarcoma masquerading as rheumatoid lung disease. *J.A.M.A.* **235**:2751-2752.

96. Sheridan, A. Q., Berger, H. W., and Taylor, T. H. (1984). Nonrheumatoid pleural effusions in patients with rheumatoid arthritis. *Mt. Sinai J. Med.* **45**:271-274.

97. Shenberger, K. N., Schend, A. R., and Taylor, T. H. (1984). Rheumatoid disease and bronchogenic carcinoma—case report and review of the literature. *J. Rheumatol.* **11**:226-228.
98. Miall, W. E. (1955). Rheumatoid arthritis in males: An epidemiological study of a Welsh mining community. *Ann. Rheum. Dis.* **14**:150-158.
99. Fallahi, S., Collins, R. D., Miller, R. K., and Halla, J. T. (1984). Coexistence of rheumatoid arthritis and sarcoidosis: Difficulties encountered in the differential diagnosis of common manifestations. *J. Rheumatol.* **11**:526-529.
100. Bonafede, R. R., and Benatar, S. R. (1987). Bronchocentric granulomatosis and rheumatoid arthritis. *Br. J. Dis. Chest* **81**:197-201.
101. Huskisson, E. C., and Hart, F. D. (1972). Severe, unusual and recurrent infections in rheumatoid arthritis. *Ann. Rheum. Dis.* **31**:118-121.
102. Kay, A. (1967). Infection in rheumatoid arthritis. *Lancet* **2**:152.
103. Vandenbroucke, J. P., Kaaks, R., Valkenburg, H. A., et al. (1987). Frequency of infections among rheumatoid arthritis patients, before and after disease onset. *Arthritis Rheum.* **30**:810-813.
104. Monson, P. R., and Hall, A. P. (1976). Mortality among arthritis patients. *J. Chron. Dis.* **29**:459-467.
105. Mowat, A. G., and Baum, J. (1971). Chemotaxis of polymorphonuclear leukocytes from patients with rheumatoid arthritis. *J. Clin. Invest.* **50**:2541-2549.

9

Systemic Lupus Erythematosus

ALLEN M. SEGAL and EDWARD V. REARDON

Cleveland Clinic Foundation
Cleveland, Ohio

Systemic lupus erythematosus (SLE) is a disease of unknown etiology characterized by the presence of multiple autoantibodies and immunologically mediated tissue damage. Many major organ systems are affected including the musculoskeletal, cutaneous, renal, and central nervous system (CNS). Although the renal and CNS complications are the most common life-threatening derangements in SLE, the pleuropulmonary manifestations still remain a significant cause of morbidity and mortality in this disease process.

The pleuropulmonary manifestations of SLE are presented in Table 1. This chapter will review only the pulmonary complications directly related to underlying SLE. Pulmonary disorders such as infection, pulmonary emboli, pneumothoraces, sarcoidosis, uremic pulmonary edema, and pseudolymphoma will not be discussed. We will detail each pulmonary manifestation including proposed pathogenic mechanisms where appropriate. The chapter will conclude with an approach to the management of the SLE related pulmonary problems.

I. Pleurisy/Pleural Effusion

Involvement of the pleura in SLE may present as pleuritic chest pain, pleural thickening, or effusion. Due to the frequent occurrence of pleuritis in SLE,

Table 1   Pulmonary Manifestations of SLE

Pleurisy with/without effusion
Acute lupus pneumonitis
Diffuse interstitial disease
Pulmonary hemorrhagic
Pulmonary hypertension
Diaphragmatic dysfunction
Atelectasis

it has been included as one of the eleven criteria of the American Rheumatism Association (ARA) Revised Criteria for the Diagnosis of SLE (1). Pleural manifestations have been reported in 30-60% of patients with SLE (2-5). The literature indicates that a clinical history of pleuritis is more common than roentgenographic abnormalities. Rothfield (5) reported that 46% of patients with SLE evaluated for pleural disease had clinical pleuritis sometime during the course of the disease compared with only 32% of the patients who had roentgenographic evidence of pleural effusion. Bulgrin et al. (6) found 35.3% of 207 chest roentgenograms (CXR) of patients with SLE had pleural changes. Ropes (7) noted that pleural rubs were found less often than both pleuritis or roentgenographic findings and were present in 22% of patients studied. Autopsy findings of pleural involvement were found in 63% of 58 patients reported by Ropes (7) and 66.6% of 54 patients with SLE studied by Purnell et al. (8). These studies demonstrate the frequent involvement of the pleura in SLE detected by both clinical and pathological evaluation.

The pleural effusion associated with active SLE may vary in size from small to massive. A summary of the characteristics of pleural effusions found in several disease entities including SLE are included in this textbook (Table 1, Chap. 1). Although these effusions share certain characteristics, important differences may be noted. Infection should always be excluded as a cause of pleural effusion in an SLE patient. A thoracentesis with examination of the pleural fluid is frequently helpful in establishing a diagnosis.

In the case of a pleural effusion secondary to infection, bacteria may be seen on gram stain or grown from culture. Leukocytosis, while noted in both types of effusions, may be much higher in the bacterially infected effusion. While the glucose and pH levels may be low in the infected pleural effusion, these values are often normal in the effusion secondary to SLE.

Differentiating the pleural effusion of SLE from that of rheumatoid arthritis (RA) may be difficult early in the course of the disease process. While the fluid in both is usually exudative, the glucose concentration in the pleural effusion secondary to SLE is greater than that noted in RA, in which the pleural fluid glucose is often less than 20 mg/100 ml (9). A pleural fluid pH may be another differentiating factor as pleural fluid acidosis (pH < 7.2) is noted in RA, while pleural fluid alkalosis (pH > 7.35) is common in SLE (10,11).

Serologic studies of the pleural fluid of SLE patients give characteristic findings. Hemolytic complement is usually depressed in the pleural fluid of SLE. Hunder et al. (12) studied pleural fluids from patients, with SLE, RA, and miscellaneous diseases. In this study, patients with RA or SLE had lower mean values for total hemolytic complement, C1q binding, and levels of C4 and C3. When compared with malignant disease, statistically significant (p < 0.01) differences were found when the total hemolytic complement, C4, and C3 levels were measured. Hunder et al. (12) hypothesized that increased complement consumption occurred in pleural effusions of SLE patients. Halla et al. (13) studied immune complexes from pleural effusions of nine SLE and twelve RA patients. Using several different assays, higher frequencies of immune complexes in RA pleural fluids than in SLE were seen. Additionally, RA pleural fluids had higher mean levels of immune complexes than did RA sera. Interestingly, there was no significant difference in SLE immune complexes in pleural fluid as compared to SLE sera. Thus the levels of immune complexes in pleural fluid in these diseases may be governed by different mechanisms (see Table 1, Chap. 1).

In comparing the utility of the lupus erythematosus (LE) cell and antinuclear antibody (ANA) as serologic tests for SLE, the LE cell is more specific while the ANA is more sensitive. The ANA is used most commonly to diagnose SLE. Several researchers have searched for LE cells and ANA in the pleural fluids of patients with idiopathic SLE or drug-induced LE. LE cells have been found infrequently (14,15) in the pleural fluid of SLE, suggesting that a search for LE cells in body effusions may only be helpful in the early or difficult diagnostic case (16).

Pleural fluid ANA was detected by Hunder et al. (12) in five of five SLE patients, but not in four patients with RA. A positive serum ANA was also noted in all five SLE patients. Chandrasekhar et al. (17) studied three patients with procainamide-induced SLE and found ANA in pleural fluids in all three patients but none in 33 other pleural effusions of various etiology. Leechawengwong et al. (18) detected pleural fluid ANA in seven patients of 100 consecutive patients with pleural effusions. All seven patients had positive serum ANAs. Although six patients were diagnosed with SLE and one was diagnosed with drug-induced SLE, only four of the seven cases reported met at least four ARA criteria for SLE. These findings may represent passive diffusion of ANA from serum into the pleural cavity.

Serum antibodies to double-stranded DNA (ds-DNA) are specific for SLE. Their presence in the pleural fluid may be helpful in differentiating pleural effusion secondary to SLE from other causes. Riska et al. (19) studied 53 pleural effusions and found that 10 were positive for antibodies to ds-DNA by a modified Farr technique (> 5 mg/l). The results included high levels of antibodies to ds-DNA in pleural fluids from five of five patients with SLE, four with lung cancer, and one with pulmonary tuberculosis. It should be noted that all patients with SLE in this study had serum values of ds-DNA antibodies that correlated with pleural fluid values. Wysenbeek et al. (20) reported an isolated case of eosinophilic pleural effusion in SLE with no detectable ds-DNA antibodies in the serum, but moderately high levels (29%) in the pleural fluid. The role of DNA-anti-DNA complexes in the pathogenesis of the pleuritis/pleural effusion of SLE is unknown.

In each patient, data should be collected which would ascertain the etiology of the pleural effusion and specifically determine if infection is present. The measurement of complement, ANA, and antibodies to ds-DNA should not be done routinely in the evaluation of pleural fluid from SLE patients. Our approach to the evaluation of pleural fluids is fully described in the section at the end of this chapter in which we discuss the management of the pleuropulmonary complications of SLE.

Nonsteroidal anti-inflammatory drugs and corticosteroids frequently provide an effective treatment for the syndrome of pleuritis/pleural effusion in SLE. It is important to note that treatment should be started only after infection and other causes of pleuritis/pleural effusion have been excluded (21).

II. Acute Lupus Pneumonitis

Acute lupus pneumonitis (ALP) is an abrupt febrile pneumonic process in an SLE patient without an infectious etiology. Matthay et al. (22) reported 12 patients, representing 11.7% of 102 patients with SLE, followed over a six year period. Of these 12 patients, six presented with ALP at the time of diagnosis of SLE. The clinical presentation was found to resemble an infectious pneumonic process with high fever, dyspnea, tachypnea, tachycardia, and cyanosis. Physical findings included only bibasilar rales in most cases. CXR findings included patchy areas of increased density, focal atelectasis, chronic interstitial infiltrates and diaphragmatic elevation. The lesions noted on CXR were most often found at the lung bases. Therapy included corticosteroids and supplemental oxygen. The more acutely ill patients received azathioprine. The mortality rate was 50%. Of the six patients who died, three had respiratory failure, one had a superimposed infection due to Nocardia, one had CNS vascular thrombosis and another had multiple pulmonary emboli. Chronic interstitial infiltrate was noted on CXR of three of the six surviving patients. All surviving patients demonstrated evidence of a persistent, restrictive ventilatory defect with a diminished diffusing capacity of carbon monoxide (DLCO).

Carett et al. (23) presented information regarding the incidence of ALP. They reported the sudden development of diffuse pulmonary infiltrates in 8 of 400 patients with SLE. Etiologic factors in their population included infection due to *Pneumocystis carinii* in one patient, congestive heart failure in one patient, and pulmonary hemorrhage in six patients. In two of these six patients with pulmonary hemorrhage, SLE was considered the only factor responsible for the hemorrhage. In the remaining patients, a combination of factors including uremia and coagulopathy, as well as congestive heart failure were implicated in addition to SLE. The findings on chest roentgenograph, as well as lung biopsy were nonspecific in all eight patients.

The pathophysiologic mechanisms responsible for the development of ALP are poorly understood. Autopsies of four of the patients in Matthay's series showed acute alveolar damage with interstitial edema and hyaline membrane formation. Acute alveolitis was present in two patients. None of the lung specimens demonstrated vasculitis. Pertschuk et al. (24) analyzed pulmonary tissue from eight patients with ALP related to SLE. Although light microscopy findings were found to be nonspecific, direct immunofluorescence demonstrated focally bound immunoglobulins and complement within pleural and/or pneumocyte nuclei in each case. Inoue et al. (25) demonstrated deposits of IgG, C3, and DNA along the alveolar walls by direct immunofluorescence in two patients with ALP. Granular deposits of IgG were noted in the interstitium of alveolar walls and along the alveolar capillary walls by immunoperoxidase studies. Lung tissue analysis by elution studies showed ANA in one patient and anti-DNA in both patients. Electron-dense deposits in alveolar walls and alveolar capillary walls were noted on electron microscopy. These data suggest that the pathogenesis of ALP may directly be related to the deposition of immune complexes in pulmonary tissue.

Differentiation between ALP and infectious pneumonia is frequently not possible on clinical grounds. All pulmonary infiltrates in SLE should be considered infectious in etiology until proven otherwise. If a definite diagnosis is not obtained after initial evaluation, additional studies such as bronchoalveolar lavage and/or transbronchial biopsy with brushing to rule out the presence of infection should be considered (see Chaps. 5 and 7). An open lung biopsy is frequently deemed more appropriate because of its greater diagnostic sensitivity. The decision when choosing between the transbronchial or open approach to a biopsy should be made based on the severity of the illness and general medical status of the patient. Broad-spectrum antibiotics as well as high-dose corticosteroids should be considered pending the outcome of diagnostic studies. A rational approach to the management of SLE-related pleuropulmonary problems is presented in the final section of this chapter.

III. Diffuse Interstitial Lung Disease

In addition to acute lupus pneumonitis, a more chronic pneumonic process occurs in SLE. It is characterized by progressive dyspnea, cough, bibasilar rales, diffuse interstitial infiltrates and a restrictive defect with reduced diffusing capacity on pulmonary function testing (PFT).

The radiographic and clinical descriptions of diffuse interstitial lung disease have been infrequently reported despite the fact that interstitial pneumonitis has been found in 56-98% of cases in large autopsy studies in patients with SLE (8,26). Ellman (27) described interstitial fibrosis in SLE which was believed to be similar to the Hamman-Rich syndrome. Grennan et al. (28), Estes and Christian (29), and Haupt et al. (30), reported cases of interstitial fibrosis attributed to SLE after exclusion of other possible etiologies.

Eisenberg et al. (31) studied 18 patients with SLE with diffuse interstitial lung infiltrates. Of these patients, 39% presented with pulmonary symptoms, 69% had a productive cough, 44% had a unilaterally elevated diaphragm, 66% had pleuritis, 66% had basilar rales, and all had dyspnea on exertion. All had diffuse interstitial infiltrates which were linear, reticulonodular, and located predominantly in the lung bases. A restrictive defect with significant reduction in DLCO was noted on pulmonary function testing. No patients had any evidence of airway obstruction. In four cases with detailed histopathology, focal fibrosis consistent with organized infarct was present in one while there was evidence of interstitial fibrosis in two. The remaining case demonstrated no evidence of interstitial fibrosis or chronic inflammation but focal epithelial hyperplasia and histiocytic desquamation was documented.

Eisenberg et al. (32) later addressed the potential role of autoimmunity in this process by studying 38 patients with varied causes of acute interstitial disease. Of these 38 patients, eight patients with active interstitial disease associated with RA and SLE demonstrated IgM, IgA, and IgG as well as complement in a diffuse focal pattern in the interstitium. These findings suggested that interstitial lung disease in patients with connective tissue disorders may involve the interaction of immune complexes and complement, and the induction of damage to the interstitium.

Hedgpeth and Boulware (33) described two patients with ANA-negative SLE and interstitial pneumonitis, both demonstrating anti-Ro (SSA) antibodies. Retrospective analysis of 12 patients with SLE and interstitial pneumonitis demonstrated 10 of 12 (83%) had anti-SSA antibodies. These findings suggest the possible association between anti-SSA antibodies and the development of pulmonary interstitial disease in SLE.

No treatment for interstitial pneumonitis in SLE has been proven effective. Attempts at treatment includes corticosteroids, which is often disappointing. Few data are available in evaluating the use of immunosuppressive therapy or plasmapheresis in this disease process. Overall, the prognosis of chronic interstitial lung disease associated with SLE is poor.

IV. Pulmonary Hemorrhage

A relatively uncommon, but often lethal, complication of SLE is massive hemorrhagic pulmonary disease. A total of over 300 patients with SLE studied by Harvey et al. (34), and Dubois and Tuffanelli (35), noted only two patients with significant pulmonary hemorrhage. Only isolated case reports of this clinical entity (36-40) existed prior to 1978. More recently, increasing numbers of reports of small clinical series and isolated case reports with detailed immunopathologic data have expanded our data base regarding pulmonary hemorrhage due to SLE.

Seven patients with SLE and pulmonary hemorrhage were reported by Mintz et al. (41). The patient population were all women with an average duration of SLE of 3.2 years (range, 2-8 years). Signs and symptoms included the acute onset of fever, dyspnea, tachycardia, and blood-tinged sputum that, within hours, progressed to massive hemoptysis and death in all but one. Postmortem examination demonstrated no evidence of vasculitis or other acute inflammatory change. Alveolar hemorrhage was noted. Immunopathologic studies were not performed.

Four cases of SLE, each with one or more episodes of acute respiratory failure secondary to massive pulmonary hemorrhage, were reported by Eagen et al. (42). Hemoptysis was absent in two of the four reported cases. The patients presented with cough, dyspnea, rales, severe hypoxemia, and sudden decreases in hematocrit levels. Pulmonary hemorrhage was suspected on clinical grounds in only two of the four patients reported. Laboratory abnormalities included depressed serum complement and elevated serum cryoglobulins in all patients. Antibodies to ds-DNA were noted in two of four patients. Three patients died from respiratory failure despite aggressive therapy. The sole surviving patient received treatment with intravenous methylprednisolone (1 g every other day) in conjunction with cyclophosphamide. Granular deposition of IgG in the alveolar septa on immunopathologic analysis was noted in all patients. Complement components, chiefly C1q, were found in association with immunoglobulin and immune aggregates in vessel walls of two of four patients.

A well-studied case of a 29-year-old woman with SLE and pulmonary hemorrhage was reported by Churg et al. (43). This patient was successfully treated with large doses of corticosteroids, only to relapse ten months later and again respond to therapy. Open lung biopsy demonstrated granular deposition of IgG in the alveolar septal walls and pulmonary vessels consistent with an immune complex process. Additional findings included widely scattered foci of polymorphonuclear leukocytes in the vessels and alveolar walls. Three patients with SLE and massive pulmonary hemorrhage, two of whom died, were described by Marino and Pertschuk (44). In two of three patients, hemorrhage was clinically unrecognized. All patients had evidence of intraalveolar hemorrhage, with prominent interstitial pneumonitis and mononuclear cell infitlrates on light microscopy. No evidence of immune complexes were noted on immunofluorescence.

Myers and Katzenstein (45) described four patients with SLE and massive pulmonary hemorrhage who underwent open lung biopsies. Acute inflammation and necrosis involving the capillaries, arterioles, and small muscular arteries was demonstrated in all biopsies. Immunofluorescence and electron microscopy demonstrated immune complexes in only two of the four patients. All patients received corticosteroids and three required mechanical ventilation. One patient received cyclophosphamide and plasmapheresis. Two patients demonstrated rapid improvement over the period of 3-4 weeks while two patients succumbed to their pulmonary hemorrhage.

Desnoyers et al. (46) reported a case of a 35-year-old female with SLE who developed acute pulmonary hemorrhage characterized by a nonproductive cough and evidence of an alveolar infiltrate on chest roentgenogram. Additional physical findings included papulovesicular eruption of the fingers, palms, and elbows. The serum creatinine level was 1.0 mg/dl with 2 + proteinuria and RBC casts were noted on urinalysis. Open lung biopsy demonstrated alveolar hemorrhage with no immunoglobulin or complement deposition. There was no evidence of vasculitis of either small or large vessels. Of interest is the fact that both percutaneous renal biopsy and biopsy of the vesiculated skin lesions demonstrated immune complex disease despite the fact that no immune complex deposition was noted in the lung disease. The patient responded to 60 mg of prednisone and was discharged to home shortly after initiation of therapy.

Miller et al. (47) and Ramirez et al. (48) reported a total of nine cases of pulmonary hemorrhage in children with SLE. Presenting symptoms included fever, dyspnea, tachypnea, cough, and malaise. Hemoptysis was noted in six of the nine patients as part of their symptoms complex. Treatment in the five patients reported by Miller et al. (47), was supportive and included the use of mechanical ventilation and immunosuppressives. To date, two of five patients reported are surviving. Of the four patients reported by Ramirez et al. (48), two are surviving with a good response to high dose corticosteroids noted in one of the surviving patients.

Pulmonary hemorrhage is an uncommon but frequently lethal complication of SLE and awareness of this possibility with high degree of clinical suspicion is necessary for prompt recognition since not all patients demonstrate hemoptysis. Massive pulmonary hemorrhage should be considered in any SLE patients with acute onset of respiratory failure in the presence of diffuse pulmonary alveolar infiltrates on CXR. Aggressive treatment, including high doses of corticosteroids, cytotoxic drugs, and plasmapheresis have been tried and have met with varying degrees of success as discussed above. Mortality in acute hemorrhagic pneumonitis approaches 80% despite the use of high-dose corticosteroids and other immunosuppressives. The exact etiology of this disease entity has yet to be determined.

V. Pulmonary Hypertension

Pulmonary artery hypertension can occur as an isolated disease (primary pulmonary hypertension) or in association with several connective tissue diseases including SLE, scleroderma, mixed connective tissue disease and RA (see Chap. 3). Pulmonary hypertension associated with SLE is extremely uncommon both pathologically and clinically.

Baehr et al. (49) studied 23 autopsy cases and found pathologic changes in the pulmonary vasculature as well as right atrial enlargement in four specimens. Necrotizing pulmonary arteritis was reported by Klemperer et al. (50) and Aitchison and Williams (51). Evidence of pulmonary hypertension in 8 of 20 autopsied cases of SLE was found by Fayemi (52). Findings noted included changes consistent with intimal fibrosis, medial hypertrophy, alteration of elastic laminae, periadventitial fibrosis as well as acute changes of fibrinoid necrosis and vasculitis. Arterioles, muscular and elastic arteries, as well as pulmonary veins demonstrated these changes. Both right ventricular hypertrophy and cor pulmonale were absent, leading the authors to hypothesize that either the process was rapid or there was little correlation between pathologic and clinical findings.

The simultaneous existence of pulmonary hypertension and SLE is well documented (53-60). Initial case reports include the 1973 Clinical Pathologic Conference of the *New England Journal of Medicine* (53) and several letters describing additional cases (54,55). Four of 43 cases of SLE in which pulmonary hypertension was the major clinical manifestation were reported by Perez and Kramer (56). Of these four patients, all had clinical signs, symptoms, echocardiographic, and cardiac catheterization findings consistent with pulmonary hypertension. More recently, Stark et al. (57), Schwartzberg et al. (58), and Quismorio et al. (59) described additional patients with both SLE and documented pulmonary hypertension.

A frequent symptom of pulmonary hypertension in SLE is breathlessness despite a normal CXR and the absence of profound hypoxemia. Pulmonary hypertension may therefore help to explain some instances of "unexplained breathlessness" in patients who have not been thoroughly evaluated for the possibility of pulmonary hypertension. Additionally, pulmonary function testing frequently demonstrates a restrictive pattern with reduced DLCO.

Interestingly, extrapulmonic findings, most specifically Raynaud's phenomenon have been found in several reported cases of SLE associated pulmonary hypertension (60). One possibility for the increased incidence of Raynaud's phenomenon is that some of the reported patients may have had an "overlap syndrome" or mixed connective tissue disease.

Treatment for severe pulmonary hypertension may include vasodilator therapy with hydralazine, calcium-channel blockers and/or cytotoxic drugs (59). From a review of the literature, it appears that the effectiveness of these agents is limited and the overall prognosis of severe pulmonary hypertension associated with SLE remains poor.

VI. Diaphragmatic Involvement

Diaphragmatic elevation with progressive loss of lung volume is a well recognized radiographic finding in patients with SLE. This syndrome has been termed the "shrinking" or "vanishing" lung syndrome and is often accompanied by progressive dyspnea in patients with SLE. In fact, Hoffbrand and Beck (61) described breathlessness without obvious cause in 8 of 24 cases of SLE. An elevated diaphragm which did not return to normal, was noted in three of their patients who had more severe dyspnea. Diaphragmatic elevation has been reported by several investigators including Holgate et al. (62) who studied 30 patients with SLE and found seven had unilateral diaphragmatic elevation and four had bilaterally elevated diaphragms. Eisenberg et al. noted that 8 of 18 patients with interstitial lung disease and SLE had unilaterally elevated diaphragms (31). Silberstein et al. found that 5% of 43 SLE patients had unilateral diaphragmatic elevation (63).

Gibson et al. (64) studied 30 consecutive unselected SLE patients of which 16 complained of breathlessness. Of these patients, seven demonstrated diaphragmatic elevation on CXR and in five it was the sole roentgenographic abnormality. Normal CXRs were noted in five of the breathless patients. Further study was performed on seven patients with the most severe volume restriction. Inability to generate normal inspiratory muscle pressures were noted in five of the seven patients. Transdiaphragmatic pressures that were considerably below normal were noted in four patients. It was speculated that a primary myopathy of the diaphragm may offer partial explanation for respiratory abnormality in SLE, especially in cases with the most severe volume restriction.

Rubin and Urowitz (65) reported a 47-year-old white female with SLE who had developed dyspnea and orthopnea during the course of her illness. Her clinical examination was found to be unremarkable, but a CXR revealed a persistently elevated left hemidiaphragm that was found to contract sluggishly when examined under fluoroscopy. Pulmonary function testing revealed a significant restrictive pulmonary defect as well as a diffusion capacity of 60% normal. The patient expired from bronchopneumonia several months later. At postmortem, thinning and fibrosis without active inflammation was seen in both hemidiaphragms. The lung parenchyma showed bilateral bronchopneumonia, minimal interstitial fibrosis, and alveolar hyaline. These findings would support the hypothesis of Gibson et al. (64), that diaphragmatic dysfunction rather than primary intrapulmonary pathology is the major contributing factor in the development of this disorder.

It has not been determined whether immunosuppressive therapy is helpful in improving diaphragmatic function in this subset of SLE patients. We have reported successful treatment of diagphragmatic dysfunction with the use of methylprednisolone pulse (1 g intravenously daily for three consecutive days) in one patient with SLE on two separate occasions (66). Gibson et al. (64) mentioned that even without specific treatment, there appeared to be a favorable prognosis as three of five untreated patients remained stable over four to six years.

VII. Atelectasis

A frequent roentgenographic finding in SLE is atelectasis. First recognized by Rakov and Taylor (67) in 1942 and Foldes (68) in 1946, it has been described frequently in pathologic, roentgenographic and clinical studies of pulmonary aspects of SLE. The linear atelectasis infiltrates are frequently basal and associated with diaphragmatic elevation and pleural effusion. As with the finding of isolated diaphragmatic elevation, the CXR findings of atelectasis alone may be disproportionately severe when compared to clinical manifestations. Pathophysiologic mechanisms of atelectasis related to SLE are poorly understood. Some researchers believe that inflammation in the alveolar walls and of perivascular and peribronchial tissue may be involved while others believe that atelectasis represents intersegmentary effusions present in lung infarction. Other theories include a deficiency of surfactant or persistent pleuritic pain and "splinting" which lead to atelectasis, as frequently seen after abdominal surgery. Specific therapy for the atelectasis associated with SLE has not been defined. Maneuvers aimed at promoting alveolar expansion, such as incentive spirometry, and to promote drainage are frequently used.

VIII. Approach to the Diagnosis and Management of the Pleuropulmonary Complications of SLE

Pulmonary involvement in SLE does not typically present diagnostic or management problems. For example, the most common pulmonary manifestation is pleuritic chest pain and/or pleural effusion. The majority of patients with SLE have mild symptoms of pleuritis or very small pleural effusions, obviating the need for any invasive diagnostic procedure such as thoracentesis or extensive medical management. However, occasionally the patient will present with a massive pleural effusion in which either diagnostic or therapeutic maneuvers are indicated. In these instances we recommend thoracentesis and an occasional pleural biopsy. Routine testing of the fluid should include general studies necessary to determine whether the fluid is an exudate or transudate. Additionally, a comparison of pleural fluid to simultaneous serum glucose is helpful in eliminating an infectious process. However, gram stain and appropriate cultures of the pleural fluid are imperative. Although, immunologic tests of pleural fluid are of academic interest, they do not significantly add to either diagnostic or therapeutic decision making. For example, both ANA and complement are nondiagnostic therefore we do not routinely perform either assay on pleural fluid. While specific, we do not perform either LE cell or anti-DNA assays especially since normal pleural fluid controls are unavailable. Furthermore, the simultaneous presence of both serum and pleural fluid ANA and anti-DNA do not yield any additional diagnostic information. After an exhaustive search of a massive pleural effusion is determined to be secondary to SLE, short-term corticosteroid treatment is usually successful.

The patient presenting with an abrupt, febrile pneumonic process with or without hemorrhage is frequently both a diagnostic dilemma and medical emergency. In a well established SLE patient, the differential diagnosis should include infection until proven otherwise. The majority of patients with acute pneumonitis will require aggressive evaluation. Bronchoalveolar lavage, transbronchial biopsy, and/or an open lung biopsy may be needed. The appropriate procedures should be performed as soon as possible for clarification of the diagnosis. After appropriate laboratory tests (including blood cultures) are obtained, empiric treatment with antibiotics and immunosuppressive agents should be considered as supportive care is continued. After an infectious process is excluded, antibiotics can be safely discontinued. Most of our patients with either acute lupus pneumonitis with or without pulmonary hemorrhage are treated initially with high doses of corticosteroids and an intravenous cytotoxic agent. Occasionally, plasmapheresis is utilized as an adjunct to immunosuppressive therapy.

Diffuse interstitial lung disease in SLE is a relatively uncommon entity characterized by progressive dyspnea, cough, bibasilar rales, and diffuse interstitial infiltrates. We find that many patients with SLE have a restrictive defect with reduced diffusing capacity on pulmonary function testing. A few develop a more chronic and progressive interstitial process. For these patients, we attempt to assess the activity of their disease by performing gallium scanning, bronchial alveolar lavage and transbronchial biopsy (see Chap. 5). An open "lung biopsy is usually not indicated as the initial diagnostic procedure for the majority of SLE patients presenting with interstitial lung disease. If an active inflammatory process is ascertained, based on the above studies, we administer a three-month course of corticosteroids at a dose of 40-60 mg per day. Patients with progressive or refractory disease are then considered for cytotoxic treatment.

On occasion, patients with SLE will demonstrate an elevated diaphragm(s) on CXR. In those patients with "unexplained breathlessness" and elevated diaphragm, we utilize transdiaphragmatic pressure recordings to document diaphragmatic dysfunction. We have utilized pulse intravenous methylprednisolone in successfully treating this lung syndrome.

While atelectasis is a frequent roentgenographic finding in SLE, we are not convinced of any pathologic relationship to the pulmonary disease process in SLE. Therefore, we do not specifically treat this roentgenographic manifestation.

References

1. Tan, E. M., Cohen, A. S., Fries, J. F., Masi, A. T., McShane, D. J., Rothfield, N. F., Schaller, J. G., Talal, N., and Winchester, R. J. (1982). The 1982 revised criteria for the classification of systemic lupus erythematosus. *Arthritis Rheum.* **25**:1271-1277.
2. Rothfield, N. F. (1981). Clinical features of systemic lupus erythematosus. In *Textbook of Rheumatology.* Edited by W. N. Kelley, E. D. Harris Jr., S. Ruddy, et al. Philadelphia, W.B. Saunders, p. 1109.
3. Davis, P., Atkins, B., Jesse, R. G., and Hughes, R. V. (1973). Criteria for classification of SLE. *Br. Med. J.* **3**:88-89.
4. Trimble, R. B., Townes, A. S., Robinson, H., Kaplan, S. B., Chandler, R. W., Hanissian, A. S., and Masi, A. T. (1974). Preliminary criteria for the classification of systemic lupus erythematosus (SLE): Evaluation in early diagnosed SLE and rheumatoid arthritis. *Arthritis Rheum.* **17**:184-188.

5. Rothfield, N. F. (1981). Clinical features of systemic lupus erythematosus. In *Textbook of Rheumatology*. Edited by W. N. Kelley, E. D. Harris Jr., S. Ruddy, et al. Philadelphia, W.B. Saunders, p. 1124.
6. Bulgrin, J. G., Dubois, E. L., and Jacobson, G. (1960). Chest roentgenographic changes in systemic lupus erythematosus. *Radiology* **74**: 42-49.
7. Ropes, M. W. (1976). Characteristics, manifestations, and pathologic findings. In *Systemic Lupus Erythematosus*, vol. 1, ed. 1. Cambridge MA, Harvard University, p. 54.
8. Purnell, D. C., Baggenstoss, A. H., and Olsen, A. M. (1955). Pulmonary lesions in disseminated lupus erythematosus. *Ann. Intern. Med.* **42**:619-628.
9. Carr, D. T., Lillington, G. A., and Mayne, J. G. (1970). Pleural fluid glucose in systemic lupus erythematosus. *Mayo Clin. Proc.* **45**:409-412.
10. Potts, D. E., Willcox, M. A., Good, J. T. Jr., Taryle, D. A., and Saha, S. A. (1978). The acidosis of low-glucose in pleural effusions. *Am. Rev. Respir. Dis.* **117**:665-671.
11. Taryle, D. A., Good, J. T. Jr., and Sahn, S. A. (1979). Acid generation by pleural fluid: Possible role in the determination of pleural fluid pH. *J. Lab. Clin. Med.* **93**:1041-1046.
12. Hunder, G. G., McDuffie, F. C., and Hepper, N. G. G. (1972). Pleural fluid complement in systemic lupus erythematosus and rheumatoid arthritis. *Ann. Intern. Med.* **76**:357-363.
13. Halla, J. T., Schronhenloher, R. E., and Volanakis, J. E. (1980). Immune complexes and other laboratory features of pleural effusions: A comparison of rheumatoid arthritis, systemic lupus erythematosus, and other diseases. *Ann. Intern. Med.* **92**:748-752.
14. Pandya, M. R., Agus, B., and Grady, R. F. (1976). In vivo LE phenomenon in pleural fluid. *Arthritis Rheum.* **19**:962-963.
15. Carel, R. S., Shapiro, M. S., Shokram, D., and Gutman, A. (1977). Lupus erythematosus cells in pleural effusion: The initial manifestation of procainamide-induced lupus erythematosus. *Chest* **72**:670-672.
16. Carel, R. S., Shapiro, M. S., Cordoba, O., et al. (1979). LE cells in pleural fluid. *Arthritis Rheum.* **22**:936-937.
17. Chandrasekhar, A., Robinson, J., and Barr, L. (1977). Antibody deposition in the pleura: A finding in drug induced lupus. *Chest* **72**:397.
18. Leechawengwong, M., Berger, H. W., and Sukumaran, M. (1979). Diagnostic significance of antinuclear antibodies in pleural effusion. *Mt. Sinai J. Med.* **46**:137-139.
19. Riska, H., Fyhrquist, F., Selander, R. K., and Hellstrom, P. E. (1978). Systemic lupus erythematosus and DNA antibodies in pleural effusion. *Scand. J. Rheum.* **7**:159-160.

20. Wysenbeek, A. J., Pick, A. I., Sella, A., Beigel, Y., and Yeshurun, D. (1980). Eosinophilic pleural effusion with high anti-DNA activity as manifestation of systemic lupus erythematosus. *Postgrad. Med. J.* **56**: 57-58.
21. Hunninghake, G. W., and Fauci, A. S. (1979). Pulmonary involvement in the collagen vascular diseases. *Am. Rev. Respir. Dis.* **119**:471-503.
22. Matthay, R. A., Schwarz, M. I., Petty, T. L., Stanford, R. E., Gupta, R. C., Sahn, S. A., and Steigerwald, J. C. (1975). Pulmonary manifestations of systemic lupus erythematosus: Review of twelve cases of acute lupus pneumonitis. *Medicine* **54**:397-409.
23. Carett, S., Macher, A. M., Nussbaum, A., and Plotz, P. H. (1984). Severe, acute pulmonary disease in patients with systemic lupus erythematosus: 10 years experience at the National Institutes of Health. *Semin. Arthritis Rheum.* **14**:52-59.
24. Pertschuk, L. P., Moccia, L. F., Rosen, Y., Lyons, H., Marino, C. M., Rashford, A. A., and Wollschlager, C. M. (1977). Acute pulmonary complications in systemic lupus erythematosus: Immunofluorescence and light microscopic study. *Am. J. Clin. Pathol.* **68**:553-557.
25. Inoue, T., Kanayama, Y., Ohe, A., Kato, N., Horiguchi, T., Ishii, M., and Shiota, K. (1979). Immunopathologic studies of pneumonitis in systemic lupus erythematosus. *Ann. Intern. Med.* **91**:30-34.
26. Gross, M., Esterly, J. R., and Earle, R. H. (1972). Pulmonary alterations in systemic lupus erythematosus. *Am. Rev. Respir. Dis.* **105**:572-577.
27. Ellman, P. (1958). Discussion on the lungs as an index of systemic disease. *Proc. Roy. Soc. Med.* **51**:654.
28. Grennan, D. M., Howie, A. D., Moran, F., and Buchanan, W. W. (1978). Pulmonary involvement in systemic lupus erythematosus. *Ann. Rheum. Dis.* **37**:536-539.
29. Estes, D., and Christian, C. L. (1971). The natural history of systemic lupus erythematosus by prospective analysis. *Medicine* **50**:85-95.
30. Haupt, H. M., Moore, G. W., and Hutchins, G. M. (1981). The lung in systemic lupus erythematosus: Analysis of the pathologic changes in 120 patients. *Am. J. Med.* **71**:791-798.
31. Eisenberg, H., Dubois, E. L., Sherwin, R. P., and Balchum, O. J. (1973). Diffuse interstitial lung disease in systemic lupus erythematosus. *Ann. Intern. Med.* **79**:37-45.
32. Eisenberg, H., Simmons, D. H., and Barnett, E. V. (1979). Diffuse pulmonary interstitial disease: An immunohistologic study. *Chest* **75**:262-264.
33. Hedgpeth, M., and Boulware, D. (1988). Interstitial pneumonitis in antinuclear antibody-negative systemic lupus erythematosus, a new clinical

manifestation and possible association with Anti-Ro (SS-A) antibodies. *Arthritis Rheum.* **31**:545-548.

34. Harvey, A. M., Shulman, L. E., Tumulty, P. A., Lockard Conley, C., and Schoenrich, E. H. (1954). Systemic lupus erythematosus: Review of the literature and clinical analysis of 138 cases. *Medicine* **33**:291-437.

35. Dubois, E. L., and Tuffanelli, D. C. (1964). Clinical manifestations of systemic lupus erythematosus. *JAMA* **190**:104-111.

36. Elliott, M. L., and Kuhn, C. (1973). Idiopathic pulmonary hemosiderosis: Ultrastructural abnormalities in the capillary walls. *Am. Rev. Respir. Dis.* **102**:895-904.

37. Gould, D. B., and Soriano, R. Z. (1975). Acute alveolar hemorrhage in lupus erythematosus. *Ann. Intern. Med.* **83**:836-837.

38. Kuhn, C. (1972). Systemic lupus erythematosus in a patient with ultrastructural lesions of the pulmonary capillaries previously reported in the *Review* as due to idiopathic pulmonary hemosiderosis. *Am. Rev. Respir. Dis.* **106**:931-932.

39. Lewis, E. J., Schur, P. H., Busch, G. J., Galvanek, E., and Merrill, J. P. (1973). Immunopathologic features of a patient with glomerulonephritis and pulmonary hemorrhage. *Am. J. Med.* **54**:507-513.

40. Menchaca, J. A., Boris, G., and Wilson, C. B. (1976). Pulmonary hemorrhage: Unusual manifestation of systemic lupus erythematosus. *Kidney Int.* **10**:505.

41. Mintz, G., Galindo, L. F., Fernandez-Diez, J., Jimenez, F. J., Robles-Saavedra, E., and Enriquez-Casillas, R. D. (1978). Acute massive pulmonary hemorrhage in systemic lupus erythematosus. *J. Rheumatol.* **5**:39-50.

42. Eagen, J. W., Memoli, V. A., Roberts, J. L., Matthew, G. R., Schwartz, M. M., and Lewis, E. J. (1978). Pulmonary hemorrhage in systemic lupus erythematosus. *Medicine* **57**:545-560.

43. Churg, A., Franklin, W., Chan, K. L., Kopp, E., and Carrington, C. B. (1980). Pulmonary hemorrhage and immune-complex deposition in the lung: complications in a patient with systemic lupus erythematosus. *Arch. Pathol. Lab. Med.* **104**:388-391.

44. Marino, C. T., and Pertschuk, L. P. (1981). Pulmonary hemorrhage in systemic lupus erythematosus. *Arch. Intern. Med.* **141**:201-203.

45. Myers, J. L., and Katzenstein, A. A. (1986). Microangiitis in lupus-induced pulmonary hemorrhage. *Am. J. Clin. Pathol.* **85**:552-556.

46. Desnoyers, M. R., Burnstien, S., Cooper, A. G., and Kopelman, R. I. (1984). Pulmonary hemorrhage in lupus erythematosus without evidence of an immunologic cause. *Arch. Intern. Med.* **144**:1398-1400.

47. Miller, R. W., Salcedo, J. R., Think, R. J., Murphy, T. M., and Magilavy, D. B. (1986). Pulmonary hemorrhage in pediatric patients with systemic lupus erythematosus. *J. Pediatr.* **108**:576-579.

48. Ramirez, R. E., Glasier, C., Kirks, D., Shackelford, G. D., and Locey, M. (1984). Pulmonary hemorrhage associated with systemic lupus erythematosus in children. *Radiology* 152:409-412.
49. Baehr, G., Klemperer, P., and Schifrin, A. (1935). A diffuse disease of the peripheral circulation (usually associated with lupus erythematosus and endocarditis). *Trans. Assoc. Am. Physicians* 50:139-155.
50. Klemperer, P., Pollack, A. D., and Baehr, G. (1941). Pathology of disseminated lupus erythematosus. *Arch. Pathol.* 32:569-631.
51. Aitchison, J. D., and Williams, A. W. (1956). Pulmonary changes in disseminated lupus erythematosus. *Ann. Rheum. Dis.* 15:26-32.
52. Fayemi, A. O. (1976). Pulmonary vascular disease in systemic lupus erythematosus. *Am. J. Clin. Pathol.* 65:284-290.
53. Castleman, B., Scully, R. E., and McNeely, B. V. (1973). Case records of the Massachusetts General Hospital (Case 4-1973). *N. Engl. J. Med.* 288:204-210.
54. Sergent, J. S., and Lockshin, M. D. (1973). Primary pulmonary hypertension and SLE. *N. Engl. J. Med.* 288:1078.
55. Cummings, P. (1973). Primary pulmonary hypertension and SLE. *N. Engl. J. Med.* 288:1078-1079.
56. Perez, H. D., and Kramer, N. (1981). Pulmonary hypertension in systemic lupus erythematosus: Report of four cases and review of the literature. *Semin. Arthritis Rheum.* 11:177-181.
57. Stark, P., Sargent, E. N., Boylen, T., and Jaramillo, D. (1987). Pulmonary arterial hypertension as a manifestation of lupus erythematosus. *Radiologe* 27:370-374.
58. Schwartzberg, M., Lieberman, D. H., Getzoff, B., and Ehrlich, G. E. (1984). Systemic lupus erythematosus and pulmonary vascular hypertension. *Arch. Intern. Med.* 144:605-607.
59. Quismorio, F. P., Sharma, O., Koss, M., Boylen, T., Edmiston, A. W., Thornton, P. H., and Tatter, D. (1984). Immunopathologic and clinical studies in pulmonary hypertension associated with systemic lupus erythematosus. *Semin. Arthritis Rheum.* 13:349-359.
60. Nair, S. S., Askari, A. D., Popelka, C. G., and Kleinerman, J. F. (1980). Pulmonary hypertension and systemic lupus erythematosus. *Arch. Intern. Med.* 140:109-111.
61. Hoffbrand, B. I., and Beck, E. R. (1965). "Unexplained" dyspnoea and shrinking lungs in systemic lupus erythematosus. *Br. Med. J.* I: 1273-1277.
62. Holgate, S. T., Glass, D. N., Haslam, P., Maini, R. N., and Turner-Warwick, M. (1976). Respiratory involvement in systemic lupus erythematosus: A clinical and immunological study. *Clin. Exp. Immunol.* 24: 385-395.

63. Silberstein, S. L., Barland, P., Grayzel, A. I., and Koerner, S. K. (1980). Pulmonary dysfunction in systemic lupus erythematosus: Prevalence, classification and correlation with organ involvement. *J. Rheumatol.* **7**:187-195.

64. Gibson, G. J., Edmonds, J. P., and Hughes, G. R. V. (1977). Diaphragm function and lung involvement in systemic lupus erythematosus. *Am. J. Med.* **63**:926-932.

65. Rubin, L. A., and Urowitz, M. B. (1983). Shrinking lung syndrome in systemic lupus erythematosus—a clinical pathologic study. *J. Rheumatol.* **10**:973-976.

66. Segal, A. M., Calabrese, L. H., Ahmad, M., Tubbs, R. R., and White, C. S. (1985). The pulmonary manifestations of systemic lupus erythematosus. *Semin. Arthritis Rheum.* **14**:202-224.

67. Rakov, H. L., and Taylor, J. S. (1942). Acute disseminated lupus erythematosus without cutaneous manifestations and with heretofore underscribed pulmonary lesions. *Arch. Intern. Med.* **70**:88-100.

68. Foldes, J. (1946). Acute systemic lupus erythematosus. *Am. J. Clin. Pathol.* **16**:160-173.

10

Systemic Sclerosis

VIRGINIA D. STEEN

University of Pittsburgh
Pittsburgh, Pennsylvania

I. Introduction

The lung is commonly involved in systemic sclerosis (scleroderma). Early investigators were aware of lung disease in scleroderma, although they frequently attributed breathing difficulty to restriction of the chest wall due to cutaneous thickening (1,2). Others felt pulmonary symptoms were secondary to the pulmonary fibrosis found at autopsy (3-5), but they did not relate the fibrosis to scleroderma. Von Notthafft in 1898 and Matsui in 1924 performed careful pathologic studies of the lung in scleroderma, describing both parenchymal fibrotic changes and vascular derangements which they felt were directly caused by scleroderma (6,7). In the 1940s the roentgenographic features of pulmonary involvement (8) and detailed physiologic studies of pulmonary function were first reported (9). Research in the past 40 years has vastly increased our knowledge and understanding of lung involvement in systemic sclerosis (10).

II. Clinical Features

Early studies found pulmonary symptoms to be infrequent. Lewin and Heller found only 6 of 509 scleroderma patients who were symptomatic (5). A more recent review (11) claimed that some evidence of pulmonary involvement was detectable in almost all scleroderma patients. Pulmonary symptoms are rarely the presenting complaint. However, individual cases have been reported in which dyspnea was the presenting symptom occurring prior to skin thickening (12-14). In our series of 1,088 consecutive systemic sclerosis patients seen at the University of Pittsburgh since 1972, only 1% had dyspnea, cough, or roentgenographic evidence of pulmonary fibrosis as an initial manifestation.

Dyspnea, particularly on exertion, is a common manifestation of lung involvement, observed in 21-80% of patients in various series (14-16). There is frequently a lack of correlation between symptoms, chest radiographs, and physiologic tests (17-19). In our series, dyspnea was present in 71% of patients with evidence of fibrosis on chest radiograph and restrictive lung disease by pulmonary function testing (17). In contrast, dyspnea was also present in 29% of patients without any evidence of lung involvement—i.e., normal chest radiograph and normal pulmonary function tests. Some patients had no pulmonary symptoms although they had objective evidence of lung disease.

In our Pittsburgh population (Table 1), 42% of patients had dyspnea on exertion at first evaluation and an additional 20% acquired this symptom at some time later in their illness. For most patients dyspnea is mild and does not interfere with daily activities. The presence of dyspnea does not predict a rapidly downhill course, as reported earlier (20), and many patients

Table 1 Clinical Features of Pulmonary Involvement in Systemic Sclerosis

	Pittsburgh scleroderma data base (n = 1,088)	
	Present at first evaluation	Developed during follow-up
Symptoms		
Dyspnea	49%	21%
Dyspnea at rest	5%	10%
Cough	11%	18%
Pleuritic chest pain	12%	9%
Physical findings		
Bibasilar rales	26%	22%
Pleural rubs	4%	5%

have stable symptoms for years without significant progression of their lung disease (21). However, a small proportion of patients progress to develop dyspnea at rest with significant hypoxemia. Severe pulmonary fibrosis, pulmonary arterial hypertension, or myocardial failure may lead to severe respiratory disability.

The cause of dyspnea in most patients is related to the loss of compliance of the lung itself from the pulmonary fibrosis rather than restriction from chest wall skin thickening (22). The interstitial fibrotic process may also lead to a reflex hyperpnea (23), as it is thought to do in other forms of interstitial lung disease. Pleural disease alone may cause dyspnea in a few patients, and myopathy of the diaphragm or intercostal muscles may rarely lead to hyperpnea (24,25). Reduced gas exchange and resultant dyspnea are more closely correlated pathologically with pulmonary vascular changes than the degree of fibrosis (26).

Cough occurs much less frequently and is usually nonproductive. The most refractory instances of cough are in association with severe pulmonary fibrosis. Bacterial infections or bronchiectasis superimposed on interstitial fibrosis are causes of purulent sputum production. However, Bjerke et al. (27) and Greenwald et al. (21) found cough present in 50% of their scleroderma patients, with smokers more likely to produce sputum. Nineteen percent of the individuals admitted to wheezing, although there was no relation to smoking or large or small airway obstruction (27). Hemoptysis has been associated with bronchial telangiectases (28). In addition, we have now seen eight patients with hemoptysis and pulmonary hemorrhage in the setting of normotensive renal crisis with microangiopathic hemolytic anemia and thrombocytopenia without documented bronchial telangiectases (29).

Pleuritic chest pain is an occasional finding (Table 1) in our Pittsburgh scleroderma population. In contrast, pathologic evidence of pleuritis or pleural effusion occurs far more frequently. It has been noted in 43-86% of patients examined in several autopsy series (14,20,30). Chest pain other than related to pleuropericarditis is distinctly unusual (18). One rare complication causing chest pain is a spontaneous pneumonothorax. This is believed to be caused from a ruptured intrapleural cyst (31).

The most frequent physical examination finding is bibasilar inspiratory rales, heard best at the bases. This sign is highly correlated with pulmonary interstitial fibrosis on chest roentgenogram. It is present only rarely in patients without pulmonary fibrosis on chest radiograph (5%) but is found in more than 50% of patients with fibrosis and restrictive disease (17). Pleural friction rubs are detected in 9% of our patients, frequently but not exclusively in patients with other evidence of pleural disease. Clubbing of digits may occur but seems to be less frequent than in other forms of interstitial fibrosis (14).

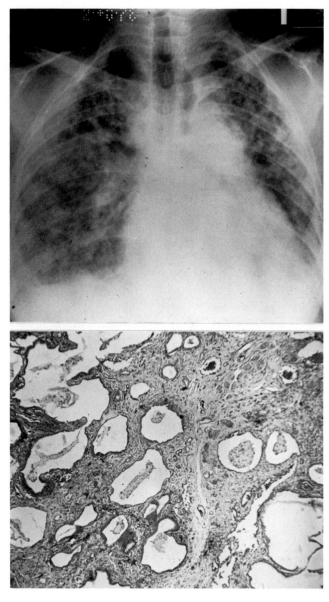

Figure 1   Chest roentgenogram and pulmonary parenchymal histology of a patient with severe pulmonary fibrosis.

III. Roentgenographic Features

The earliest roentgenographic description of pulmonary fibrosis in systemic sclerosis was reported by Murphy et al. in 1941 (8). Most commonly one finds increased fine interstitial markings in the lung bases. Severe fibrosis results in more extensive and denser markings symmetrically in the lower two thirds of the lung. The apices are usually spared. Progression of the disease may lead to a honeycomb pattern of fibrosis, which is indistinguishable from other forms of pulmonary fibrosis. The pattern of fibrosis is most commonly reticulonodular, although reticular and nodular changes alone may be seen (Fig. 1; Table 2).

Radiographic evidence of pleural disease is not found as frequently as pathologic evidence (30). Radiographic pleural thickening and/or pleural effusions are found in 11-56% of patients. Microcalcification of the lung parenchyma were described but believed to be quite rare (32). In our series of 165 nonsmoking systemic sclerosis patients, calcifications or calcified granulomata were found in 67% of patients with the Calcinosis, Raynaud's, Esophageal dysmotility sclerodactyly, Telangiectasia (CREST) syndrome, but in only 14% of patients with diffuse scleroderma (33). However, there was

Table 2 Roentgenographic Findings in 165 Nonsmoking Systemic Sclerosis Patients

	Diffuse scleroderma (n = 77)	CREST syndrome (n = 88)
Pulmonary fibrosis	40%	33%
Severity		
mild	26%	16%
moderate	14%	17%
Pattern		
reticulonodular pattern	35%	18%
reticular pattern	0	10%
nodular pattern	5%	5%
Pulmonary artery enlargement	0	6%
Pleural effusion	7%	11%
Pleural thickening	7%	21%
Calcified granulomata	14%	67%
Superior rib notching	17%	0

Source: Owens et al. (33).

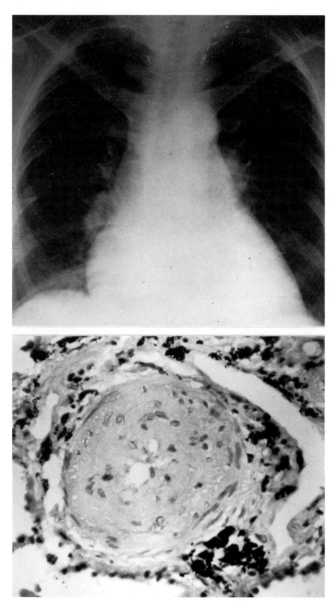

Figure 2   Chest roentgenogram and pulmonary artery histology of a patient who
died with isolated pulmonary hypertension.

no association of these pulmonary calcifications with the presence of more typical peripheral subcutaneous calcifications in these CREST syndrome patients (17). Pulmonary artery enlargement and right heart enlargement can be seen in patients with pulmonary hypertension (Fig. 2). Superior rib notching initially described by Steigerwald et al. (34) appears to be exclusive to patients with diffuse scleroderma and has been identified in 17% of patients with this disease variant (33). Patients with this abnormality frequently have distal phalangeal tuft resorption as well (17). Table 2 summarizes radiographic findings of 165 consecutive nonsmoking systemic sclerosis patients reported by Owens et al. (33).

IV. Pulmonary Function

Physiological studies demonstrating a restrictive pattern in patients with pulmonary fibrosis and systemic sclerosis were first reported by Baldwin et al. in 1947 (9). Since then, numerous studies have confirmed the frequent occurrence of restrictive lung disease in systemic sclerosis, which varies from 30% to 60% depending on the type of patients studied. Extent and duration of disease as well as confounding factors such as smoking, asthma, and congestive heart failure may affect the frequency of abnormalities (11,19,27,35, 36). The best evaluation of pulmonary function abnormalities purely related to systemic sclerosis is Owens' series of 165 consecutive nonsmoking patients without other known lung disease (33). Table 3 summarizes the patterns of pulmonary function abnormalities in this study. Only 33% had entirely normal lung function, and 28% had restrictive lung disease. There were no significant differences in the frequency of restrictive disease, obstructive pattern, or isolated reduction of diffusing capacity in patients with diffuse scleroderma and CREST syndrome.

Table 3 Pulmonary Function Abnormalities in 165 Nonsmoking Systemic Sclerosis Patients

	Diffuse scleroderma (n = 77)	CREST syndrome (n = 88)
Normal	37%	28%
Restrictive	34%	23%
Obstructive	8%	16%
Small airways	3%	7%
Isolated reduction of DLCO	18%	26%

Source: Owens et al. (33).

Obstruction of air flow in scleroderma was reported initially by Spain and Thomas (37), who felt it was related to peribronchial fibrosis. Obstructive disease was considered an unusual and relatively late finding in systemic sclerosis until recently (38,39). Large airway obstruction as manifested by decreased forced expiratory volume in 1 s/forced vital capacity ratio (FEV_1/FVC) is often attributable to smoking. The relatively high prevalence of obstructive abnormalities reported may reflect the effect of smoking (19,35). Nevertheless, an obstructive pattern was found in 8% of diffuse scleroderma patients and 16% of CREST syndrome patients who had never smoked (33), suggesting that it can be due to scleroderma alone. In the more recent series, prolonged disease duration was not associated with obstructive changes, as suggested by earlier investigators. Small airways obstruction independent of smoking, evidenced primarily by a markedly decreased forced expiratory flow rate between 25% and 75% of vital capacity (FEF_{25-75}) with other parameters normal, is another abnormality that may be present in a small proportion of systemic sclerosis patients (33).

Impairment of the diffusing capacity for carbon monoxide (DLCO) is a well-recognized and frequent abnormality in systemic sclerosis (10). DLCO is a function of lung volumes and parallels the severity of restrictive lung disease. It can also accompany obstructive disease (16,19,39). However, an *isolated* reduction in the diffusing capacity in patients with otherwise normal pulmonary function tests occurs commonly and is a sensitive marker in systemic sclerosis (15).

Some authors have felt this was the most sensitive and earliest abnormality of lung function (15,16,20,39,40). Others have found only an infrequent patient with such an isolated abnormality (19,32,38). Owens et al. detected an isolated reduction of DLCO in 24% of their patients (33). These patients did not have early disease, and in many of the limited scleroderma (CREST syndrome) patients disease duration was over 10 years (17). Longitudinal studies show that patients with the isolated reduction in DLCO infrequently progress to serious restrictive lung disease (35,41). Of note, a severe isolated reduction in DLCO (less than 45% predicted normal) is a recognized precursor of isolated pulmonary arterial hypertension (42).

There have been numerous studies trying to determine the natural history of pulmonary involvement in systemic sclerosis (40,43,44). Colp et al. restudied 16 patients 2-8 years after their initial abnormal pulmonary function tests (PFTs) (43). The results remained relatively unchanged over time, and there was less deterioration than in patients with idiopathic pulmonary fibrosis. Bagg and Hughes studied only nine patients but found that PFT abnormalities can occur late in disease and that the overall course is variable (40).

There have been four recent reports of serial pulmonary function tests in systemic sclerosis (21,35,36,45). All authors have found a striking variability in the course of longitudinal pulmonary function abnormalities. Some patients show marked deterioration, others demonstrate impressive improvement, and some may have no changes over time. Thus, because of this substantial variability, no drug-associated improvement can be claimed without an adequate control group (35,36).

In three retrospective studies (35,36,45), there was no greater deterioration in vital capacity or diffusing capacity than one would expect in normal persons in a 3-to-5-year follow-up period. Nor was there a tendency to develop obstructive disease. This is particularly important since in retrospective series one might intuitively suspect that those having repeat testing would have more severe and progressive disease. In the only prospective study by Greenwald et al. (21), there was a twofold greater than expected decline in forced vital capacity and an eightfold greater than expected fall in diffusing capacity independent of smoking. The subset of patients destined to have rapidly progressive and disabling lung disease has not yet been adequately characterized.

Smoking has a deleterious effect on the lung involvement in scleroderma. In addition to the expected increased frequency of obstructive disease, we have also found that patients who smoke and have restrictive lung disease had significantly lower vital capacity and diffusing capacity than otherwise similar patients with restrictive disease who did not smoke. Likewise, smoking patients with an isolated reduction of the DLCO had markedly decreased DLCOs compared to the nonsmoking group with this type of abnormality (17). Schneider et al. found a greater serial decline in lung volumes in his smoking patients than in the nonsmoking ones (36). Similar results have been reported in rheumatoid arthritis (46). Whether the inhalation injury from smoking initiates, aggravates, or contributes independently to the fibrotic process in systemic sclerosis is not known. Alternatively, vasoconstriction due to nicotine may have an additive effect on the vascular changes.

Risk factors for more progressive deterioration in lung function other than smoking include male sex (21), new onset of scleroderma with an initially normal vital capacity (21,35), and severe Raynaud's phenomenon (35). Race, age, and initial degree of pulmonary impairment were unassociated with significant deterioration. Symptoms do not necessarily progress in direct relation to pulmonary function tests (21).

Respiratory failure accounts for a small number of deaths in most series of systemic sclerosis (30,47)—6% of deaths in our experience. Despite the rarity of death due to respiratory failure, the mere presence of lung disease is associated with reduced survival. Medsger et al. (48) identified pulmonary disease as the third most important prognostic feature after renal and cardiac disease, and this has been confirmed by others (49,50). An increased frequency of pneumonia or congestive heart failure in patients with limited pulmonary reserve may account for this finding. Peters-Golden et al. (51) and Steen et al. (17) show similar decreased survival in patients with restrictive or obstructive disease. Likewise, a marked reduction in diffusing capacity, whether associated with pulmonary fibrosis (51) or pulmonary hypertension (42,52), predicts a dismal survival.

V. Pulmonary Arterial Hypertension

Pulmonary arterial hypertension (PHT) is a well-recognized complication in systemic sclerosis. Several series of selected patients undergoing cardiac catheterization have shown that elevated pulmonary artery pressure occurs in 33-67% of patients (22,52,53). Many of these patients had only minimal evidence of pulmonary hypertension, and no follow-up reports of these patients have indicated whether they developed clinically significant pulmonary hypertension. The significance of a mildly elevated pulmonary artery pressure is not known. In an unselected population pulmonary hypertension identified clinically was found in only 9% of 673 systemic sclerosis patients, but there was no attempt to identify patients with marginal elevations in pulmonary artery pressure (42). The true frequency of pulmonary hypertension lies between these two figures but has not yet been accurately determined.

Although pulmonary hypertension (PHT) may certainly develop in the setting of a patient with severe interstitial fibrosis and severe restrictive disease, Sackner et al. found that seven out of eight patients with PHT had only a mild reduction in vital capacity (22). Salerni et al. described the syndrome of isolated pulmonary hypertension in 10 patients with long-standing limited scleroderma (CREST syndrome) and very little or no radiographic or pathologic evidence of pulmonary interstitial fibrosis (54). In a careful autopsy study of the lung in 30 systemic sclerosis patients, eight patients had marked intimal and medial hyperplasia of the pulmonary arteries, five of them had only slight or no interstitial fibrosis and three had a clinical syndrome of "malignant pulmonary hypertension" with a rapidly downhill course (26). This distinct clinical pathologic entity of malignant pulmonary hypertension is akin to that of malignant systemic hypertension from involvement of the renal arteries in diffuse scleroderma patients.

In keeping with the paucity of significant pulmonary fibrosis in PHT, pulmonary functions tests most often show mild or no restrictive disease (42,54). However, the diffusing capacity in such cases is usually severely depressed. Several authors have found that a DLCO less than 45% of the predicted normal was the single most sensitive indicator of pulmonary arterial hypertension (42,52) and a poor prognostic sign (51). It also may be the best predictor of PHT, since six PHT patients had a severely depressed DLCO (mean 44%) 1-6 years prior to the appearance of clinically evident pulmonary hypertension (42). The degree of DLCO reduction is greater in PHT associated with systemic sclerosis than in idiopathic primary PHT. A recent study of 187 patients with primary PHT found a mean DLCO of 69% predicted (73% predicted in females) (55) compared with a mean of 39% in systemic sclerosis patients (42). This difference may be accounted for by the presence of long-standing vascular changes present in systemic sclerosis (56) rather than the more acute plexiform or angiomatoid lesions seen in primary pulmonary hypertension (26).

Systemic sclerosis patients at greatest risk for developing this form of isolated pulmonary hypertension are those with limited scleroderma (or the CREST syndrome). First noted by Trell and Lindstrom (57), Salerni subsequently described 10 CREST syndrome patients with this clinical syndrome (54). Stupi et al. (42) in a large series of CREST syndrome patients identified 9% who had isolated pulmonary hypertension. Another 4% had pulmonary hypertension associated with either severe pulmonary fibrosis or severe cardiac disease. Only 5% of the diffuse scleroderma patients were felt to have PHT, and in none of them was if felt to be isolated PHT. Although anticentromere antibody is highly associated with limited cutaneous scleroderma (CREST syndrome) (58) and is found in patients with PHT, it is not an additional marker in predicting the development of PHT within patients with the CREST syndrome (42). Anti-Scl 70 antibody, which is associated with pulmonary interstitial fibrosis (59,60), has not been found in any of our patients with isolated pulmonary hypertension, although it may be associated with PHT secondary to pulmonary fibrosis.

The natural history of this type of isolated pulmonary hypertension in systemic sclerosis is almost always one of continued deterioration and death within 5 years. Patients with severe pulmonary fibrosis (forced vital capacity less than 55% predicted) and secondary pulmonary hypertension also have a decreased survival. However, as Figure 3 shows, isolated PHT has the worst prognosis. Numerous vasodilators have been unsuccessful in altering survival. It seems likely that structural changes in pulmonary arteries are more important than the vasospastic contribution (26,56). The natural history of patients with mildy increased pulmonary artery pressures on cardiac catheterization is unknown. Our recent autopsy study of the morphometry of pulmonary arteries in scleroderma demonstrates that significant thickening of pulmonary arteries occurs in CREST syndrome patients prior to development of clinical pulmonary hypertension (56). Further pathophysiologic and therapeutic studies are needed in the subset of patients with CREST syndrome and a severely reduced diffusing capacity.

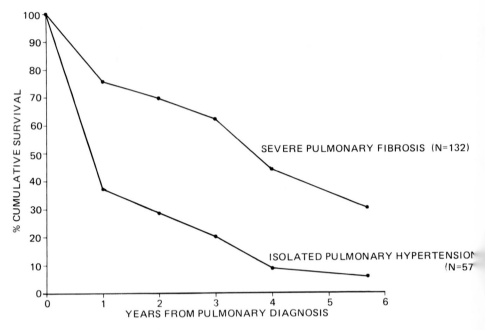

Figure 3 Cumulative survival rates of 132 patients with severe pulmonary fibrosis and 57 patients with isolated pulmonary hypertension.

VI. Pathogenesis

The etiology of systemic sclerosis is unknown. There have been several environmental and occupational exposures that have been implicated as potential causes of sclerodermalike illnesses (61). These include vinyl chloride (62), rapeseed oil (63), epoxy resins (64), silicone (65), and carbidoba (66), which cause a sclerodermalike illness. Workers exposed to gold dust (67) and silica (68) have an exceptionally high prevalence of systemic sclerosis. Several reports of scleroderma from exposure to solvents including trichlorethylene (69), a perchlorethylene (70), are particularly interesting. One recent report described two men with exposure to metaphenylenediamine (71) who had moderate to severe pulmonary fibrosis. Although chemically induced scleroderma may account for only a small number of cases, the recognition of these syndromes may ultimately lead to improved understanding of the pathogenesis of the disease.

A variety of nonpulmonary etiologies of lung involvement in systematic sclerosis have been suggested without convincing support. These include skin thickening of the thorax (37), sclerodermatous fibrosis of the diaphragm (24,25), and chronic aspiration from esophageal dysmotility and reflux (72). These may enhance or aggravate pulmonary fibrosis, just as there is a deletarious effect from smoking. However, intrinsic lung pathophysiologic abnormalities appear to be the most plausible explanation for tissue damage. Recent research in pulmonary fibrosis and pulmonary hypertension in scleroderma is directed at the two theories underlying the pathogenesis of entire disease—i.e., the immunologic and vascular theories. Although it is not known whether the fibrotic process in the lung is similar to that occuring in the skin and other organs in scleroderma, it is possible that research efforts in the lung will lead to an overall understanding of systemic sclerosis.

Pulmonary fibrosis is the most common pathologic finding in the lung with the bases most strikingly involved (Fig. 1). Early changes include edema and widening and hypercellularity of the alveolar walls (20), leading to diffuse alveolar fibrosis and obliteration of capillaries. In the most severe stages extensive interstitial fibrosis, peribronchial fibrosis, and derangement of lung tissue with cystic changes occur. Although few studies have demonstrated striking inflammatory change, alveolitis may be the first step of the fibrotic process, as is hypothesized for other interstitial lung diseases (73). The current concepts of the pathophysiology of pulmonary fibrosis are reviewed in Chapter 1.

Gallium scanning, a noninvasive technique of monitoring alveolitis, has been abnormal in more than half of the systemic sclerosis patients studied (74-78). Most studies have been unable to show any correlation with disease duration, pulmonary symptoms, chest roentgenograms, or pulmonary function tests. However, in one study, gallium scan positivity closely correlated with symptoms of recent onset (78). Gallium scan positivity is thought to represent an increase in pulmonary-activated alveolar macrophages, which may contribute to the fibrotic process (73).

Bronchoalveolar lavage (BAL), another method of evaluating alveolitis in interstitial lung diseases, has been reported in a number of studies in systemic sclerosis (Table 4). Abnormalities have been observed frequently (44-93%), but, unlike idiopathic pulmonary fibrosis, which is characterized by a high proportion of neutrophils and sarcoidosis in which lymphocytes are significantly increased, no consistent pattern for the differential cell count was found in scleroderma patients (76-81). Increased lymphocytes (76,80), neutrophils (77-81), and eosinophils (77-79,81) have all been found. In two studies, lung biopsy confirmed the BAL findings of alveolitis (77,82).

Generally, BAL results have not correlated particularly well with the degree of pulmonary involvement except for an association of neutrophils (82) and macrophages (78) with decreased DLCO.

Table 4 Results of Bronchoalveolar Lavage in Systemic Sclerosis

	Silver (79) (n = 24)	Konig (80) (n = 20)	Edelson (76) (n = 25)	Rossi (77) (n = 11)	Owens (78) (n = 14)	Pesci (81) (n = 7)
Abnormal results	60%	45%	44%		93%	86%
Cell type						
Macrophage						
Neutrophil	↑↑	↑		↑	↑	
Lymphocyte		↑	↑↑		↑	↑
Eosinophil	↑			↑	↑	↑
Other findings	↑Immune complexes	↑Collagenase activity	↑Release of interleukin 1	↑Fibronectin ↑AMDGF[a]		CREST syndrome patients

[a]AMDGF = alveolar macrophage-derived growth factor.

The significance and relationship of these BAL abnormalities to the pathogenesis of lung disease in scleroderma are unknown. It is possible that these inflammatory changes may only be a secondary process, that of a reparative nature rather than an initiating injury (83), or that they could lead to endothelial cell damage. However, increased immunoglobulins (82), immune complexes (79), collagenase activity (80), enhanced release of interleukin 1 (76), fibronectin, and alveolar macrophage-derived growth factor (77,84) have all been found in BAL fluid. These observations have led to a variety of theories concerning the etiology of the fibrotic process in scleroderma. Further investigations and a better understanding of these findings are necessary before BAL can be used routinely in the clinical setting.

Immunologic abnormalities found in the sera of patients with serious lung involvement also support the "immunologic" theories of pathogenesis. Pisko et al. (85), Furst et al. (74), and Seibold et al. (86) found increased levels of immune complexes in patients with lung disease. Several authors have detected an increased frequency of anti-Scl-70 antibody in patients with pulmonary fibrosis (59,60) and a reduced frequency of anticentromere antibody (58). The relationship between these antibodies and the pathogenesis of lung disease is unknown.

The suggestion of "visceral" Raynaud's phenomenon in the kidney (87) and heart (88) has led to the question of a similar occurrence in the lung. Emmanuel et al. (89) found that the DLCO was lower in the colder months than in the warm months in scleroderma patients. Increases in pulmonary artery pressures during episodes of Raynaud's phenomenon, either spontaneous or cold-induced (90-92), have been observed in patients with pulmonary hypertension. Furst et al. reported evidence of decreased lung perfusion in five of nine patients in response to cold challenge using Krypton lung scanning (74). However, cardiac catheterization in nine scleroderma patients failed to show any evidence of or increased pulmonary artery pressures during cold challenge (93). Diffusing capacity has not been significantly altered by cold challenge in scleroderma patients (94-96), suggesting that they are unable to distend or recruit pulmonary vessels. However, findings in Raynaud's patients without scleroderma have been contradictory, with some patients showing an increased DLCO during cold challenge (94,95) and others with striking decreases in DLCO during cold challenge (96). Different laboratory techniques and patient selection may explain these discrepancies, but no conclusions are justified at this time.

Several authors have suggested that repeated episodes of pulmonary vasospasm may lead to later fixed changes (90,91). Our recent study of the morphometry of pulmonary arteries suggests that the opposite occurs (56). Some patients without evidence of pulmonary hypertension had significantly thickened pulmonary arteries and may be the patients who would exhibit pulmonary Raynaud's. This may be predictive of future pulmonary hypertension. Again, more extensive studies in this group of patients are necessary to understand the pathogenesis of the isolated pulmonary hypertension.

VII. Treatment

There is little evidence that any therapeutic agent significantly alters pulmonary involvement in systemic sclerosis. Corticosteroids have been felt to be ineffective in the pulmonary fibrosis of scleroderma (97), but this lack of response could be due to failure to use them in early disease. When used during an alveolitis stage, corticosteroids have been demonstrated to improve pulmonary function (98), gallium-67 scans (77), and BAL findings (77,90). Prospective studies of patients with early inflammatory pulmonary changes are needed. The majority of patients with pulmonary fibrosis do not have progressive deterioration, and therapeutic intervention may not be necessary.

D-penicillamine has been shown to be associated with a beneficial effect in idiopathic pulmonary fibrosis (99) and in systemic sclerosis (45,100). Although vital capacity did not change in these two studies, there was significant improvement in diffusing capacity. Stabilization of pulmonary symptoms and radiographic findings was also seen in D-penicillamine-treated patients compared to untreated patients (45). The patient with deteriorating pulmonary symptoms and lung function who has no evidence of alveolitis may be a candidate for D-penicillamine therapy, although dramatic improvement in severe restrictive disease should not be anticipated.

Vasodilators have been used in attempts to ameliorate pulmonary hypertension. Numerous reports of vasodilating drugs have suggested that they may be effective (94,101-104), either in the catheterization lab or transiently in the clinical setting. One recent study using very high doses of calcium channel blockers in patients with primary pulmonary hypertension resulted in a significant decrease in pulmonary artery pressure over a 1-year period (105). However, no study has shown a significant alteration in the dismal downhill course of pulmonary hypertension in scleroderma. The severe degree of histologic intimal thickening of pulmonary arteries seen in patients with pulmonary hypertension is not likely to be easily reversed by ordinary amounts of vasodilators. Earlier intervention, prior to the development of fixed arterial changes, with vasodilators or other agents that have the potential to reverse the intimal changes may be more successful in preventing pulmonary hypertension.

VIII. Conclusions

Pulmonary involvement in the form of pulmonary fibrosis, pleural thickening, and pulmonary hypertension is an integral part of systemic sclerosis. A wide spectrum of clinical manifestations occurs. Although the majority of patients have a mild nonprogressive course, some have severe fibrosis and respiratory failure, and others have pulmonary hypertension. Further clinical, pathologic, and serologic studies will be necessary to identify patients at high risk for serious involvement so that appropriate therapeutic intervention can be determined. Recent advances in our understanding of the pathogenesis of interstitial lung disease may help achieve these goals, but it is likely that an understanding of overall disease pathogenesis will be necessary to achieve them fully.

References

1. Day, W. (1870). Case of scleroderma or sclerema with the autopsy and remarks. *Am. J. Med. Sci.* **59**:350-359.
2. Finlay, D. W. (1891). Abstracts of exceptional cases. *Middlesex Hosp. Rep.* **29**.
3. Harley, J. (1877). A case of slowly advancing scleroderma attended by cardiac and gastric disorders. *Br. Med. J.* **1**:107.
4. Dinkler, M. (1891). Zur Lehre von die Sklerodermia. *Dtsch. Arch. Klin. Med.* **48**:514.
5. Lewin, G., and Heller, J. (1895). Quoted by Church, R. E., and Ellis, A. R. P.: Cystic pulmonary fibrosis in generalized scleroderma. *Lancet* **1**: 392-394.
6. Von Notthafft, A. (1898). Neure Arbeiten und Anschihten uber Sklerodermia. *Zentralbl. Allg. Pathol. Pathol. Anat.* **9**:870.
7. Matsui, S. (1924). Ober die Pathologie und Pathogenese von Sklerodermia Universalis. *Mitteilungen Medizxinischen Fakultat Univ. Tokyo* **31**:55-116.
8. Murphy, J. R., Krainin, P., and Gerson, M. J. (1941). Scleroderma with pulmonary fibrosis. *J.A.M.A.* **116**:499-501.
9. Baldwin, E., Cournand, A., and Richards, D. W. Jr. (1949). Pulmonary insufficiency. II. A study of thirty-nine cases of pulmonary fibrosis. *Medicine* **28**:1-25.
10. Alton, E., and Turner-Warwick, M. (1988). Lung involvement in scleroderma. In Systemic Sclerosis: Scleroderma. Edited by Jayson, M. I. V., and Black. John Wiley & Sons, New York, pp. 181-205.

11. Guttadauria, M., Ellman, H., and Kaplan, D. (1979). Progressive systemic sclerosis: Pulmonary involvement. *Clin. Rheum. Dis.* **5**:151-166.
12. Hayman, L. D., and Hunt, R. E. (1952). Pulmonary fibrosis in generalized scleroderma. *Dis. Chest* **21**:691-704.
13. Opie, L. H. (1955). The pulmonary manifestations of generalized scleroderma. *Dis. Chest* **28**:665-680.
14. Sackner, M. A. (1966). *Scleroderma*. Grune and Stratton, New York.
15. Wilson, R. J., Rodnan, G. P., and Robin, E. D. (1964). An early pulmonary physiologic abnormality in progressive systemic sclerosis (diffuse scleroderma). *Am. J. Med.* **36**:361-369.
16. Adhikari, P. K., Bianchi, F. A., Boushy, S. F., Sakamoto, A., and Lewis, B. M. (1962). Pulmonary function in scleroderma: Its relation to changes in chest roentgenogram and in the skin of the thorax. *Am. Rev. Respir. Dis.* **86**:823-831.
17. Steen, V. D., Owens, G. R., Fino, G. J., Rodnan, G. P., and Medsger, T. A. Jr. (1985). Pulmonary involvement in systemic sclerosis (scleroderma). *Arthritis Rheum.* **28**:759-767.
18. DeMuth, G. R., Furstenberg, N. A., Dabick, L., and Zarafonetis, C. J. D. (1968). Pulmonary manifestations in scleroderma. *Am. J. Med. Sci.* **255**:94-104.
19. Guttadauria, M., Ellman, H., Emmanuel, G., Kaplan, D., and Diamond, H. (1977). Pulmonary function in scleroderma. *Arthritis Rheum.* **20**:1071-1079.
20. Weaver, A. L., Divertie, M. B., and Titus, J. L. (1968). Pulmonary scleroderma. *Dis. Chest* **54**:490-498.
21. Greenwald, G. I., Tashkin, D. P., Gong, H., et al. (1987). Longitudinal changes in lung function and respiratory symptoms in progressive systemic sclerosis. *Am. J. Med.* **83**:83-92.
22. Sackner, M. A., Akgun, N., Kimbel, P., and Lewis, D. H. (1964). Pathophysiology of scleroderma involving the heart and respiratory system. *Ann. Intern. Med.* **60**:611-630.
23. Baldwin, E., Cournand, A., and Richards, D. W. Jr. (1949). Pulmonary insufficiency. I. Physiological classification, clinical methods of analysis, standard values in normal subjects. *Medicine* **27**:243-278.
24. Iliffe, G. D., and Pettigrew, N. M. (1983). Hypoventilatory respiratory failure in generalised scleroderma. *Br. Med. J.* **286**:337-338.
25. Chausow, A. M., Kane, T., Levinson, D., and Szidon, J. P. (1984). Reversible hypercapnic respiratory insufficiency in scleroderma caused by respiratory muscle weakness. *Am. Rev. Respir. Dis.* **130**:142-144.
26. Young, R. H., and Mark, G. J. (1978). Pulmonary vascular changes in scleroderma. *Am. J. Med.* **64**:998-1004.

27. Bjerke, R. D., Tashkin, D. P., Clements, P. J., Chopra, S. K., Gong, H. Jr., and Bein, M. (1979). Small airways in progressive systemic sclerosis. *Am. J. Med.* **66**:201-208.
28. Kim, J. H., Follett, J. V., Rice, J. R., and Hampson, N. B. (1988). Endobronchial telangiectases and hemoptysis in scleroderma. *Am. J. Med.* **84**:173-174.
29. Helfrich, D. J., Banner, B., Steen, V. D., and Medsger, T. A. Jr. (1989). Normotensive renal failure in systemic sclerosis (scleroderma). *Arthritis Rheum.* **32**:1128-1134.
30. D'Angelo, W. A., Fries, J. F., Masi, A. T., and Shulman, L. E. (1969). Pathologic observations in systemic sclerosis. *Am. J. Med.* **46**:428-440.
31. Israel, M. S., and Harley, B. J. S. (1956). Spontaneous pneumothorax in scleroderma. *Thorax* **11**:113-118.
32. Ashba, J. K., and Ghanem, M. H. (1965). The lungs in systemic sclerosis. *Dis. Chest* **47**:52-64.
33. Owens, G. R., Fino, G. J., Herbert, D. L., et al. (1983). Pulmonary function in progressive systemic sclerosis. Comparison of CREST syndrome variant with diffuse scleroderma. *Chest* **84**:546-550.
34. Steigerwald, J., Seifert, M., Cliff, M., and Neff, T. (1975). Bone resorption of the ribs and pulmonary function in progressive systemic sclerosis. *Chest* **68**:838-840.
35. Peters-Golden, M., Wise, R. A., Schneider, P., Hochberg, M., Stevens, M. B., and Wigley, F. (1984). Clinical and demographic predictors of loss of pulmonary function in systemic sclerosis. *Medicine* **63**:221-231.
36. Schneider, P. D., Wise, R. A., Hochberg, M. C., and Wigley, F. M. (1982). Serial pulmonary function in systemic sclerosis. *Am. J. Med.* **73**:385-394.
37. Spain, D. M., and Thomas, A. G. (1950). The pulmonary manifestations of scleroderma. An anatomic physiological correlation. *Ann. Intern. Med.* **32**:152-161.
38. Ritchie, B. (1964). Pulmonary function in scleroderma. *Thorax* **19**:28-36.
39. Catterall, M., and Rowell, N. R. (1963). Respiratory function in progressive systemic sclerosis. *Thorax* **18**:10-15.
40. Bagg, L. R., and Hughes, D. T. D. (1979). Serial pulmonary function tests in progressive systemic sclerosis. *Thorax* **34**:224-228.
41. Graham, G. E., Steen, V., Owens, G., and Medsger, T. A. Jr. (1984). Followup of patients with an isolated diffusing capacity abnormality in progressive systemic sclerosis (PSS). *Arthritis Rheum.* **27**:S75.
42. Stupi, A. M., Steen, V. D., Owens, G. R., Barnes, E. L., Rodnan, G. P., and Medsger, T. A. Jr. (1986). Pulmonary hypertension in the CREST syndrome variant of systemic sclerosis. *Arthritis Rheum.* **29**:515-524.

43. Colp, C. R., Riker, J., and Williams, H. Jr. (1973). Serial changes in scleroderma and idiopathic interstitial lung disease. *Arch. Intern. Med.* **132**:506-515.
44. Hughes, D. T. D., and Lee, F. (1963). Lung function in patients with systemic sclerosis. *Thorax* **18**:16-20.
45. Steen, V. D., Owens, G. R., Redmond, C., Rodnan, G. P., and Medsger, T. A. Jr. (1985). The effect of D-penicillamine on pulmonary findings in systemic sclerosis. *Arthritis Rheum.* **28**:882-888.
46. Walker, W. C., and Wright, V. (1968). Pulmonary lesions and rheumatoid arthritis. *Medicine* **47**:501-519.
47. Trostle, D. C., Bedetti, C. D., Steen, V. D., Al-Sabbagh, M. R., Zee, B., and Medsger, T. A. Jr. (1988). Renal vascular histology and morphometry in systemic sclerosis: A case-control autopsy study. *Arthritis Rheum.* **31**:393-400.
48. Medsger, T. A. Jr., Masi, A. T., Rodnan, G. P., Benedek, T. G., and Robinson, H. (1971). Survival with systemic sclerosis (scleroderma). *Ann. Intern. Med.* **75**:369-376.
49. Bennett, R., Bluestone, R., Holt, P. J. L., and Bywaters, E. G. L. (1971). Survival in scleroderma. *Ann. Rheum. Dis.* **30**:581-588.
50. Eason, R. J., Tan, P. L., and Gow, P. J. (1981). Progressive systemic sclerosis in Auckland: A ten year review with emphasis on prognostic features. *Aust. N.Z. J. Med.* **11**:657-662.
51. Peters-Golden, M., Wise, R. A., Hochberg, M. V. C., Stevens, B. M., and Wigley, F. M. (1984). Carbon monoxide diffusing capacity as predictor of outcome in systemic sclerosis. *Am. J. Med.* **77**:1027-1034.
52. Ungerer, R. G., Tashkin, D. P., Furst, D., et al. (1983). Prevalence and clinical correlates of pulmonary arterial hypertension in progressive systemic sclerosis. *Am. J. Med.* **75**:65-74.
53. Germain, B. F., Howard, T. P., Solomon, D. A., Vagesh, M., Espinoza, L. R., Spoto, E. Jr., Vasey, F. B., and Goldman, A. L. (1981). Cardiopulmonary function in the CREST syndrome. *Clin. Res.* **29**:164A.
54. Salerni, R., Rodnan, G. P., Leon, D. F., and Shaver, J. A. (1977). Pulmonary hypertension in the CREST syndrome variant of progressive systemic sclerosis (scleroderma). *Ann. Intern. Med.* **86**:394-399.
55. Rich, S., Dantzker, D. R., Ayres, S. M., et al. (1987). Primary pulmonary hypertension: A national prospective study. *Ann. Intern. Med.* **107**:216-223.
56. Al-Sabbagh, M. R., Zee, B., Nalesnik, M., Trostle, D. C., and Medsger, T. A. Jr. (1986). Pulmonary arterial morphometry in systemic sclerosis: A case-control autopsy study. *Arthritis Rheum.* **29**:S52.
57. Trell, E., and Lindstrom, C. (1971). Pulmonary hypertension in systemic sclerosis. *Ann. Rheum. Dis.* **30**:390-400.

58. Steen, V. D., Ziegler, G. L., Rodnan, G. P., and Medsger, T. A. Jr. (1984). Clinical and laboratory associations of anticentromere antibody in patients with progressive systemic sclerosis. *Arthritis Rheum.* **27**: 125-131.
59. Catoggio, L. J., Bernstein, R. M., Black, C. M., Hughes, G. R. V., and Maddison, P. J. (1983). Serological markers in progressive systemic sclerosis: Clinical correlations. *Ann. Rheum. Dis.* **42**:23-27.
60. Steen, V. D., Powell, D. L., and Medsger, T. A. Jr. (1988). Clinical correlations and prognosis based on serum autoantibodies in systemic sclerosis. *Arthritis Rheum.* **31**:196-203.
61. Haustein, U. F., and Ziegler, V. (1985). Environmentally induced systemic sclerosis-like disorders. *Int. J. Dermatol.* **24**:147-151.
62. Veltman, G., Lange, C., Juhe, S., Stein, G., and Bachner, V. (1975). Clinical manifestations and course of vinyl chloride disease. *Ann. N.Y. Acad. Sci.* **246**:6-17.
63. Alonzo-Ruiz, A., Zea-Mendoza, A., Salazar-Vallinas, J., and Rocamore-Ripoll, A. (1986). Toxic oil syndrome: A syndrome with features overlapping those of various forms of scleroderma. *Semin. Arthritis Rheum.* **15**:200-212.
64. Yamakage, A., Ishikawa, H., Saito, Y., and Hattori, A. (1980). Occupational scleroderma-like disorder occurring in men engaged in the polymerization of epoxy resins. *Dermatologica* **161**:33-40.
65. Kumagai, Y., Shiokawa, Y., Medsger, T. A. Jr., and Rodnan, G. P. (1984). Clinical spectrum of connective tissue disease after cosmetic surgery. *Arthritis Rheum.* **27**:1-12.
66. Sternberg, E., Van Woent, M., Young, S., Maghussen, I., Baker, H., Gauthier, S., and Osterland, C. K. (1980). Development of a scleroderma-like illness during therapy with L-5-hydroxytryptophan and cardiopa. *N. Engl. J. Med.* **303**:782-787.
67. Erasmus, L. (1957). Scleroderma in gold miners in the Witwatersrand with particular reference to pulmonary manifestations. *S. Afr. J. Lab. Clin. Med.* **3**:209-231.
68. Rodnan, G., Benedek, T., Medsger, T., and Cammerata, R. (1967). The association of progressive systemic sclerosis (scleroderma) with coal miners' pneumoconiosis and other forms of silicosis. *Ann. Intern. Med.* **66**:323-334.
69. Lockey, J., Kelly, C., Cannon, G., Colby, T., Aldrich, V., and Livingston, G. (1987). Progressive systemic sclerosis associated with exposure to trichloroethylene. *J. Occup. Med.* **29**:493-496.
70. Sparrow, G. (1977). A connective tissue disorder similar to vinyl chloride disease in a patient exposed to perchlorethylene. *Clin. Dermatol.* **2**:17-22.

71. Owens, G. R., and Medsger, T. (1988). Systemic sclerosis secondary to occupational exposure. *Am. J. Med.* **85**:114-116.

72. Denis, P., Ducrotte, P., Pasquis, P., and Lefrancois, R. (1981). Esophageal motility and pulmonary function in progressive systemic sclerosis. *Respiration* **42**:21-24.

73. Crystal, R. G., Gadek, J. E., Ferrans, V. J., Fulmer, J. D., Line, B. R., and Hunninghake, G. W. (1981). Interstitial lung disease: Current concepts of pathogenesis, staging and therapy. *Am. J. Med.* **70**:542-567.

74. Furst, D. E., Davis, J. A., Clements, P. J., Chopra, S. K., Theofilopoulos, A. N., and Chia, D. (1981). Abnormalities of pulmonary vascular dynamics and inflammation in early progressive systemic sclerosis. *Arthritis Rheum.* **24**:1403-1408.

75. Baron, M., Feiglin, D., Hyland, R., Urowitz, M. B., and Shiff, B. (1983). [67]Gallium lung scans in progressive systemic sclerosis. *Arthritis Rheum.* **26**:969-974.

76. Edelson, J. D., Hyland, R. H., Ramsden, M., et al. (1985). Lung inflammation in scleroderma: Clinical, radiographic, physiologic and cytopathological features. *J. Rheumatol.* **12**:957-963.

77. Rossi, G. A., Bitterman, P. B., Rennard, S. I., Ferrans, V. J., and Crystal, R. G. (1985). Evidence for chronic inflammation as a component of the interstitial lung disease associated with progressive systemic sclerosis. *Am. Rev. Respir. Dis.* **131**:612-617.

78. Owens, G. R., Paradis, I. L., Gryzan, S., et al. (1986). Role of inflammation in the lung disease of systemic sclerosis: Comparison with idiopathic pulmonary fibrosis. *J. Lab. Clin. Med.* **107**:253-260.

79. Silver, R. M., Metcalf, J. F., and LeRoy, E. C. (1986). Interstitial lung disease in scleroderma: Immune complexes in sera and bronchoalveolar lavage fluid. *Arthritis Rheum.* **29**:525-531.

80. Konig, G., Luderschmidt, C., Hammer, C., Adelmann-Grill, B. C., Braun-Falco, O., and Fruhmann, G. (1984). Lung involvement in scleroderma. *Chest* **85**:318-324.

81. Pesci, A., Bertorelli, G., Manganelli, P., and Ambanelli, U. (1986). Bronchoalveolar lavage analysis of interstitial lung disease in CREST syndrome. *Clin. Exp. Rheum.* **4**:121-124.

82. Silver, R. M., Metcalf, J. F., Stanley, J. H., and LeRoy, E. C. (1984). Interstitial lung disease in scleroderma. *Arthritis Rheum.* **27**:1254-1262.

83. Owens, G. R., and Follansbee, W. P. (1987). Cardiopulmonary manifestations of systemic sclerosis. *Chest* **91**:118-127.

84. Moore, S. A., Gryzan, S., Paradis, I. L., et al. (1987). Alveolar macrophage modulation of fibroblast growth in patients with systemic sclerosis. *Am. Rev. Respir. Dis.* **135**:A67.

85. Pisko, E., Gallup, K., Turner, R., Parker, M., Numeir, A., Box, J., Davis, J., Box, P., and Rothberger, H. (1979). Cardiopulmonary mani-

festations of progressive systemic sclerosis: Association with circulating immune complexes and fluorescent antinuclear antibodies. *Arthritis Rheum.* **22**:518-523.

86. Seibold, J. R., Medsger, T. A. Jr., Winkelstein, A., Kelly, R. H., and Rodnan, G. P. (1982). Immune complexes in progressive systemic sclerosis (scleroderma). *Arthritis Rheum.* **25**:1167-1173.
87. Cannon, P. J., Hassar, M., Case, D. B., Casarella, W. J., Sommers, S. C., and LeRoy, E. C. (1974). The relationship of hypertension and renal failure in scleroderma (progressive systemic sclerosis) to structural and functional abnormalities of the renal cortical circulation. *Medicine* **53**:1-46.
88. Alexander, E. L., Firestein, G. S., Heuser, R. R., et al. (1986). Reversible cold-induced abnormalities in myocardial perfusion and function in systemic sclerosis. *Ann. Intern. Med.* **105**:661-668.
89. Emmanuel, G., Saroja, D., Gopinathan, K., Gharpure, A., and Stuckey, J. (1976). Acute and chronic fibrotic states. Environmental factors and the diffusing capacity of the lung in progressive systemic sclerosis. *Chest* **69(2)**:304-309.
90. Naslund, M. J., Pearson, T. A., and Ritter, J. M. (1981). A documented episode of pulmonary vasoconstriction in systemic sclerosis. *Johns Hopkins Med. J.* **148**:78-80.
91. Rozkovec, A., Bernstein, R., Asherson, R. A., and Oakley, C. M. (1983). Vascular reactivity and pulmonary hypertension in systemic sclerosis. *Arthritis Rheum.* **26**:1037-1040.
92. Ohar, J. M., Robichaud, A. M., Fowler, A. A., and Glauser, F. L. (1986). Increased pulmonary artery pressure in association with Raynaud's phenomenon. *Am. J. Med.* **81**:361-362.
93. Shuck, J. W., Oetgen, W. J., and Tesar, J. T. (1985). Pulmonary vascular response during Raynaud's phenomenon in progressive systemic sclerosis. *Am. J. Med.* **78**:221-227.
94. Wise, R. A., Wigley, F., Newball, H. H., and Stevens, M. B. (1982). The effect of cold exposure on diffusing capacity in patients with Raynaud's phenomenon. *Chest* **81**:695-698.
95. Miller, M. J. (1983). Effect of the cold pressor test on diffusing capacity. Comparison of normal subjects and those with Raynaud's disease and progressive systemic sclerosis. *Chest* **84**:264-266.
96. Fahey, P. J., Utell, M. J., Condemi, J. J., Green, R., and Hyde, R. W. (1984). Raynaud's phenomenon of the lung. *Am. J. Med.* **76**:263-269.
97. Rodnan, G. P., Black, R. L., Bollet, A. J., and Bunim, J. J. (1956). Observations on the use of prednisone in patients with progressive systemic sclerosis (diffuse scleroderma). *Ann. Intern. Med.* **44**:16-29.
98. Kallenberg, C. G. M., Jansen, H. M., Elema, J. D., and The, T. H. (1984). Steroid-responsive interstitial pulmonary disease in systemic sclerosis. Monitoring by bronchoalveolar lavage. *Chest* **86**:489-492.

99. Goodman, M., and Turner-Warwick, M. (1978). Pilot study of penicillamine therapy in corticosteroid failure patients with widespread pulmonary fibrosis. *Chest* **74**:338.

100. deClerck, L. S., Dequeker, J., Francx, L., and Demedts, M. (1987). D-penicillamine therapy and interstitial lung disease in scleroderma. A long-term followup study. *Arthritis Rheum.* **30**:643-650.

101. Morrison, D., Goldman, S., and Alepa, F. P. (1984). Unloading the right ventricle in the CREST syndrome variant of progressive systemic sclerosis (scleroderma). *Clin. Cardiol.* **7**:49-53.

102. Ohar, J., Polatty, C., Robichaud, A., Fowler, A., Vetrovec, G., and Glauser, F. (1985). The role of vasodilators in patients with progressive systemic sclerosis. Interstitial lung disease and pulmonary hypertension. *Chest* **88**:263S-265S.

103. O'Brien, J. T., Hill, J. A., and Pepine, C. J. (1985). Sustained benefit of verapamil in pulmonary hypertension with progressive systemic sclerosis. *Am. Heart J.* **109**:380-383.

104. Prouse, P. J., Gumpel, J. M., and Lahiri, A. L. (1984). The CREST syndrome—successful reduction of pulmonary hypertension by captopril. *Postgrad. Med. J.* **60**:672-674.

105. Rich, S., and Brundage, B. H. (1987). High-dose calcium channel-blocking therapy for primary pulmonary hypertension: Evidence for long-term reduction in pulmonary arterial pressure and regression of right ventricular hypertrophy. *Circulation* **76**:135-141.

11

Inflammatory Muscle Disease

IRA N. TARGOFF

University of Oklahoma Health Science Center
Oklahoma Medical Research Foundation, and
Veterans Administration Medical Center
Oklahoma City, Oklahoma

I. Introduction

This chapter will discuss pulmonary involvement in the autoimmune inflammatory myopathies, polymyositis (PM) and dermatomyositis (DM), the major forms of inflammatory myopathy facing the rheumatologist (1). Other forms of inflammatory myopathy may occur [viral, parasitic, etc. (2)], and these could affect the lungs in some cases (e.g., a viral syndrome affecting both the lungs and the muscle). These conditions should be considered in the differential diagnosis but will not be discussed in this section.

Pulmonary complications of a variety of types are of major concern in patients with PM/DM. They may be the source of significant morbidity and may contribute to mortality. Of particular interest is interstitial lung disease (ILD), which appears to result from the expression of the disease in the lungs, with inflammation leading to fibrosis. This complication is being recognized with increasing frequency, in part, as a result of the association of ILD in PM/DM with the subgroup of patients defined by the Jo-1 family of myositis-specific antibodies.

II. Polymyositis and Dermatomyositis

PM or DM may be difficult to diagnose at times and may be confused with other conditions. The criteria of Bohan and Peter (1) have been accepted and employed by most workers for establishing the diagnosis and are useful for defining the condition. Patients satisfying four criteria are considered to have definite PM or DM, and three criteria "probable" PM or DM (Table 1).

As in most primary myopathies, the cardinal clinical feature of PM/DM is proximal muscle weakness. Patients have difficulty with activities, such as rising from a chair without the aid of the arms, walking upstairs, combing the hair, etc., that require the large proximal muscles around the shoulders, hips, thighs, etc. The trunk muscles and neck muscles are also prominently affected. The disease may affect the muscles of respiration (diaphragm, intercostals, and accessory muscles) as well as the muscles of swallowing (see below). Pharyngeal muscles and the muscles of speech may become weak, with a change in speech to a more nasal quality (3).

The creatine kinase (CK) level is elevated in the overwhelming majority of patients at some point in the course of disease [over 90% in most series (4,5)] and in most patients on presentation. CK elevation may be a very helpful marker, warning of impending exacerbation or persisting disease. The third criterion after proximal muscle weakness and elevated muscle enzyme levels is the characteristic pattern on electromyography. PM/DM patients

Table 1 Major Criteria for Diagnosis of Polymyositis and Dermatomyositis

1. Symmetrical weakness of the limb-girdle muscles and anterior neck flexors, progressing over weeks to months.
2. Elevation in serum of skeletal muscle enzymes.
3. Electromyographic abnormalities characteristic of inflammatory muscle disease.
4. Muscle biopsy evidence of fiber necrosis, phagocytosis, regeneration, inflammation, and other characteristic findings.
5. Dermatologic features including the heliotrope discoloration of the eyelids with periorbital edema, Gottron's patches, or erythematous dermatitis over the knees, elbows, medial malleoli, face, neck, and upper torso.

Confidence Limits Definition:
  Four criteria = Definite disease.
  Three criteria = Probable disease.
Source: Bohan and Peter (1).

show the myopathic potentials but may in addition show insertional irritability, attributed to diffuse damage to the sarcolemma (6). The muscle biopsy is important for ruling out other conditions and should show the usual findings of PM/DM (the fourth criterion), including inflammation, mononuclear cell infiltration, and necrosis and regeneration. A characteristic pattern of perifascicular atrophy is often seen (7), particularly in childhood DM. The fifth criterion is the presence of the DM rash, which may be highly characteristic, including the "heliotrope," a lilac discoloration that appears most frequently over the eyelids, often accompanied by periorbital edema, and the Gottron's patches, erythematous scaly eruptions over the extensor surfaces of the joints of the fingers, with similar patches over other extensor surfaces.

Even if these criteria are satisfied, it is important to know that no other condition is present that may account for these findings before concluding that PM or DM is present (1). Evidence of any form of endocrinopathy should be excluded, particularly thyroid disease. Certain forms of muscular dystrophy may present late in life, including limb-girdle and fascioscapulohumeral dystrophy, and great care must be taken in making the diagnosis of PM/DM in any patient with a family history of myopathy. The muscle biopsy should be examined for evidence of other myopathies. Evidence should be sought of infections that may present with a PM-like picture [including toxoplasmosis (8,9), certain viruses (10,11), and AIDS (12)]. Certain neuropathies, especially those that have minimal sensory manifestations such as amyotrophic lateral sclerosis (13), may also be confused with PM.

The most common classification scheme is that of Bohan and Peter, which separates patients into five groups (1). The distinction between types I (PM) and II (DM) is based on the presence of the DM rash in type II. Types I and II include adults without malignancy or overlap syndromes. The myositis is usually considered to be similar, although some have described pathological differences between them (2,7). Type III includes patients with a malignancy in association with their PM or DM, about 15% of PM/DM patients, and is more common in DM than PM (14). Malignancy found recently antecedent or concurrent with the diagnosis of PM or DM is most likely to be related (15). The sites of the primary tumors are usually felt to have the same distribution as those in the general population. Type IV includes children with myositis (16). The DM rash (>90%), vasculitis, and subcutaneous calcifications are more common in children than in adults. Type V includes patients with overlap syndromes, who satisfy criteria for PM/DM as well as a second connective tissue disease, most commonly scleroderma, systemic lupus erythematosus, and Sjogren's syndrome. Certain features that are found in other connective tissue diseases, such as Raynaud's phenomenon and arthritis, may also occur in patients with PM/DM and do not necessarily imply the presence of an overlap syndrome. ILD is usually not considered an overlapping disease but another manifestation of the underlying condition.

III. Pulmonary Involvement in PM/DM

The major forms of pulmonary involvement in PM/DM include those related to muscle weakness (ventilatory failure and aspiration pneumonia), those related to treatment (opportunistic infection and hypersensitivity pneumonitis), and those related to the disease process (interstitial pneumonitis and fibrosis). All are serious and potentially life-threatening. Dickey and Myers (17) found lung infections to be the most common form of clinical involvement (29% of 42 patients), half of which (14% overall) were due to aspiration. Overall, pulmonary complications occurred in 45% of their patients, contributing directly to death in 10%. Even in the absence of evidence of pulmonary involvement, the physician must always be alert for the development of such complications in caring for a patient with PM/DM.

A. Respiratory Muscle Weakness

Any condition leading to widespread muscle weakness can result in respiratory compromise, and PM/DM is no exception. This form of pulmonary involvement is similar to that seen with other myopathies (18). Respiratory muscle weakness occurred in 4% of the patients of DeVere and Bradley (19), and ventilatory failure occurred in 7% of the patients of Dickey and Myers (17).

Braun et al. (18) found that abnormalities of respiratory muscle strength (RMS) [the average of the percent of predicted maximal static inspiratory pressure (Pi) and expiratory pressure (Pe)] occurred in 37 of 47 patients with myopathies referred for pulmonary function testing, with an equal prevalence among patients with PM/DM and with other myopathies (the average RMS was lower in other myopathies). Both inspiratory and expiratory muscles may become involved in PM/DM, including the diaphragm, the accessory muscles, the intercostals, and the abdominal muscles (19). While some other conditions (such as myasthenia gravis and amyotrophic lateral sclerosis) have been associated with greater expiratory than inspiratory weakness, the inspiratory and expiratory muscles in PM/DM were found by Braun et al. to be equally affected (18), reflected by a normal ratio of Pi to Pe.

In addition to decreases in Pi%, Pe%, and RMS, PM/DM patients showed decreased total lung capacity (TLC), vital capacity (VC), and maximal voluntary ventilation (MVV), with VC and MVV strongly correlated with RMS. Residual volume (RV) is often normal or increased, because of expiratory muscle weakness [inversely correlated with Pe (18)]. Interpretation of pulmonary function tests may be complicated by coexisting interstitial lung disease (ILD) (20). Respiratory insufficiency with hypercapnia may result from respiratory weakness. Braun et al. found that pCO_2 elevations were not observed until the RMS fell below 40%, and hypercapnia became severe only with RMS below 30% and the VC below 55%. They felt that the RMS was the best test for identifying those with significant respiratory muscle weakness.

Respiratory failure requiring intubation and assisted ventilation may develop. Mechanical ventilation was required for two of 42 patients of Dickey and Myers (17); with treatment, the number of patients who require a respirator is small, and most will improve sufficiently to ventilate independently, although chronic CO_2 retention has been reported after such an episode (17). Diaphragmatic atrophy was observed at autopsy in three cases (21). Ventilatory failure may develop rapidly, and early signs of respiratory weakness may be subtle or unrecognized (17,18), emphasizing the need to be alert for this possible complication. Patients with severe weakness elsewhere or pharyngeal weakness should be tested for evidence of respiratory muscle weakness. Most patients who eventually develop overt ventilatory failure also have involvement of the pharyngeal, facial, and tongue muscles, with dysphagia and impaired speech. Respiratory muscle weakness can lead to impairment of episodic deep breathing; to weakness of the chest wall, with lower resting lung volumes; and to impairment of expiration and of cough. These abnormalities can predispose to atelectasis and secondary infection, as well as aspiration.

B. Aspiration Pneumonia

About 10-15% of patients may develop weakness in the muscles involved in swallowing (4) (pharyngeal muscles, tongue, soft palate, and muscles of the upper esophagus), resulting in dysphagia, which poses significant risk of aspiration. Dickey and Myers (17) found dysphagia to be more common (43%). Regurgitation of material into the nose may occur when swallowing is attempted. Speech may also be impaired. Dysphagia and difficulty with speech should be taken as warning signs of the possibility of aspiration, and efforts to avoid this complication should be instituted. Dysphagia in PM/DM may also result from dysfunction of the cricopharyngeal muscles with spasm and improperly timed contraction (22). This can be corrected surgically if necessary. Swallowing impairment may be documented by barium swallow (although aspiration of the barium may occur) or by esophageal manometry. Dickey and Myers (17) were able to document pharyngeal dysfunction in five of six who aspirated, and all six complained of dysphagia.

Dysphagia has been associated with a poor prognosis in many studies (5,23,24) and may be a marker of a higher 1-year mortality. However, it is generally associated with more severe disease, and recent studies have been unable to show an independent contribution of dysphagia to increased mortality with multivariate analysis (5). Dysphagia was common among PM/DM patients with lung involvement who came to autopsy at the Mayo Clinic (34 of 65 cases) whether pneumonia was absent or present, but five of six with clear-cut aspiration pneumonia had a history of dysphagia (21). As noted, the intercostal, pharyngeal, and abdominal muscles may be involved in PM/DM, which can impair cough and thus predispose to aspiration. Weakness of the trunk muscles is common and may lead to difficulty with turning on the side, also promoting aspiration, particularly after vomiting. Aspiration pneumonia is treated as in other situations.

C. Other Infections

Patients with PM/DM treated with corticosteroids and immunosuppressive agents are at higher risk for infections. In addition to increased risk from common organisms, they are at risk for opportunistic infections (gram-negative bacteria, fungi, parasites, etc.). Patients with respiratory muscle weakness are particularly at risk for pulmonary infections because of atelectasis and difficulty with clearing secretions. Infection is the most common immediate cause of death in patients with PM/DM (5). Bronchopneumonia was also the most common finding (35 of 65 cases) in an autopsy study from the Mayo Clinic of all cases of PM/DM with pulmonary involvement (21). These cases included a variety of opportunistic organisms such as *Cryptococcus, Candida, Nocardia,* and *Pneumocystis.*

D. Other Forms of Pulmonary Involvement

Interstitial pneumonitis will be discussed below. The most common immunosuppressive drug other than corticosteroids used in PM/DM is methotrexate. Hypersensitivity pneumonitis has been reported with this drug in most of the conditions in which it has been used, including PM/DM (25). It usually presents with acute illness marked by fever, cough, dyspnea, bilateral interstitial infiltrates on chest X-ray, and lymphocytic infiltrates on biopsy sometimes characterized by giant cells and noncaseating granulomata (25). This condition can lead to fibrosis but usually responds to withdrawal of the drug, sometimes also requiring corticosteroids. Cyclophosphamide, also used for treatment of PM/DM, has also been associated with this complication.

PM/DM may occur in association with malignancies, including lung tumors (14,21,26,27). Some of these patients have had other forms of lung involvement, including ILD (27) and pneumonia (21). In patients presenting with lung and muscle disease, the possibility of PM/DM associated with a lung tumor should be considered. Patients with PM/DM may develop congestive heart failure related to cardiac involvement of the myositis, or from unrelated causes, which must be differentiated from pulmonary disease. Pulmonary edema was observed in 28 of 65 autopsy cases of PM/DM with lung involvement, usually related to associated cardiac or renal disease (21). Pleural effusions in PM/DM are usually due to other coexistent (such as congestive heart failure) or overlapping conditions. Other medical complications manifested in the lung may also occur [pulmonary emboli, chronic obstructive pulmonary disease, and adult respiratory distress syndrome (21)].

IV. Interstitial Lung Disease in PM/DM

A. Prevalence

The first case of ILD in PM/DM was reported by Mills and Mathews in 1956 (28), and since then it has become a well-recognized complication. The actual frequency of this complication is hard to assess. A review in 1984 (17) noted that 65 cases had been previously reported in the English literature, and many cases and series including such cases have been reported since that time (20,29-38). There has not been an extensive prospective study using reliable techniques for the detection of ILD to determine its statistical prevalence, and the rates in large series have been remarkably divergent. Early studies did not report this complication despite large numbers of patients collected (39,40). ILD was also very rare among 153 patients with PM/DM studied by Bohan et al. (4) and was absent among those patients without overlap syndromes.

Frazier and Miller (41) found ILD by X-ray in 10 of 213 cases of PM/ DM studied retrospectively from the Mayo Clinic in 1974 and considered this to be a high rate. However, Hochberg et al. (5) from Baltimore reported pulmonary fibrosis in 26% initially, with a cumulative rate of 37% of adult patients. Tymms and Webb (37) from Australia found ILD in 28%; Bernstein et al. (29) from London found it in 26% of 72 PM/DM patients; and Songcharoen et al. (42) found ILD in 7 of 15 cases in a referral center in Mississippi. Other studies showed a more moderate rate, including that of Salmeron et al. (43), who reported a rate of 9%, and Dickey and Myers (17), who found radiologic ILD in 10%.

A recent series of reports indicates an even higher rate among PM/DM patients in Japan. Takizawa et al. (35) found ILD in 9 of 14 patients (64.3%) 13 of whom had DM). Their report cited five additional series of PM/DM patients from the Japanese literature since 1980 with rates of ILD ranging from 46% to 80%. Yoshida et al. (44) also found a high rate of ILD (43.8%)

in PM/DM in Japan. However, Hidano et al. (31), using data from a survey of Japanese dermatologists, found pulmonary fibrosis in only 85 (15%) of 637 DM patients. Overall, it appears that ILD is more frequent than the early studies suggested, at least 10% of patients overall and higher in Japan. Dickey and Myers (17) also studied a small group of patients prospectively for evidence of lung disease by lung volumes and diffusing capacity, and found abnormalities that suggested ILD in 31% of patients. Similarly, Hochberg et al. (5) found a decrease in diffusing capacity (DLCO) in 65% of patients tested (not prospectively selected), as well as a high frequency of decreased lung volumes. Although some of these pulmonary function abnormalities could have been due to respiratory muscle weakness, the frequency of ILD is likely to be higher than that which is apparent by X-ray.

B. Clinical Presentation

The presentation of ILD in PM/DM is similar to that of idiopathic ILD, but may be complicated by the other types of pulmonary involvement in PM/DM (20). Some patients with ILD apparently remain without pulmonary symptoms, with the lung disease manifested only by abnormalities on chest X-ray or pulmonary function tests. The size of this group has yet to be definitively established, but it may be the largest (17). On the other hand, a number of patients will present with ILD, and it may be the dominant feature of the disease. Symptomatic ILD in PM/DM has been separated into two groups. Some patients, apparently a small proportion, present with fulminant lung disease with fever, nonproductive cough, and rapidly progressive dyspnea. This form may be fatal within weeks or months. A second group has a more chronic course, with gradually developing dyspnea, although it can still dominate the clinical picture in some cases.

The physical findings in ILD in PM/DM are similar to those in idiopathic and other forms of ILD and may include bibasilar inspiratory rales and tachypnea. Clubbing is unusual but has been observed. The chest X-ray typically shows a reticulonodular pattern, which may be limited to or more prominent in the bases (41,42,45), with a superimposed diffuse alveolar pattern in the more fulminant, acute cases. Pleural effusion is not a part of this picture (45). Pulmonary function tests are usually consistent with ILD, showing restrictive lung disease with decreased TLC and VC, usually without impairment of the FEV_1/FVC. The DLCO is a useful measurement in ILD, which can decrease before chest X-ray abnormalities develop. It can be used to quantitate and follow the course of the functional abnormality in ILD. Hypoxemia with exercise is another early sign. Lung compliance can decrease. Pulmonary function testing may be complicated by respiratory muscle weakness, which can also lead to decreased lung volumes (although RV is preserved).

Pi, Pe, RMS, and the MVV should be decreased in patients with respiratory muscle weakness, while diffusing capacity should be decreased in ILD.

C. Features of PM in Patients with Complicating ILD

In general, the myositis in patients with PM/DM complicated by ILD is similar to the myositis in other patients with PM/DM. ILD may occur in PM/DM of any type, including myositis with malignancy (46,47) and childhood myositis (48). There is no consistent relationship between the severity of the myositis and the ILD (45), and the myositis or the ILD may be asymptomatic, with the other dominating the clinical picture. The muscle weakness may even be entirely overlooked; it may be mild, or attributed to the fatigue brought on by hypoxemia, or masked by decreased activity imposed by the lung disease. Patients may present with ILD with evidence of elevation of the muscle enzymes without recognized muscle weakness, even by direct examination. Although these patients do not satisfy clinical criteria for PM/DM, they may have myositis-specific autoantibodies of the Jo-1 group that could support the diagnosis (see below). In other cases, there is no evidence of myositis at the time of onset of the ILD, but the myositis develops later. The lung disease may precede the muscle disease (33,38,49), occasionally by as much as 3 years, in up to 40% of cases (45), although they tend to be closer in onset. In one reported case (50), a patient with the DM rash developed rapidly progressive fatal fibrosing alveolitis without developing apparent myositis even at autopsy. In some cases, treatment with corticosteroids directed at the ILD may suppress the myositis before it becomes evident. Duncan et al. (49), Wasicek et al. (38), and others reported patients whose PM became evident only after tapering the dosage of the prednisone that was being administered for ILD.

Although differences in absolute CK levels between patients do not necessarily reflect the relative severity of PM/DM or of weakness, Songcharoen et al. (42) found that all those with PM/DM with ILD had CK and aldolase levels were higher than PM/DM patients without ILD, and more patients with ILD had severe inflammation on biopsy. However, a study of a small series of patients with documented PM/DM without any elevation in CK levels found them to have a higher than expected frequency of ILD and a poorer than expected prognosis (51). Similarly, Fergusson et al. (52) reported two cases of DM with fatal ILD, both of whom had normal CK levels with elevated LDH levels. Also, Takizawa et al. (35,53) found the mean CK level in those PM/DM patients without ILD (874 U) to be higher than in those with ILD (201 U), and that four of six patients who died of ILD had low CK levels including two with normal levels.

Arthritis is common in case reports and series of ILD with PM/DM (21,28,31,33,50,49,52) and may precede other manifestations of PM/DM (including myositis) or be the presenting symptom. It appears to be more common in the group with ILD than in other PM/DM patients. Arthritis was present in four of five patients with ILD and pulmonary vasculitis studied by Lakhanpal et al. (21). Schumacher et al. (54) studied nine cases with objective arthritis among patients with pure PM/DM without overlap syndromes. All nine had evidence of ILD, usually with pulmonary fibrosis. Rheumatoid factor may occur in these patients (41,49), as it may in idiopathic ILD, but does not necessarily correlate with the presence of arthritis (45). Some have found Raynaud's phenomenon to be more common in patients with ILD (31).

D. Pathology of the Lung

The lung pathology in these patients is also similar to ILD in other connective tissue diseases and in other situations. Particularly in acute cases, an inflammatory infiltrate may be seen in the interstitium, mostly composed of mononuclear cells (particularly lymphocytes, but also macrophages and plasma cells), with a small number of neutrophils and eosinophils. This involvement may be patchy (21,35,43) and, as with the X-ray findings, predominate in the lower lobes (43). Some fibrosis is usually present, which may vary from minimal in acute fulminant disease to extensive in chronic progressive cases (49). Alveoli show loss of type I cells, proliferation of type II cells, and increased numbers of free alveolar macrophages (35,43). Schwarz et al. (45) found evidence of bronchiolitis obliterans with organizing pneumonia in three of six cases in addition to the interstitial pneumonitis and alveolar cell hyperplasia with desquamation. These three cases had alveolar infiltrates on X-ray and other features of acute disease but no evidence of aspiration or infectious pneumonia. Schwarz et al. suggested that the pathological process proceeds from the acute stage characterized by bronchiolitis, interstitial pneumonitis, and desquamation to pulmonary fibrosis over time. Bronchiolitis obliterans was not reported in other series (21,35,43).

There may be medial and/or intimal thickening of small pulmonary arteries or arterioles suggesting pulmonary hypertension (45,49). Lakhanpal et al. (21) found pulmonary vasculitis in 5 of 35 patients with PM/DM and ILD at autopsy but in none of 30 PM/DM patients with other forms of pulmonary involvement. One of these patients presented with pulmonary hypertension (55), which is otherwise rare in PM/DM (19). Multifocal dystrophic calcifications were reported in the lung of one patient (45). Histological evidence of pleural inflammation may be observed in some cases (43,45) despite the lack of clinical pleural involvement. Unlike SLE (56) and idiopathic ILD (57), direct immunofluorescence has been negative for immunoglobulin and complement deposition in the lung (35,45,58), and electron microscopy does not show evidence of immune complexes (43).

Tubuloreticular structures have been reported in endothelial cells in the lung (59), but alveolar capillary endothelial cells were reported to be normal in another study (43). Tubuloreticular structures have also been found in endothelial cells of the muscle in PM/DM (60), particularly in DM patients, as well as the synovial vascular endothelial cells in patients with arthritis, PM/DM, and ILD (54). They are believed to represent evidence of endothelial cell damage, rather than viruses, which was suspected to be the primary abnormality in DM (60).

E. Aspects of Management of Lung Disease in PM

Many reports in the literature indicate that ILD in PM/DM can respond to corticosteroid therapy, particularly if treatment is begun early, in an active inflammatory stage. Clinical, radiological, and functional improvement has been demonstrated in some cases after therapy of acute disease (38,41,42). The studies of Duncan et al. (49) and Schwarz et al. (45) found that treatment was more effective in cases in which interstitial pneumonitis with active inflammation was the major finding on lung biopsy rather than interstitial fibrosis. Songcharoen et al. (42) felt that the acute form of ILD in PM/DM may be amenable to steroid therapy, but if delayed, pulmonary fibrosis ensues, which is unresponsive to treatment.

The acute fulminant form cannot always be successfully treated, however. Fergusson et al. (52) reported two cases of rapidly progressive fibrosing alveolitis, both associated with DM, that were unresponsive despite early therapy, both dying of lung disease within 6 months. The fulminant form of ILD may result in death within weeks (46), emphasizing the need for prompt diagnosis and treatment. Although the more chronic form of ILD, dominated by fibrosis on biopsy, is felt to be more resistant to therapy (49), Frazier and Miller (41) felt that therapy in this situation could prevent progression. It is possible that the active, treatable stage can be differentiated from the chronic, unresponsive stage by gallium scan or by bronchoalveolar lavage (61). In prednisone-resistant cases of uncomplicated PM/DM, cytotoxic agents are frequently used. While methotrexate is frequently used in that situation, it has the potential to cause pneumonitis and should therefore probably be avoided if possible in patients with PM/DM with ILD. Two DM patients with ILD treated with methotrexate (in late stages) did not respond (45), while methotrexate was successful in another patient (with features of overlap) despite previous failure on azathioprine (62). Azathioprine can be successful in this condition, however (63). Cyclophosphamide has also been used successfully in DM with ILD (64), but experience is limited.

Reports of prognosis of ILD in PM/DM have shown wide variation. Schwarz et al. (45) note that in collected case reports, half the patients have responded favorably to therapy, and that the major factors determining response were histology (as above) and age with responders averaging 43 years and nonresponders 52. Three of their six new patients died of respiratory failure related to ILD. Hidano et al. (31) found that 38 of 85 patients with ILD and DM died of their ILD, and Takizawa et al. (35) found that six of nine patients (66.7%) died of ILD. However, Songcharoen et al. (42) found that all patients subjectively improved, and only one of seven died. Salmeron et al. (43) had only one death from respiratory insufficiency among 10 patients with ILD and PM/DM, with improvement in five. Even if the ILD does not respond to steroid therapy, the myositis may respond, which can be important in improving lung function is respiratory muscle weakness is a contributing factor. Exacerbations of ILD and myositis may occur together (42,45) or separately (38,45).

V. Autoantibodies and Their Relationship to ILD in PM/DM

Most of the features of ILD in PM/DM noted above are similar to ILD in other connective tissue diseases. The unique feature of ILD in PM/DM is its association with specific, defined autoantibody reactions. These represent autoantibody markers of a greatly increased risk for ILD, one of the few such markers available in any situation. This association has evident clinical significance, and it may be important in understanding the mechanisms behind the ILD as well as the PM/DM itself.

A. Autoantibodies in PM/DM

Autoantibodies are common in patients with PM/DM. They may be divided into antibodies directed at muscle specific antigens and antibodies directed at nuclear and cytoplasmic antigens that are fundamental constituents of all cells. Many studies have been unable to associate antibodies to muscle-specific antigens with PM/DM (65,66), but recent studies with purified antigens have found antibodies to myosin (67) and myoglobin (68) more commonly and in higher titer in patients with PM/DM than in controls (although they are not specific for PM/DM). Their significance in PM/DM is unclear. No studies have associated antibodies to any muscle-specific component with the presence or absence of ILD. There have been no reports of circulating antilung antibodies in PM/DM patients with ILD, and as noted above, deposition of antibody in the lung has not been found.

Antinuclear and anticytoplasmic antibodies have also been associated with PM/DM. The larger series from the older literature often reported low frequencies of positive antinuclear antibody tests, such as the 12% reported by Bohan et al. (4). Generally these studies used insensitive methods, and most now find autoantibodies of this type in over half of PM/DM patients. One recent survey (69) using a combination of indirect immunofluorescence on HEp-2 cells and Ouchterlony immunodiffusion found autoantibodies in 89% of patients. These antibodies occur frequently in patients with all types of PM/DM, but they are probably most common in overlap patients.

Studies using immunodiffusion and immunoprecipitation have now defined the predominant antigenic specificities of these antibodies. The antigenic specificities are heterogeneous across the spectrum of PM/DM patients, but individuals tend to have autoantibodies of one or a few specificities. Certain of these antibody specificities are found exclusively or predominantly in patients satisfying criteria for PM/DM (PM/DM-specific) (70) and tend to be associated with characteristic clinical subgroups. The PM/DM-specific antibodies include anti-Jo-1 (71,72), anti-PL-7 (73), anti-PL-12 (74), anti-Mi-2 (75), and anti-PM-Scl (76). Other antibodies have been described in PM/DM and may prove to be PM/DM specific with further study, such as the antibody to signal recognition particle (77) and antibodies to unidentified tRNA-related antigens (78). Anti-UlnRNP (79) has an association with PM/DM (80) but is also common in other connective tissue diseases (81). Anti-Ku (82) is associated with polymyositis/scleroderma overlap in Japanese patients, but is rare in this syndrome in U.S. patients.

B. Antibodies to Aminoacyl-tRNA Synthetases

Anti-Jo-1 is the best-studied PM/DM-specific antibody. It was first described by Nishikai and Reichlin in 1980 (71) as the most common Ouchterlony precipitin line found in PM/DM sera. It was later noted (83) that immunoprecipitates formed between this serum and HeLa cell extracts contain a single type of transfer RNA (tRNA), the tRNA for histidine. Mathews and Bernstein (72) showed that the Jo-1 antigen, known to be a protein, was in fact the enzyme histidyl-tRNA synthetase, since anti-Jo-1 sera specifically inhibited this enzyme. Histidyl-tRNA synthetase is the enzyme that attaches histidine to its cognate tRNA. This enzyme thus plays a crucial role in protein synthesis and must be present in every living cell (84).

Twenty separate cytoplasmic aminoacyl-tRNA synthetases catalyze a tRNA charging reaction (aminoacylation), one for each of the amino acids. In general, sera with anti-Jo-1 show no antibody activity by any test toward any of the aminoacyl-tRNA synthetases other than histidyl-tRNA synthetase. However, sera with antibodies to threonyl-tRNA synthetase (anti-PL-7) (73) and sera with antibodies to alanyl-tRNA synthetase (anti-PL-12) (74) have been described, occurring predominantly in patients with PM/DM. Again, each serum reacts with only one synthetase in almost every case. While anti-Jo-1 and anti-PL-7 react only with the synthetase enzyme, anti-PL-12 sera react both with the enzyme and with the tRNA[ala] itself (74).

Anti-Jo-1 is highly specific for PM/DM. Almost all patients with this antibody have had PM/DM (44,71,83,85). In most studies, the antibody is found in approximately 20-30% of patients satisfying criteria for PM/DM (69,71,85,86) and is found in less than half of patients with adult PM, the group in which it is most commonly found. However, anti-Jo-1 seems to be associated with patients with certain characteristic features and may define a particular subgroup or syndrome. The most distinctive feature is the high frequency of ILD. A significant association between anti-Jo-1 and ILD in PM/DM has been documented in studies of at least four different patient populations. Yoshida et al. (44) in Japan found radiographic pulmonary fibrosis in all nine patients with anti-Jo-1 but in only 22% of patients without anti-Jo-1 (P < .001) (64% of patients with ILD had anti-Jo-1). There was no relationship between the anti-Jo-1 titer and the severity of ILD. Bernstein et al. (29) from London found anti-Jo-1 in 68% of 19 patients with ILD and PM/DM but in only 7.5% of 53 patients with PM/DM alone (thus 76.5% of patients with anti-Jo-1 had ILD while 10.9% of anti-Jo-1-negative patients had ILD). Bernstein et al. also tested 62 patients with ILD without PM/DM for the anti-Jo-1 antibody and found it in two patients. Hochberg et al. (32) from Baltimore looked for evidence of ILD retrospectively by findings on chest X-ray and diffusing capacity. They found ILD in 50% of patients with anti-Jo-1 but in only 14.7% of patients without this antibody (P = 0.05) (50% of patients with ILD had anti-Jo-1). Walker et al. (87) from Australia also found a significantly higher frequency of anti-Jo-1 in patients with PM/DM with ILD (88%) than in PM/DM patients without ILD (35%). Thus, the association of this antibody with ILD among PM/DM patients is well established. While not all PM/DM patients with ILD have anti-Jo-1, in most studies they are the majority. As with ILD in PM/DM in general, the ILD associated with anti-Jo-1 may be severe and dominate the clinical picture, or it may be an incidental finding on chest X-ray that never causes symptoms.

Other characteristics have been ascribed to the subgroup defined by anti-Jo-1 antibodies. Most studies have found that the DM rash occurs in a small minority of patients with anti-Jo-1. Anti-Jo-1 was found in 47% of adult PM patients by Hochberg et al. (5) but was not found in DM. Only one of nine patients with anti-Jo-1 of Yoshida et al. (44) had DM, while 16 of 23 without the antibody had DM. Even by the sensitive ELISA technique (86), anti-Jo-1 was more common (36%) and of higher titer in adult PM than adult DM (10%). However, Walker et al. found anti-Jo-1 in 38% of DM patients. Surprisingly, a predominance of PM over DM has not been reported for ILD itself, and DM is common in case reports and series of PM/DM and ILD. Almost all patients with anti-Jo-1 have been adults, and anti-Jo-1 has not been reported in typical juvenile dermatomyositis (88).

Anti-Jo-1 also has not been reported in PM/DM with malignancy [unlike anti-Mi-2, a DM associated antibody (75)]. ILD, however, has clearly been reported in patients with PM/DM with malignancy (27,46,47).

A higher frequency of arthritis has been found in PM/DM with anti-Jo-1 than in patients with PM/DM without anti-Jo-1 by at least two groups (44,89) but not by a third (87). This is interesting in view of the association of ILD in PM/DM with arthritis as discussed above. Nash et al. (33) found anti-Jo-1 and later PM/DM in their patient with ILD after finding inflammatory arthritis. Bernstein and Mathews (89) observed Raynaud's phenomenon in 90% of patients with anti-Jo-1, and Walker et al. (87) found it in 56% with anti-Jo-1 but only 18% without the antibody. Anti-Jo-1 may occur in type V PM/DM (overlap syndromes) as well as type I (adult PM); at least one study found the most common overlapping condition in patients with anti-Jo-1 to be Sjogren's syndrome (69). The production of antibody to Jo-1 was also found to be linked to HLA type. While HLA DR-3 was found in only 22% of anti-Jo-1-negative PM/DM patients, it was found in 64% of anti-Jo-1-positive patients ($P < .05$), and all anti-Jo-1 patients had either HLA DR-3 or HLA DR-6 or both (90).

From the picture that emerges, Bernstein and Mathews (89) describe a "Jo-1 syndrome," consisting of a high frequency of myositis (90%), ILD (80%), arthralgias or arthritis (60-100%), Raynaud's phenomenon (90%), sicca syndrome (55%), and sclerodactyly (20%), and a low frequency of rash and malignancy. Of great interest is the finding that patients with antibodies to PL-7 and PL-12 have a generally similar syndrome. Bernstein and Mathews (89) indicate that all three antisynthetases mark a similar subgroup, specifically finding a high frequency of ILD in patients with anti-PL-7 and with anti-PL-12. We have found a high frequency of ILD in our patients with anti-PL-7 and particularly with anti-PL-12, the latter including patients with ILD without myositis or with CK elevations alone (91). Other features of the Jo-1 syndrome also appear in patients with PL-7 and PL-12. Arthritis has been a prominent feature of patients with antibodies to PL-7 and PL-12, and some have presented with this symptom. The combination of myositis, ILD, and Raynaud's phenomenon occurs frequently in these patients (89). Thus, patients who have antibodies to functionally analogous enzymes develop the same clinical syndrome.

C. Other Antibodies to Cytoplasmic Antigens

The group of antibodies that are part of this association may be broader than just these three antisynthetases. Mathews et al. (78) have reported other antibodies to tRNA-related antigens in PM, although not yet in ILD, including anti-Fer, anti-Mas, and anti-Cam. Thus, it was suggested that PM/DM has a general association with antibodies to tRNA-related antigens. However, we have recently found another anticytoplasmic antibody associated with a syndrome very similar to that described for the antisynthetases, but we could not demonstrate an association of the antigen with tRNA (Fig. 1)(36). The KJ antibody was found in two patients, both had ILD with PM, including one in whom ILD dominated the clinical picture along with Raynaud's phenomenon. Despite the absence of tRNA from immunoprecipitates with this antibody, it could be demonstrated that the antigen was involved in the process of protein synthesis and therefore functionally related to the synthetases.

It is possible that PM/DM with ILD has a general association with antibodies to antigens involved in protein synthesis. In this regard, it is of interest that antibodies directed at the 54-kD protein of the signal recognition particle (SRP) have been reported in PM patients (77,92). The SRP is involved in the synthesis of certain proteins, directing nascent proteins with certain signal sequences into the endoplasmic reticulum. However, unlike the antisynthetases, anti-SRP does not appear to be associated with pulmonary fibrosis (92). Another antibody, called anti-Alu, has also been reported to react with the signal recognition particle but with the 68-kD protein (93). This antibody has been found in PM and in ILD, but was also found in other conditions (94).

D. ILD and Other Autoantibodies

ILD is said to be more common (50%) in patients with anti-PM-Scl than in PM/DM patients without this antibody (89). While most patients with anti-PM-Scl have PM/DM, about half of the cases have overlap with scleroderma (76), which can sometimes overshadow the PM/DM. In a few cases, no evidence of PM/DM is found. Seven of the 22 patients with antibodies to PM-Scl in one study (76) had bilateral pulmonary infiltrates, and most were among the 10 with features of scleroderma overlap. Since ILD is common in scleroderma, further study would be needed to determine whether there is an independent association of anti-PM-Scl with ILD. ILD is also said to be more common in PM/DM patients with anti-nRNP than in PM/DM patients without this antibody (80,89). This association has not been well studied, and the antibody is most commonly associated with overlap syndromes with SLE and other conditions.

E. Relationship of PM/DM-Specific Autoantibodies to Etiology and Pathogenesis

The reason for the association of a group of related antibodies with PM/DM with ILD is a matter of speculation, but it is likely to have some relationship to the underlying etiologic and pathogenetic factors responsible for the development of the disease, in view of the disease specificity of the

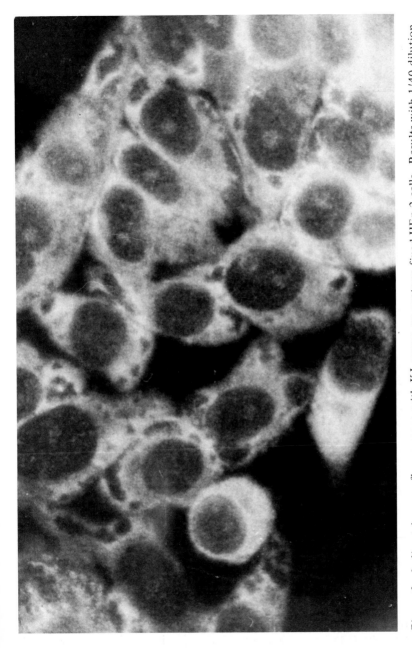

Figure 1. Indirect immunofluorescence with KJ serum on acetone fixed HEp-2 cells. Results with 1/40 dilution are shown, but this sample could be titered to 1/3,240. (Reproduced with permission of the *Journal of Clinical Investigation*.)

antibodies. It has been suggested that a virus acts as an etiologic agent in at least some cases of PM/DM. The most common virus implicated has been Coxsackievirus. Various lines of evidence for this have been presented (95-98). including the recent report of Coxsackievirus genetic material in extracts of PM/DM muscle (99). One hypothesis suggests that the Jo-1 antigen is selected as target because of specific interactions between the viral protein or nucleic acid and the host histidyl-tRNA synthetase enzyme. In genetically susceptible patients, antibodies develop owing to the altered appearance of the host protein (72) or through an antiidiotypic mechanism (100). An alternative hypothesis proposes that the antibody develops because of epitopes on viral proteins that are shared by the Jo-1 antigen ("molecular mimicry") (101), although this would require similar, independent cross-reactions to explain the other antisynthetases. The mechanism by which the lung and muscle diseases are linked is not known and could theoretically by due to infection of both lung and muscle by the inciting virus or to a shared autoimmune reaction. Thus, the autoantibodies may be marking a subgroup of PM/DM triggered by a particular virus or group of viruses.

A separate question relates to whether these antibodies participate directly in the pathogenesis of lung or muscle disease. This cannot be answered with certainty at this time. The lack of evidence of deposition of antibody or immune complexes in the lung speaks against a role for these antibodies in the generation of the lung lesion. There appears to be more evidence for participation of antibody-mediated mechanisms in the pathogenesis of the muscle disease in DM than in PM [deposition of the membrane attack complex (102), more consistent deposition of immunoglobulins (103), and more prominent vasculitis (104) and capillary disease (60)]. Since the antisynthetases have been more closely associated with PM than with DM, and evidence is in favor of antigen-directed cell-mediated muscle damage in PM (105, 106), any possible role of anti-Jo-1 in muscle disease remains to be defined.

F. Clinical Significance

Tests for these specific antibodies can hold diagnostic usefulness for the clinican. These antibodies can be useful in distinguishing PM/DM from other myopathies or neuropathies, and the PM/DM-specific antibodies may help differentiate PM/DM from other connective tissue diseases. The presence of an antisynthetase antibody (anti-Jo-1, anti-PL-7, or anti-PL-12), and probably other antibodies to tRNA-related antigens, in a patient with myositis should raise the possibility that complicating ILD may be present, even in the absence of symptoms. ILD may respond best when treated early, and the presence of antisynthetases or related antibodies may be a valuable part of early recognition of the disease. Early recognition of ILD is also important when considering initiating therapy with drugs such as methotrexate; with the potential for lung toxicity that could resemble complicating ILD, these antibodies might suggest caution with such therapy. In patients presenting with ILD, these antibodies can help in recognizing the underlying disease as PM/DM, even before any manifestation of PM/DM occurs in the muscle. These antibodies may occur in ILD before the appearance of myositis (29,33,89), and consideration should be given to testing for these antibodies in all patients with ILD of unclear origin, particularly if the CK is elevated. Thus, antisynthetases may be used as markers of ILD in PM/DM patients, or as markers of PM/DM in ILD patients, but they mark only a portion of each group. Although anti-Jo-1 antibody titer tends to fall with treatment and remission of the myositis (44), it has not been shown to correlate with the activity of the myositis or the ILD (29) and is usually not used for assessing disease activity.

References

1. Bohan, A., and Peter, J. B. (1975). Polymyositis and dermatomyositis. Parts 1 and 2. *N. Engl. J. Med.* **292**:344-347;403-407.
2. Mastaglia, F. L., and Ojeda, V. J. (1985). Inflammatory myopathies. Parts 1 and 2. *Ann. Neurol.* **17**:216-227;317-323.
3. Kagen, L. J. (1985). Polymyositis/dermatomyositis. In *Arthritis and Allied Conditions*, 10th ed. Edited by D. J. McCarty. Lea and Febiger, Philadelphia, pp. 971-993.
4. Bohan, A., Peter, J. B., Bowman, R. L., and Pearson, C. M. (1977). A computer-assisted analysis of 153 patients with polymyositis and dermatomyositis. *Medicine* **56**:255-286.
5. Hochberg, M. C., Feldman, D., and Stevens, M. B. (1986). Adult onset polymyositis/dermatomyositis: An analysis of clinical and laboratory features and survival in 76 patients with a review of the literature. *Semin. Arthritis. Rheum.* **15**:168-178.
6. Bradley, W. G. (1985). Diagnostic tests in neuromuscular disease. In *Textbook of Rheumatology,* 2d ed. Edited by Kelley, W. N., E. D. Harris, S. Ruddy, and C. B. Sledge. W. B. Saunders, Philadelphia, pp. 707-716.
7. Carpenter, S., and Karpati, G. (1981). The major inflammatory myopathies of unknown cause. *Pathol. Annu.* **16**:205-237.
8. Kagen, L. J. (1984). Less common causes of myositis. In *Inflammatory Disorders of the Muscle.* Edited by B. M. Ansell. *Clin. Rheum. Dis.* **10**:175-186.
9. Greenlee, J. E., Johnson, W. D. Jr., Campa, J. F., Adelman, L. S., and Sande, M. A. (1975). Adult toxoplasmosis presenting as polymyositis and cerebellar ataxia. *Ann. Intern. Med.* **82**:367-371.

10. Kallen, P. S., Louie, J. S., Nies, K. M., and Bayer, A. S. (1982). Infectious myositis and related syndromes. *Semin. Arthritis Rheum.* **11**:421-439.

11. Gamboa, E. T., Eastwood, A. B., Hays, A. P., Maxwell, J., and Penn, A. S. (1979). Isolation of influenza virus from muscle in myoglobinuric polymyositis. *Neurology* **29**:1323-2335.

12. Dalakas, M. C., Pezeshkpour, G. H., Gravell, M., and Sever, J. L. (1986). Polymyositis associated with AIDS retrovirus. *J.A.M.A.* **256**:2381-2383.

13. Harrington, T. M., Cohen, M. D., Bartleson, J. D., and Ginsburg, W. (1983). Elevation of creatine kinase in amyotrophic lateral sclerosis. Potential confusion with polymyositis. *Arthritis Rheum.* **26**:201-205.

14. Callen, J. P. (1984). Myositis and malignancy. *Clin. Rheum. Dis.* **10**:117-130.

15. Manchul, L., Jin, A., Pritchard, K. J., Tenenbaun, J., Boyd, N. F., Lee, P., Germanson, T., and Gordon, D. A. (1985). The frequency of malignant neoplasms in patients with polymyositis and dermatomyositis. *Intern. Med.* **145**:1835-1839.

16. Pachman, L. (1986). Juvenile dermatomyositis. *Pediatr. Clin. North Am.* **33**:1097-1117.

17. Dickey, B. F., and Myers, A. R. (1984). Pulmonary disease in polymyositis/dermatomyositis. *Semin. Arthritis Rheum.* **14**:60-76.

18. Braun, N. M., Arora, N. S., and Rochester, D. F. (1983). Respiratory muscle and pulmonary function in polymyositis and other proximal myopathies. *Thorax* **38(8)**:616-623.

19. Devere, R., and Bradley, W. G. (1975). Polymyositis: Its presentation, morbidity and mortality. *Brain* **98**:637-666.

20. Schiavi, E. A., Roncoroni, A. J., and Puy, R. J. (1984). Isolated bilateral diaphragmatic paresis with interstitial lung disease. *Am. Rev. Respir. Dis.* **129**:337-339.

21. Lakhanpal, S., Lie, J. T., Conn, D. L., and Martin, W. J. II (1987). Pulmonary disease in polymyositis/dermatomyositis: A clinicopathological analysis of 65 autopsy cases. *Ann. Rheum. Dis.* **46**:23-29.

22. Dietz, F., Logeman, J. A., Sahgal, V., and Schmid, F. R. (1980). Cricopharyngeal muscle dysfunction in the differential diagnosis of dysphagia in polymyositis. *Arthritis Rheum.* **23**:491-495.

23. Medsger, T. A., Robinson, H., and Masi, A. T. (1971). Factors affecting survivorship in polymyositis: A life-table study of 124 patients. *Arthritis Rheum.* **14**:249-258.

24. Benbassat, J., Gefel, D., Larholt, K., Sukenik, S., Morgenstern, V., and Zlotnick, A. (1985). Prognostic factors in polymyositis/dermatomyositis. *Arthritis Rheum.* **28**:249-255.

25. Arnett, F. C., Whelton, J. C., Zizic, T. M., and Stevens, M. B. (1973). Methotrexate therapy in polymyositis. *Ann. Rheum. Dis.* **32**:536-546.
26. Barnes, B. E. (1976). Dermatomyositis and malignancy—a review of the literature. *Ann. Intern. Med.* **84**:68-76.
27. Tang, W. Y., Singh, D., and Chuan, P. S. (1980). Diffuse interstitial pulmonary fibrosis, dermatomyositis and lung cancer—a case report. *Singapore Med. J.* **21**:778-780.
28. Mills, E. S., and Mathews, W. H. (1956). Interstitial pneumonitis in dermatomyositis. *J.A.M.A.* **160**:1467-1470.
29. Bernstein, R. M., Morgan, S. H., Chapman, J., Bunn, C. C., Matthews, M. B., Hughes, G. R. V., and Turner-Warwick, M. (1984). Anti-Jo-1 antibody: A marker for myositis with interstitial lung disease. *Br. Med. J.* **289**:151-152.
30. Biswas, T., Miller, F. W., Takagaki, Y., and Plotz, P. H. (1987). An enzyme-linked immunosorbent assay for the detection and quantitation of anti-Jo-1 antibody in human serum. *J. Immunol. Methods* **98**:243-248.
31. Hidano, A., Kaneko, K., and Arai, Y. (1985). Survey of the association of dermatomyositis and pulmonary fibrosis. *Arerugi* **34**:245-251.
32. Hochberg, M. C., Feldman, D., Stevens, M. B., Arnett, F. C., and Reichlin, M. (1984). Antibody to Jo-1 in polymyositis/dermatomyositis: Association with interstitial pulmonary disease. *J. Rheumatol.* **11**:663-665.
33. Nash, P., Schrieber, L., and Webb, J. (1987). Interstitial lung disease as the presentation of anti-Jo-1 positive polymyositis. *Clin. Rheumatol.* **6**:282-286.
34. Phillips, T. J., Leigh, I. M., and Wright, J. (1987). Dermatomyositis and pulmonary fibrosis associated with anti-Jo-1 antibody. *J. Am. Acad. Dermatol.* **17**:381-382.
35. Takizawa, H., Shiga, J., Moroi, Y., Miyachi, S., Nishiwaki, M., and Miyamoto, T. (1987). Interstitial lung disease in dermatomyositis: Clinicopathological study. *J. Rheumatol.* **14**:102-107.
36. Targoff, I. N., ARnett, F. C., Berman, L., O'Brien, and Reichlin, M. (1989). Anti-KJ: A new antibody associated with the syndrome of polymyositis and interstitial lung disease. *J. Clin. Invest.* **84**:162-172.
37. Tymms, K. E., and Webb, J. (1985). Dermatopolymyositis and other connective tissue diseases: A review of 105 cases. *J. Rheumatol.* **12**:1140-1148.
38. Wasicek, C. A., Reichlin, M., Montes, M., and Raghu, G. (1984). Polymyositis and stitial lung disease in a patient with anti-Jo-1 prototype. *Am. J. Med.* **76**:538-544.
39. Pearson, C. M. (1966). Polymyositis. *Annu. Rev. Med.* **17**:63-82.

40. Rose, A. L., and Walton, J. N. (1966). Polymyositis: A survey of 89 cases with particular reference to treatment and prognosis. *Brain* **89**:747-768.
41. Frazier, A. R., and Miller, R. D. (1974). Interstitial pneumonitis in association with polymyositis and dermatomyositis. *Chest* **65**:403-407.
42. Songcharoen, S., Raju, S. F., and Pennebaker, J. B. (1980). Interstitial lung disease in polymyositis and dermatomyositis. *J. Rheumatol.* **7**:353-360.
43. Salmeron, G., Greenberg, S. D., and Lidsky, M. D. (1981). Polymyositis and diffuse interstitial lung disease. *Arch. Intern. Med.* **141**:1005-1010.
44. Yoshida, S., Akizuki, M., Mimori, T., Yamagata, H., Inada, S., and Homma, M. (1983). The precipitating antibody to an acidic nuclear protein antigen, the Jo-1, in connective tissue disease. A marker for a subset of polymyositis with interstitial pulmonary fibrosis. *Arthritis Rheum.* **26**:604-611.
45. Schwarz, M. I., Matthay, R. A., Sahn, S. A., Stanford, R. E., Marmorstein, B. L., and Scheinhorn, D. J. (1976). Interstitial lung disease in polymyositis and dermatomyositis: Analysis of six cases and review of the literature. *Medicine* **55**:89-104.
46. Holmes, R., Black, M. M., Farebrother, M. J. B., and Van Grutten, M. (1980). Malignancy associated dermatomyositis with fibrosing alveolitis. *Clin. Exp. Dermatol.* **5**:415-420.
47. Perlman, S. G., and Barth, W. F. (1980). Polymyositis, breast carcinoma and interstitial lung disease. *J. Rheumatol.* **7**:348-352.
48. Dubowitz, L. M., and Dubowitz, V. (1964). Acute dermatomyositis presenting with pulmonary manifestations. *Arch. Dis. Child.* **39**:293-296.
49. Duncan, P. E., Griffin, J. P., Garcia, A., and Kaplan, S. B. (1974). Fibrosing alveolitis in polymyositis. *Am. J. Med.* **57**:621-626.
50. Fernandes, L., and Goodwill, C. J. (1979). Dermatomyositis without apparent myositis, complicated by fibrosing alveolitis. *J. R. Soc. Med.* **72**:777-779.
51. Fudman, E. J., and Schnitzer, T. J. (1986). Dermatomyositis without creatine kinase elevation: A poor prognostic sign. *Am. J. Med.* **80**:329-332.
52. Fergusson, R. J., Davidson, N. M., Nuki, G., and Crompton, G. K. (1983). Dermatomyositis and rapidly progressive fibrosing alveolitis. *Thorax* **38**:71-72.
53. Takizawa, H., Hidaka, N., and Akiyama, K. (1985). Clinicopathological studies on interstitial lung disease in polymyositis-dermatomyositis. *Kyobu Geka* **23**:528-536.

54. Schumacher, H. R., Schimmer, B., Gordon, G. V., Bookspan, M. H., Brogadir, S., and Dornart, B. B. (1979). Articular manifestations of polymyositis and dermatomyositis. *Am. J. Med.* **67**:287-292.
55. Bunch, T. W., Tancredi, R. G., and Lie, J. T. (1981). Pulmonary hypertension in polymyositis. *Chest* **79**:105-107.
56. Inoue, T., Kanayama, Y., Ohe, A., Kato, N., Horiguchi, T., Ishi, M., and Shiota, K. (1979). Immunopathologic studies of pneumonitis in systemic lupus erythematosus. *Ann. Intern. Med.* **91**:30-34.
57. Schwarz, M. I., Dreisin, R. B., Pratt, D. S., and Stanford, R. E. (1978). Immunofluorescent patterns in the idiopathic interstitial pneumonias. *J. Lab. Clin. Med.* **91**:929-938.
58. Thompson, P. L., and Mackay, I. R. (1970). Fibrosing alveolitis and polymyositis. *Thorax* **25**:504-507.
59. Hammar, S. P., Winterbauer, R. H., Bockus, D., Remington, F., Sale, G. E., and Meyers, G. D. (1983). Endothelial cell damage and tubuloreticular structures in interstitial lung disease associated with collagen vascular disease and viral pneumonia. *Am. Rev. Respir. Dis.* **127**:77-84.
60. Crowe, W. E., Bove, K. E., Levinson, J. E., and Hilton, P. K. (1982). Clinical and pathogenetic implications of histopathology in childhood polydermatomyositis. *Arthritis Rheum.* **25**:126-139.
61. Crystal, R. G., Codek, J. E., Ferrans, V. J., Fulmer, J. D., Line, B. R., and Hunninghake, G. W. (1981). Interstitial lung disease: Current concepts of pathogenesis, staging and therapy. *Am. J. Med.* **70**:542-568.
62. Scott, D. G., and Bacon, P. A. (1980). Response to methotrexate in fibrosing alveolitis associated with connective tissue disease. *Thorax* **35 (10)**:725-732.
63. Rowen, A. J., and Reichel, J. (1983). Dermatomyositis with lung involvement, successfully treated with azathioprine. *Respiration* **44(2)**: 143-146.
64. Plowman, P. N., and Stableforth, D. E. (1977). Dermatomyositis with fibrosing alveolitis: Response to treatment with cyclophosphamide. *Proc. R. Soc. Med.* **70**:738-740.
65. Caspary, E. A., Gubbay, S. S., and Stern, G. M. (1964). Circulating antibodies in polymyositis and other muscle-wasting disorders. *Lancet* **2**:941.
66. Pachman, L. M., Friedman, J. M., Maryjowski-Sweeney, M. L., Johnason, D., Radvang, R. A., Sharp, G. C., Cobb, M. A., Battles, N. D., Crowe, W. E., Fink, C. W., Hanson, V., Levinson, J. E., Spencer, G. H., and Sullivan, D. B. (1985). Immunogenetic studies of juvenile dermatomyositis. III. Study of antibody to organ-specific and nuclear antigens. *Arthritis Rheum.* **8**:151-157.
67. Wada, K., Ueno, S., Hazama, T., Ogasahara, S., Kang, J., Takahasni, M., and Tqrui, S. (1983). Radioimmunoassay for antibodies to human

skeletal muscle myosin in serum from patients with polymyositis. *Clin. Exp. Immunol.* **52**:297-304.

68. Nishikai, M., and Homma, M. (1977). Circulating autoantibody against human myoglobin in polymyositis. *J.A.M.A.* **237**:1842-1844.

69. Reichlin, M., and Arnett, F. C. (1984). Multiplicity of antibodies in myositis sera. *Arthritis Rheum.* **27**:1150-1156.

70. Reichlin, M. (1984). Seroreactivity in myositis patients. *J. Rheumatol.* **11**:591-592.

71. Nishikai, M., and Reichlin, R. (1980). Heterogeneity of precipitating antibodies in polymyositis. Characterization of the Jo-1 antibody system. *Arthritis Rheum.* **23**:881-888.

72. Mathews, M. B., and Bernstein, R. M. (1983). Myositis autoantibody inhibits histidyl-tRNA synthetase: A model for autoimmunity. *Nature* **304**:177-179.

73. Mathews, M. B., Reichlin, M., Hughes, G. R. V., and Bernstein, R. M. (1984). Anti-threonyl-tRNA synthetase, a second myositis-related autoantibody. *J. Exp. Med.* **160**:420-434.

74. Bunn, C. C., Bernstein, R. M., and Mathews, M. B. (1986). Autoantibodies against ananyl-tRNA synthetase and tRNA[ala] coexist and are associated with myositis. *J. Exp. Med.* **163**:1281-1291.

75. Targoff, I. N., and Reichlin, M. (1985). The association between Mi-2 antibodies and dermatomyositis. *Arthritis Rheum.* **28**:796-803.

76. Reichlin, M., Maddison, P. J., Targoff, I. N., Bunch, T., Arnett, F., Sharp, G., Treadwell, E., and Tan, E. M. (1984). Antibodies to nuclear/nucleolar antigen in patients with polymyositis-overlap syndrome. *J. Clin. Immunol.* **4**:40-44.

77. Reeves, W. H., Nigam, S. K., and Blobel, G. (1986). Human autoantibodies reactive with the signal-recognition particle. *Proc. Natl. Acad. Sci. USA* **84**:9507-9511.

78. Mathews, M. B., Bunn, C. C., and Bernstein, R. M. (1985). Autoantibodies to Jo-1 and other tRNA-related antigens in myositis. In *Rheumatology-85*. Edited by Brooks, P. M., and J. R. York. Elsevier Science, New York, pp. 189-192.

79. Lerner, M. R., and Steitz, J. A. (1979). Antibodies to small nuclear RNAs with proteins are produced by patients with systemic lupus erythematosus. *Proc. Natl. Acad. Sci. USA* **76**:5495-5499.

80. Venables, P. J. W., Mumford, P. A., and Maini, R. N. (1981). Antibodies to nuclear antigens in polymyositis: Relationship to autoimmune "overlap syndromes" and carcinoma. *Ann. Rheum. Dis.* **40**:271-223.

81. Reichlin, M. (1985). Antinuclear antibodies. In *Textbook of Rheumatology*, 2d ed. Edited by Kelly, W. N., H. Harris, and C. B. Sledge. W.B. Saunders, Philadelphia, pp. 690-707.

82. Mimori, T., Akizuki, M., Yamagata, H., Inada, S., and Homma, M. (1981). Characterization of a high molecular weight acidic nuclear protein recognized by autoantibodies in sera from patients with polymyositis-scleroderma overlap. *J. Clin. Invest.* **68**:611-620.

83. Hardin, J. A., Rahn, D. R., Shen, D., Lerner, M. R., Wolin, S. L., Rosa, M. D., and Steitz, J. A. (1982). Antibodies from patients with connective tissue disease bind specific subsets of cellular RNA-protein particles. *J. Clin. Invest.* **70**:141-147.

84. Dang, C. V., and Dang, C. V. (1986). Higher eukaryotic aminoacyl-tRNA synthetases in physiologic and pathologic states. *Mol. Cell Biochem.* **71**:107-120.

85. Bernstein, R. M., Bunn, C. C., Hughes, G. R. V., Francoeur, A. M., and Mathews, M. B. (1984). Cellular protein and RNA antigens in autoimmune disease. *Mol. Biol. Med.* **2**:105-120.

86. Targoff, I. N., and Reichlin, M. (1987). Measurement of antibody to Jo-1 by ELISA and comparison to enzyme inhibitory activity. *J. Immunol.* **138**:2874-2882.

87. Walker, E. J., Tymms, K. E., Webb, J., and Jeffrey, P. D. (1987). Improved detection of anti-Jo-1 antibody, a marker for myositis, using purified histidyl-tRNA synthetase. *J. Immunol. Methods* **96**:149-156.

88. Pachman, L. M., Hardin, J. A., Cobb, M. A., and Arroyave, C. M. (1984). The anti-nuclear antibody (ANA) in juvenile dermatomyositis (JDMS) is not Jo-1, suggesting that JDMS and polymyositis (PM) are different diseases. *Arthritis Rheum.* **27**:S45 (Abstract A21).

89. Bernstein, R. M., and Mathews, M. B. (1985). Jo-1 and other myositis antibodies. In *Rheumatology-85*, Excerpta Med. Int. Congr. Ser. Edited by Brooks, P. M., and J. R. York. Elsevier, New York, pp. 273-278.

90. Arnett, F. C., Hirsch, T. J., Bias, W. B., Nishikai, M., and Reichlin, M. (1981). The Jo-1 antibody system in myositis: Relationships to clinical features and HLA. *J. Rheum.* **8**:925-930.

91. Targoff, I. N., and Arnett, F. C. Clinical manifestations in patients with anti PL-12 antibody (ananyl-tRNA synthetase). Submitted for publication.

92. Targoff, I. N., Johnson, A. E., and Miller, F. W. Antibodies to signal recognition particle in polymyositis. Submitted for publication.

93. Andrews, G. A., and Kole, R. (1987). Alu RNA transcribed in vitro binds the 68-kDa subunit of the signal recognition particle. *J. Biol. Chem.* **262**:2908-2912.

94. Kole, R., Fresco, L. D., Keene, J. D., Cohen, P. L., Eisenberg, R. A., and Golden Andrews, P. (1985). Alu RNA-protein complexes formed in vitro react with a novel lupus autoantibody. *J. Biol. Chem.* **260**:11781-11786.

95. Whitaker, J. N. (1982). Inflammatory myopathy: A review of etiologic and pathogenetic factors. *Muscle Nerve* **5**:573-592.
96. Pearson, C. M. (1975). Myopathy with viral-like structures. (Editorial.) *N. Engl. J. Med.* **292**:641-642.
97. Strongwater, S. L., Dorovini-Zis, K., Ball, R. D., and Schnitzer, T. J. (1984). A murine model of polymyositis induced by Coxsackievirus B1 (Tucson strain). *Arthritis Rheum.* **27**:433-442.
98. Christensen, M. L., Pachman, L. M., Schneiderman, R., Patel, D. C., and Friedman, J. M. (1986). Prevalence of Coxsackie B virus antibodies in patients with juvenile dermatomyositis. *Arthritis Rheum.* **29**: 1365-1370.
99. Bowles, N. E., Dubowitz, V., Sewry, C. A., and Archard, L. C. (1987). Dermatomyositis, polymyositis and Coxsackie-B-virus infection. *Lancet* **1**:1004-1007.
100. Plotz, P. H. (1983). Autoantibodies are anti-idiotype antibodies to antiviral antibodies. *Lancet* **2**:824-826.
101. Walker, E. J., and Jeffrey, P. D. (1986). Polymyositis and molecular mimicry, a mechanism of autoimmunity. *Lancet* **2**:605-607.
102. Kissel, J. T., Mendell, J. R., and Rammohan, K. W. (1986). Microvascular deposition of complement membrane attack complex in dermatomyositis. *N. Engl. J. Med.* **314**:329-334.
103. Whitaker, J. N., and Engel, W. K. (1972). Vascular deposits of immunoglobulin and complement in idiopathic inflammatory myopathy. *N. Engl. J. Med.* **286**:333-338.
104. Feldman, D., Hochberg, M. C., Zizic, T. M., and Stevens, M. B. (1983). Cutaneous vasculitis in adult polymyositis/dermatomyositis. *J. Rheumatol.* **10**:85-89.
105. Arahata, K., and Engel, A. G. (1984). Monoclonal antibody analysis of mononuclear cells in myopathies. I. Quantitation of subsets according to diagnosis and sites of accumulation and demonstration and counts of muscle fibers invaded by T cells. *Ann. Neurol.* **16**:193-208.
106. Engel, A. G., and Arahata, K. (1984). Monoclonal antibody analysis of mononuclear cells in myopathies. II. Phenotypes of polymyositis and inclusion body myositis. *Ann. Neural.* **16**:209-215.

12

Systemic Vasculitis

STEVEN MATHEWS

Jacksonville, Florida

THOMAS R. CUPPS

Georgetown University Medical Center
Washington, DC

I. Introduction

A vasculitis is a clinicopathologic process characterized by inflammation and necrosis of the blood vessels. The clinical spectrum ranges from a primary disease process involving blood vessels exclusively to an involvement of vessels as a relatively insignificant component of another underlying systemic disease (1). No unifying concept of pathogenesis or cause has been confirmed. Hence, the approach to classification has been, of necessity, clinicopathologic or syndromic (2). Although virtually any organ system can be involved by a vasculitis, the lung is commonly affected for several reasons: (a) the extensive vascular network in the lung; (b) sensitizing antigens can reach the lung through the respiratory tract; and (c) the presence of large numbers of vasoactive cells in the lungs (3).

The true nature of the pathogenesis of pulmonary vasculitis is unknown. The most widely accepted mechanism is the deposition of antigen-antibody immune complexes on the vessel walls with subsequent activation of the complement cascade (1,4,5). Polymorphonuclear leukocytes are brought by chemotaxis to the vessel wall with subsequent release of lysosomal enzymes, resulting in necrosis (6). The lung, because of its high concentration of B lymphocytes which are brought into close proximity with the wide variety of inhaled antigens, allows for the formation of antigen-antibody complexes (6). These immune complexes can be deposited along the extensive pulmonary vasculature (7).

In this chapter we will discuss the vasculitides that may involve the lung, including (a) Wegener's granulomatosis, (b) allergic angiitis and granulomatosis (Churg-Strauss disease), (c) lymphomatoid granulomatosis, and (d) Takayasu's arteritis. Other disease entities that may be associated with vasculitic process, such as rheumatoid arthritis, systemic lupus erythematosus, Behcet's syndrome, and sarcoidosis, are discussed in other chapters.

II. Wegener's Granulomatosis

Wegener's granulomatosis is characterized as a necrotizing, granulomatous vasculitis involving the upper and lower respiratory tract together with glomerulonephritis and variable degrees of disseminated small vessel vasculitis (4,5,8). Wegener's granulomatosis was first described by Klinger (9) in 1931 but was characterized as a clinicopathological entity in 1936 by Wegener (10).

The etiology of Wegener's granulomatosis is unknown. One possible etiology is that it is the result of hyperactivity of the immune system. The inhalation of an antigen could easily explain the primary involvement of the respiratory tract in this disease; however, an inciting antigen or infectious agent has not been identified.

A. Clinical Presentation

Various presenting signs and symptoms may be seen in Wegener's granulomatosis, from nonspecific fever and weight loss to classical hemoptysis and sinusitis. The presenting signs and symptoms as noted in 85 patients with Wegener's granulomatosis are listed in Table 1). Wegener's granulomatosis most commonly presents with upper respiratory tract signs and symptoms, including sinusitis, nasal obstruction, otitis, epistaxis, and gingival inflammation. The lower respiratory tract accounts for approximately one third of the initial symptoms, including cough, sputum production, dyspnea, pleurisy, chest pain, and hemoptysis. Nonspecific complaints of fever, weight loss, and maliase are less commonly seen at presentation. Musculoskeletal symptoms of myalgias, arthralgias, and even frank arthritis are seen in a small percentage of people as a presenting complaint. Orchitis and skin lesions are rarely seen as the initial manifestation of this disease.

Although the lower respiratory tract manifests the presenting sign or symptom in only one third of the patients, the lung is involved in essentially

Table 1 Presenting Signs and Symptoms in 85 Patients with Wegener's Granulomatosis[a]

Presenting sign or symptom	Percentage
Head and neck (total)	85
Sinusitis/nasal obstruction	53
Ear (otitis, hearing loss, pain)	15
Gingival inflammation	6
Epistaxis	6
Sore throat/laryngitis	5
"Saddle nose" deformity	4
Lower respiratory tract (total)	34
Cough/sputum production	16
Dyspnea	8
Pleurisy/chest pain	6
Hemoptysis	4
Fever	12
Extremity involvement (total)	9
Arthralgia/arthritis	6
Myalgias	3
Systemic symptoms (i.e., weight loss, malaise)	5

[a]Data summarized from Walton (18) and Fahey et al. (29).

all patients with Wegener's granulomatosis (11). Asymptomatic lung involvement may be evident by pathological or radiological abnormalities. No other organ system shows such complete involvement. Rarely, patients with Wegener's granulomatosis will present with a clinical picture of adult respiratory distress syndrome and hemoptysis. This unusual presentation must be distinguished from Goodpasture's syndrome.

The upper airways are involved in 95% of all patients with Wegener's granulomatosis. The paranasal sinuses are frequent sites of inflammation. The order of involvement of the paranasal sinuses in descending order of frequency is maxillary, sphenoid, and ethmoid sinuses (12). A superimposed bacterial infection may sometimes be seen with lesions of the paranasal sinuses. This increased incidence of infection is felt to be secondary to the damage of the mucosal barrier with secondary obstruction and failure to clear secretions. The most common bacterial organism isolated in these episodes of sinusitis is *Staphylococcus aureus*. Another lesion that is seen in the upper airways is the "saddle nose" deformity. This is caused by the destruction and loss of the nasal cartilage due to the inflammation associated with the vasculitic lesions. Although aphthous lesions have also been reported on the oral mucosa, perforation of the hard and soft palates is not generally seen in Wegener's granulomatosis. Gingivitis, epistaxis, and sore throat are also seen secondarily to upper respiratory tract involvement. Tracheal and bronchial stenoses have also been described and may be significant management problems (13).

Kidney involvement with focal segmental glomerulonephritis is a hallmark of generalized Wegener's granulomatosis and has significant bearing on prognosis and therapy. Clinical evidence of renal involvement is not generally apparent at presentation.

Although uncommon as a presenting complaint, there is significant musculoskeletal involvement with Wegener's granulomatosis later in the course of the disease. Joint signs and symptoms were seen in 58% of patients in one study with 28% having frank arthritis (14). A nonerosive polyarticular arthritis is the most commonly recognized pattern of joint involvement. Deforming and erosive changes are rarely reported.

Cutaneous manifestations of Wegener's granulomatosis are quite common with involvement in 40-50% of cases (8,15). The skin lesions may be purpuric, hemorrhagic, vesicular, nodular, or ulcerative.

Ocular manifestations are seen in 43% of the cases of Wegener's granulomatosis (11). The most common eye finding is proptosis. The proptosis is caused by a retroorbital mass lesion, which usually consists of acute and chronic inflammation (16). Inflammation of the anterior structures of the eye is also commonly seen (12). A less frequently seen ocular manifestation is vasculitis of the retinal arteries and veins.

Cardiovascular involvement in Wegener's granulomatosis may be quite extensive, including pericarditis, coronary arteritis, myocarditis, valvulitis, and endocarditis (17,18). Palpitations, chest pain, and cough have all been seen in patients with Wegener's granulomatosis of the cardiovascular system. Serious complications, such as cardiac dysrythmias, may be secondary to vasculitis-induced ischemia (8).

The nervous system is also subject to involvement in Wegener's granulomatosis, with involvement reported in a quarter of all patients (11). The clinicopathological findings are varied, including contiguous invasion of the cranial vault by a granulomatous process in the paranasal sinuses and vasculitis of the vasa nervosum, causing cranial arteritis or mononeuritis multiplex. Diffuse cerebral vasculitis leading to cerebral vascular thrombosis and intracerebral or subarachnoid hemorrhage is less commonly reported (19).

B. Laboratory Findings

The laboratory findings in Wegener's granulomatosis reflect an active immune system. The erythrocyte sedimentation rate is invariably elevated, frequently to greater than 100 mm/h (20). A routine CBC will most likely reveal a leukocytosis and thrombocytosis. This elevation of the platelet count is believed to reflect the increased acute-phase reactants (8). The hematocrit and red cell indices, on the other hand, are usually consistent with a mild to moderate normochromic, normocytic anemia. It has been thought that this is the anemia of chronic disease (16). Leukopenia and thrombocytopenia have been reported but are extremely unusual findings in untreated patients. Hypergammaglobulinemia is a common finding, with elevations of IgG and IgA being well documented (16). Although elevations of IgE have been reported (13), this has not been found by all investigators (21). A positive rheumatoid factor is often reported by the latex fixation method (16). This is most likely secondary to the increased number of circulating immune complexes that have been reported in some patients. The urinalysis is a very simple but important source of information in evaluating a patient with Wegener's granulomatosis. An abnormal urinary sediment is seen in as many as 80% of patients (8). These abnormalities may include hematuria, proteinuria, and red cell casts. Since renal involvement is often clinically silent, these laboratory findings may be the first indication of kidney involvement.

Recent observations suggest that the presence of antineutrophil cytoplasmic antibodies may be a sensitive marker for Wegener's granulomatosis (22). Although this test may be useful as a screen in patients in whom the diagnosis is suspected, careful clinical correlation with biopsy confirmation should be obtained prior to the institution of treatment. It has also been noted that the level of antineutrophil cytoplasmic antibodies falls and returns to the background range in correlation to the disappearance of disease activity (22). The role of antineutrophil cytoplasmic antibodies in the diagnosis and management of patients with Wegener's granulomatosis is currently undergoing much research and shows promise for the future (22a,22b).

Radiologic studies are also important in Wegener's granulomatosis (Table 2). Frequent lower respiratory tract lesions are demonstrated radiologically. The most common pattern on routine chest X-ray are solitary or multiple nodular densities or infiltrates. These lesions may be unilateral or bilateral. The infiltrates may vary in size from less than 1 cm to greater than 9 cm in diameter (23). Cavitation of these infiltrates can occur, and occasionally air-fluid levels are found (23,24). The cavities have been described by some investigators as being thick-walled (25), whereas others state that they are really thin-walled and that the wall of the cavities only appear thickened owing to the infiltration of the surrounding lung parenchyma. The infiltrates are often transient and may be associated with areas of atelectasis

Table 2 Radiologic Manifestations in 80 Patients with Wegener's Granulomatosis[a]

Unilateral	55%
Bilateral	45%
Infiltrate	63%
(cavitation)	(8%)
Nodules	31%
(cavitation)	(10%)

[a]Summarized from Fahey et al. (29),
Flye et al. (78), and Pinching et al.
(79).

(23). Radiologic studies of the paranasal sinuses may be helpful in
Wegener's granulomatosis. As noted earlier, sinusitis is seen in the majority
of patients. One of the earliest radiologic abnormalities seen in the nasopharynx is thickening of the maxillary antra, which can progress to complete
opacification of the sinus (1). It is important to remember that these findings, although consistent with the diagnosis, are not specific for the diagnosis
of Wegener's granulomatosis.

Pulmonary function tests have been reported to be abnormal in some
patients. The results are consistent with a restrictive lung defect and can be
quite severe (26). Since most of these patients have been treated with cyclophosphamide, it is unclear whether the abnormality is due to the Wegener's
granulomatosis itself or secondary to the treatment (27).

C. Pathology

The pathologic pattern of Wegener's granulomatosis is a necrotizing granulomatous vasculitis of small veins and arteries. The granulomas characteristically have multinucleated giant cells, which may or may not be in close
proximity of vasculitic lesions or areas of necrosis. The classic renal lesion
in Wegener's granulomatosis is a focal and segmental glomerulonephritis
which is highly variable in severity and is sometimes accompanied by a necrotizing vasculitis (17). Severe glomerular involvement with crescent formation is also reported. Electron microscopy studies on these renal biopsies
may demonstrate subepithelial basement membrane densities, suggesting immune complex deposition (20). The typical findings on renal biopsy in Wegener's granulomatosis are consistent with but not diagnostic of this disease. A
lung biopsy, on the other hand, has a high yield for pathologic diagnosis in

this disease. An open lung biopsy is the preferred procedure because transbronchial biopsy by fiberoptic bronchoscopy does not provide an adequate tissue sample to demonstrate the granulomatous vasculitis. Although biopsies from lesions in the nasopharynx and skin can be diagnostic in 10-15% of cases, the most common pattern reported is acute and chronic inflammation with or without granulomas, which is a nonspecific pattern.

D. Therapy and Prognosis

The prognosis of untreated Wegener's granulomatosis is very poor, with a mean survival time of only 5 months and a 93% mortality at 2 years (10). The response to therapy with corticosteroids alone is marginal. In one study only 32% of the patients treated with steroids alone did better than patients who received no treatment at all (28).

Nitrogen mustard was the first cytotoxic drug reported successful in the treatment of Wegener's granulomatosis (29). Since that initial therapeutic trial, numerous cytotoxic agents have been used either alone or in combination with steroids with various degrees of response. Cyclophosphamide has clearly established itself as the drug of choice in classic Wegener's granulomatosis (8,30). In a prospective study of 85 patients with Wegener's granulomatosis treated with combined cyclophosphamide and prednisone, a complete remission was achieved in 93% of the patients, with a mean duration of 48.2 ± 3.6 months (30). The recommended regimen is 2 mg/kg of body weight by mouth per day. Corticosteroids are a useful adjunct; therefore, prednisone 1 mg/kg of body weight by mouth per day is started concomitantly. The daily prednisone is continued at this dose for 10-14 days, until the patient begins to respond to the cyclophosphamide.

Care should be taken to avoid suppressing the total white blood cell count below 3,000/mm^3 or an absolute polymorphonuclear leukocyte count below 1,500 cells/mm^3 (20). Once the patient has been treated for 2-4 weeks with cyclophosphamide, the prednisone should be quickly tapered over 1-2 months to an alternate-day dosage schedule. Then the prednisone should be gradually tapered until it can be discontinued. The cyclophosphamide should be continued at full dose for 1 year after the patient has gone into complete remission. At that time the cyclophosphamide dose should be lowered by 25-mg decrements every 2-3 months until the drug is discontinued or a minimum dosage is reached, below which there is a reactivation of the disease. If there is a reactivation of the Wegener's granulomatosis after treatment with this protocol, repeat induction is just as effective as the initial treatment. Cyclophosphamide is the treatment of choice for this disorder; however, there are reports of treatment failure in some patients (31,32). Other cytotoxic agents, such as chlorambucil or azathioprine, have been used in patients who do not tolerate cyclophosphamide. These agents do not appear to be as effective as cyclophosphamide in the treatment of Wegener's granulomatosis. Trimethoprim-sulfamethoxazole has been used as an adjuvant agent with some success in the treatment of this disease (33). The role of trimethoprim-sulfamethoxazole in the treatment of generalized Wegener's granulomatosis needs to be more clearly defined.

E. Limited Forms of Wegener's Granulomatosis

The limited form of Wegener's granulomatosis was first described by Carrington and Liebow (34) in 1966, when they identified 16 patients who had pulmonary lesions suggestive of "classic" Wegener's granulomatosis but without the renal glomerular lesions. Some cases of presumed limited disease are infact cases of generalized Wegener's granulomatosis. Studies have shown that clinically silent glomerulonephritis could go undiagnosed if a renal biopsy is not done. The findings on routine chest X-rays usually consist of multiple, bilateral, frequently cavitating, thin-walled lesions. It should be reemphasized that although the glomerulus is spared in the limited form, there is renal involvement with necrotizing granulomas found within the kidneys (34). Prior to the use of cytotoxic therapy, patients with the limited form of Wegener's granulomatosis were felt to have a better prognosis (34). Despite corticosteroid therapy, deaths secondary to respiratory insufficiency, massive hemoptysis, or a complication from therapy have been reported (4).

III. Allergic Angiitis and Granulomatosis

Allergic angiitis and granulomatosis (Churg-Strauss disease) was first described as a subset of polyarteritis nodosa (35). This association is based on the observation that vascular lesions identical to those seen in classic polyarteritis nodosa may be seen in this disease. However, there are major differences between the two entities. The features that differentiate allergic angiitis and granulomatosis from polyarteritis nodosa are (a) the high frequency of pulmonary involvement, (b) the involvement of small to medium-size arterioles and venules, (c) intra- and extravascular granuloma formation, (d) the peripheral eosinophilia and eosinophilic infiltrates, and (e) the high incidence of asthma (2).

The pathophysiology of this entity (6) is still not known. It may be similar to that of classic polyarteritis nodosa, being associated with immune complex deposition. However, hypocomplementemia and cryoglobulins are seen less commonly in allergic angiitis and granulomatosis (36). The significance of the eosinophilia and the role it plays in the pathogenesis of this disease are not understood.

A. Clinical Manifestations

Almost all patients with allergic angiitis and granulomatosis exhibit some type of pulmonary finding. Asthma is a very common initial presentation. In fact, it may precede any evidence of systemic involvement by as much as 30 years (37). The length of this period may have some prognostic significance. Evaluation of the relationship between mortality and the length of time from onset of asthma and the first evidence of additional pulmonary involvement suggests that the brevity of this period is an unfavorable prognostic sign (38). The presence of asthma may be transient. It has been reported that in up to 58% of cases asthma goes into remission with the onset of vasculitis (36). During the treatment for the vasculitis the asthma tends not to be a significant clinical problem. The disappearance of the asthma may be secondary to the treatment of the vasculitis with corticosteroids. The asthma, however, may recur when vasculitis therapy is discontinued.

Another common sign is pulmonary infiltrates. Radiologically, these are usually transient, and patchy in appearance. The infiltrates lack lobar or segmental distribution but may be symmetrical (37,38). Unlike the infiltrates seen in Wegener's granulomatosis, these rarely cavitate. Pleural effusions have also been described and are characterized as having a large concentration of eosinophils in the fluid (39).

The gastrointestinal tract is involved in approximately 40% of patients with allergic angiitis and granulomatosis. Eosinophilic infiltration of the bowel wall can produce obstructive lesions (40). Involvement of the mucosal layer can lead to diarrhea and bleeding (41). Ascitic fluid with a large concentration of eosinophils may result from serosal involvement (39). Other common presentations of gastrointestinal involvement include bowel perforation, gastric ulcers, and ulcerative colitis (37).

Cardiac involvement is present in over 50% of patients with allergic angiitis and granulomatosis. The spectrum of manifestations includes acute and constrictive pericarditis (39). The incidence of cardiac failure and myocardial infarction is also well described (37). Cardiac involvement has a significant impact on patient morbidity and mortality, accounting for 23% of deaths seen with this disease (20).

Cutaneous involvement is a common feature of allergic angiitis and granulomatosis. Skin lesions may present with purpura (often palpable), urticaria, or subcutaneous nodules. The etiologies of these lesions are varied from leukocytoclastic vasculitis, in the case of the purpuric lesions (42), to extravascular granulomas, in the case of the subcutaneous nodules (35). Livido reticularis and cutaneous infarction have also been reported.

The neurologic involvement in allergic angiitis and granulomatosis is very similar to the neurological manifestations of polyarteritis nodosa. The characteristic pattern is a mononeuritis multiplex which may progress to a symmetrical sensorimotor peripheral neuropathy (36). Central nervous system involvement is also common, the importance of which is illustrated by the fact that cerebral hemorrhage and infarction are major causes of death (43).

There is clinical evidence of renal involvement in 33% of patients with allergic angiitis and granulomatosis (20). The characteristic glomerular lesion is a focal segmental glomerulonephritis, with necrotizing features including crescents in some cases (36). Renal failure in allergic angiitis and granulomatosis secondary to poorly controlled malignant hypertension has been reported. Hypertension, secondary to high renin levels caused by kidney ischemia, is the most common clinical manifestation of kidney involvement.

B. Laboratory Findings

No laboratory finding is diagnostic for allergic angiitis and granulomatosis. An elevated erythrocyte sedimentation rate and leukocytosis are common, but both are nonspecific. One characteristic abnormality is peripheral eosinophilia. Approximately 85% of cases will exhibit an elevated eosinophil count (generally exceeding $5 \times 10^9/L$) at some point in the course of their disease (35). However, this eosinophilia may not be of long duration, and it will resolve rapidly once steroid therapy has been instituted. Other findings that have been reported include a positive low-titer rheumatoid factor by latex fixation (36).

C. Pathology

The histopathological pattern in allergic angiitis and granulomatosis may vary with the tissue site. Not all histological features (i.e., eosinophilic infiltration, intra- or extravascular granulomas, or necrotizing vasculitis) need to be present at the same pathological site (44,45). As stated previously, small to medium-size arterioles and venules are affected in this disease. Vascular involvement ranges from perivascular cuffing by eosinophils to a panmural necrotizing arteritis (36). Aneurysm formation, infarction, thrombosis, and fibrinoid necrosis may also be present (20).

D. Therapy and Prognosis

Prior to the use of steroids, the prognosis of allergic angiitis and granulomatosis was quite poor. In one study, 50% of patients had died by 3 months after the onset of vasculitis, and the 5-year survival rate was only 4% (46). The response to glucocorticosteroids is well documented and often quite dramatic. The recommended treatment for vasculitic disease is high-dose steroids (40-60 mg of prednisone by mouth per day) for several weeks, followed by a tapering schedule dictated by the patient's clinical response (47). The use of topical steroid preparations in the upper and lower respiratory tracts has been shown to be useful in reducing systemic steroid requirements (36). A subset of patients, particularly those with severe visceral involvement, will be resistant to corticosteroids and will require immunosuppressive therapy. Although azathioprine has been used with success in some cases, it is not effective in inducing remissions in all corticosteroid-resistant cases (36). Cyclophosphamide has been used successfully in treating corticosteroid-resistant patients with allergic angiitis and granulomatosis (47).

Another important aspect in the treatment of these patients is the control of the systemic hypertension. Poorly controlled hypertension may result in the progression to chronic renal failure. The use of angiotensin-converting enzyme inhibitors may be particularly effective in the management of hypertension.

IV. Lymphomatoid Granulomatosis

Lymphomatoid granulomatosis, described in 1972 by Liebow et al. (48), is an angiocentric and angiodestructive lymphoreticular proliferative and granulomatous disease involving predominantly the lungs. It is an uncommon disease, with approximately 200 cases reported in the literature. Lymphomatoid granulomatosis usually presents during middle age, and there is a slightly higher prevalence in males.

The exact pathogenesis of lymphomatoid granulomatosis is unknown. It has been postulated that lymphomatoid granulomatosis may, in fact, represent a lymphoproliferative process in a patient with an impaired immune system. This is based on the observation that many patients with this disease are anergic, and some will progress to a frank neoplastic process (49).

A. Clinical Manifestations

The most common presenting signs and symptoms are systemic in nature (i.e., fever, malaise, and weight loss) and lack diagnostic specificity. Symptoms related to specific organ system involvement including cough, dyspnea, neurologic dysfunction, and skin lesions are present in a significant number of patients at presentation.

Pulmonary involvement is universal in lymphomatoid granulomatosis. Although unusual, airway involvement can be extensive and include bronchiolitis obliterans and bronchial ulceration as well as destruction and occlusion of bronchioles by masses of inflammatory cells and fibrous tissue (50). Pulmonary lesions have been shown to be a significant cause of death in this disease due to respiratory insufficiency and hemoptysis (50,48).

Central nervous system involvement may be present in approximately a quarter of patients (48). Neurologic lesions may be noted on presentation with such symptoms as ataxia, hemiparesis, blindness, and dizziness (48). The infiltration of the walls of cerebral blood vessels has been associated with thrombosis, obstruction, and aneurysm formation in this disease (51). Spinal cord as well peripheral nerve involvement has been reported (52).

Clinically apparent cutaneous involvement is present in almost half of the patients with lymphomatoid granulomatosis (48). The most frequently seen lesions are erythematous, macular, or plaquelike lesions, which are typically found on the lower extremities (53). Histologically, a granulomatous reaction with infiltration of atypical lymphocytes and plasmacytoid cells is characteristically seen with frequent mitoses and occasional vasculitis (52).

Although histological renal involvement is common, clinically apparent renal disease is rare in lymphomatoid granulomatosis (48,50,53). Liebow et al. (48) first described what appeared to be rounded or wedge-shaped masses of tissue which reflected infiltration around the renal vessels with focal necrosis. The glomerulus is characteristically spared in this disease.

The presence of hepatomegaly has been described on clinical exam of patients with lymphomatoid granulomatosis (54). Liebow et al. (48) noted scattered areas of focal infiltration of lymphocytes and plasmacytoid cells on histological examination of the liver. Although the presence of hepatomegaly is not a clinically dominant feature of this disease, it has been associated with a worse prognosis.

B. Laboratory Findings

There is no consistent laboratory abnormality that is seen in lymphomatoid granulomatosis. The white blood cell count is not helpful in this disease. Katzenstein et al. (50), in their review of 152 cases, reported a leukocytosis in 30% of patients, a leukopenia in 20%, and normal values in 50% of all cases. A mild anemia may also be seen in a small percentage of cases (48,50). The erythrocyte sedimentation rate may be normal or slightly elevated (50). A polyclonal increase in serum IgG or IgM levels is present in less than half the cases (50). Antinuclear antibodies, LE prep, and rheumatoid factor are generally negative (48). The urinary sediment in these patients is typically normal.

Routine diagnostic radiologic studies of the chest are often very helpful in lymphomatoid granulomatosis. They may reveal characteristic abnormalities in a clinically asymptomatic patient. The most common radiological pattern seen is that of multiple bilateral nodular lesions that are predominantly in the peripheral and lower lung fields, similar to the pattern seen with

Table 3 Radiologic Manifestations in 173 Patients with Lymphomatoid Granulomatosis[a]

Multiple bilateral nodes	80%
(cavitation)	(30%)
Air bronchograms	35%
Pleural effusion	33%
Atelectasis	30%
Pneumonic/masslike lesion	30%
Pneumothorax	5%

[a]Summarized from Liebow et al. (48) and Katzenstein et al. (50).

metastatic disease (48). Other radiographic abnormalities are summarized in Table 3.

C. Pathology

The histopathology of lymphomatoid granulomatosis is characterized by an angiocentric angiodestructive infiltration of atypical-appearing lymphocytoid and plasmacytoid cells. The atypical lymphoreticular cells have a characteristic morphology. They are larger and contain more cytoplasm than normal mature lymphocytes, and some of these cells show plasmacytoid features which resemble immunoblasts (50). Mitotic figures are frequently present (48,50,53). Although the description of the above-stated cell population shares some characteristics of a lymphoproliferative malignancy, there are several important features that distinguish it from a lymphoma including (a) polyclonal origin of the infiltrative cells, (b) the location of vasculitic lesions distant from sites of parenchymal involvement, and (c) the marked lack of involvement of the lymphatic system (48,50,53). A significant number of cases of lymphomatoid granulomatosis have been noted to progress to a frankly neoplastic process. In one retrospective study that looked at this disturbing occurrence, 12% of patients developed a lymphoreticular neoplasm which was most commonly a non-Hodgkin's lymphoma (50). This figure may be a conservative estimate. A prospective study was done in which the occurrence was reported to be a 50% rate of progression to malignancy (20).

D. Prognosis and Treatment

Lymphomatoid granulomatosis most likely represents a spectrum of clinical entities ranging from benign lymphocytic angiitis and granulomatosis through the true lymphomatoid granulomatosis form of the disease to malignant lymphoma. Obviously, the overall prognosis is significantly different for each of these entities. In the preliminary studies the prognosis was rather poor, with a mortality rate of 67% and a median survival of 14 months. A subsequent prospective study by Fauci et al. (55) reported on 13 patients who were treated with cyclophosphamide and prednisone. These patients exhibited a relatively excellent response to this protocol, with seven patients achieving complete remissions lasting 5.2 ± 0.6 years. Cyclophosphamide was initiated at 2 mg/kg of body weight by mouth per day. The total white blood cell count must be monitored closely to ensure that it remains above 3,000 cells/mm^3. Prednisone was started at a dose of 1 mg/kg body weight orally each day for the first 1-2 months of therapy and then rapidly tapered to an alternate-day schedule. Once on an alternate-day schedule, the corticosteroid is gradually tapered until the patient is completely off the medicine or is maintained at the lowest dosage level to sustain a remission.

As was stated before, lymphomatoid granulomatosis does not appear to be one disease, but rather a spectrum of closely related clinical entities. It is clearly known that the more advanced stages of the disease are very difficult to treat and have a very low response rate. Therefore, it is imperative to identify patients with lymphomatoid granulomatosis early and begin therapy promptly. It would also be advisable that all patients with presumptive diagnosis of lymphomatoid granulomatosis be systematically evaluated for the presence of lymphoma. Tissue from any site of involvement may have a pattern of lymphomatoid granulomatosis, while tissues from a second site may be frankly neoplastic. Biopsies of multiple sites of disease activity may be required.

V. Takayasu's Arteritis

Takayasu's arteritis (pulseless disease, aortic arch syndrome, or reversed coarctation) is a disease characterized by inflammation and stenosis of intermediate to large-size arteries with frequent involvement of the aortic arch and its branches (56-59). Takayasu's arteritis tends to be a disease of young women. There is an 8.5:1 female-to-male ratio, and 80% of the patients are between 11 and 30 years of age (58).

The etiology of Takayasu's arteritis is unknown. A possible association with tuberculosis infection has been noted, and some authors have felt that this might have been of great significance in the pathogenesis of the disease (58,60,61). However, no clear cause-and-effect relationship has been established, and this mechanism is no longer widely supported. The possibility of an immune-mediated etiology for Takayasu's arteritis has also been suggested. In support of this hypothesis is the observation that serum immunoglobulins are elevated in patients with this disease (62). The acute-phase reactants erythrocyte sedimentation rate and C-reactive protein are both very sensitive markers of disease activity in Takayasu's arteritis. High titers of antibodies against the aortic wall antigen have been reported (63). There may be a genetic predisposition to the development of Takayasu's arteritis. Numano et al. (64) presented a case of monozygotic twins who developed Takayasu's arteritis, supporting the possibility of genetic influence in this disease. Several studies report an increased incidence of certain HLA markers in patients with this disease (65).

A. Clinical Manifestations

Two clinical stages of Takayasu's arteritis are recognized. The first stage is marked by acute inflammation and is clinically characterized by nonspecific symptoms including fever, malaise, myalgias, weight loss, arthralgias, and night sweats (66). Frank arthritis has been reported to occur in this first stage of the disease (67). Transient pleuritic chest pain and pericarditis are also sometimes present. The presence of skin lesions, which are similar to erythema multiforme and erythema nodosum, has been noted during this period (68). This first stage of Takayasu's arteritis may be relatively brief, with a total duration of approximately 1 month. Recurrent episodes of inflammation may be seen in some patients. The symptoms of the inflammatory stage gradually subside (69). The second clinical stage of Takayasu's arteritis, also known as the chronic or ischemic stage, has specific signs and symptoms which are the result of the ischemia of various organs. The time period between these two clinical stages is quite variable, with a range from a few months to decades with a mean duration of 8 years (70).

Vascular manifestations of Takayasu's arteritis are often quite dramatic. There may be involvement of any medium to large-size artery. The radial, ulnar, and carotid arteries are frequently involved and are easily evaluated on physical exam. Absent or decreased pulse, tenderness to palpation, or the presence of a bruit suggests clinical involvement.

Systemic hypertension has been reported to be present in 50% of patients with Takayasu's arteritis (71). Because of the frequent involvement of the aortic arch, upper extremity blood pressure determination may not reliably reflect the central blood pressure; consequently, the blood pressure in all extremities in these patients should be measured. Several mechanisms for the etiology of the observed hypertension in Takayasu's have been suggested, including renal artery stenosis with a secondary hypertensive state (68), atypical coarctation of the aorta (72), and blunting of the normal reflexes of the carotid and aortic arch baroreceptors in this disease.

The fundal findings that were first described by Takayasu (73) in 1908 are found in only 33% of all patients with this disease (20). It is felt that these arteriovenous anastomoses are secondary to ischemia and not vasculitis (20). Another ocular manifestation, which is much more commonly seen, is the "face-down" posture (74). The head is maintained in the flexed position to avoid a transient impairment of vision, which is frequently experienced by patients with Takayasu's arteritis when the head is held in a "face-up" or upright position.

The neurological manifestations of Takayasu's arteritis are the result of arterial hypertension or central nervous system ischemia (75). These manifestations include parasthesias, seizures, headaches, dizziness, and syncope.

Palpitations and dyspnea are common symptoms indicative of cardiac involvement. Congestive heart failure has been noted in over one third of patients with Takayasu's arteritis (20). The left-sided heart failure is generally accepted to be secondary to systemic hypertension, whereas right-sided heart failure is most likely secondary to pulmonary vascular disease. The complaint of atypical chest pain represents a complex diagnostic problem. All possible etiologies, including hypertension, myocardial ischemia, and aortic dissection, must be systematically evaluated.

Pulmonary artery involvement has been reported to be present in up to 50% of all patients with Takayasu's arteritis (60). Clinically, the pulmonary involvement is usually silent, although cough and dyspnea are sometimes seen early in the disease. Even though there is a paucity of symptoms, it has been shown that pulmonary involvement signifies a poor prognosis (69).

B. Laboratory Findings

In the first stage of Takayasu's arteritis the laboratory results reflect the acute inflammatory processes. The erythrocyte sedimentation rate is moderately elevated initially in the majority of patients, which is followed by a gradual return to normal limits. A routine complete blood count will most likely reveal a mild leukocytosis with a hypochromic or normochromic normocytic anemia (59). Serum immunoglobulins are often elevated, but the rheumatoid factor and antinuclear antibodies are usually not found to be significantly elevated (62).

Radiographic studies are an important tool in the evaluation of patients with Takayasu's arteritis. Findings on routine chest films that are suggestive of the diagnosis of Takayasu's arteritis include an irregular descending aorta, a calcified aortic wall, an ectatic aortic arch, and cardiomegaly (76). Rib notching on the chest X-ray, secondary to the collateral circulation, is also suggestive of the diagnosis (see Table 4). In one study 68% of the patients had abnormalities on aortography, with stenosis being the most common finding followed by occlusion, aneurysm, and dilatation (11). Pulmonary angiograms are often abnormal, showing occlusion of the main vessels of the pulmonary circulation (60). The importance of pulmonary perfusion scan-

Table 4 Radiologic Manifestations in 166 Patients with Takayasu's Arteritis[a]

Cardiomegaly	47%
Irregular descending aorta	45%
Normal	37%
Calcified aorta	17%
Pulmonary edema	6%
Rib notching	6%
Pleural effusion	4%

[a]Summarized from Lupi-Herrera et al. (58) and Yomato et al. (76).

ning has also been noted in screening patients for perfusion abnormalities (77).

C. Pathology

The pathology of Takayasu's arteritis is characterized by a panarteritis of medium to large-size arteries with mononuclear cell infiltrates with or without giant cell formation (68). After the inflammatory stage, which is often recurrent, there is significant fibrosis of the vessel wall, causing stenosis and occlusion of the vessel lumen. This, in turn, causes the second stage of the disease, which reflects the ischemic damage of the various organ systems.

D. Prognosis and Treatment

The prognosis of Takayasu's arteritis varies significantly among investigators. One study reports a 75% mortality rate at 2 years (56), whereas another study reports only a 17% mortality at 5 years (57). The leading cause of death in Takayasu's arteritis in descending order of frequency is congestive heart failure, myocardial infarction, and cerebral vascular accident (57-59).

Treatment with corticosteroids is the first line of therapy. Ideally, treatment should be started during the initial inflammatory stage of the disease. A starting dose of 30 mg by mouth per day of prednisone for 9 weeks followed by a maintenance of 5-10 mg by mouth per day for several years has been recommended (56). This treatment approach is generally effective in suppressing signs and symptoms of the inflammatory component of the disease and may prevent progression of the occlusive phase of Takayasu's arteritis. A subset of patients may progress despite corticosteroid therapy. Cyclophosphamide started at 2 mg/kg body weight orally combined with corticosteroid therapy may be effective in preventing progression in some corticosteroid-resistant cases (66). Vascular reconstructive surgery has also been shown to reduce the morbidity and mortality of this disease by avoiding ischemic conditions (66). Reconstructive surgery should be undertaken only when the inflammatory component of the disease has been adequately treated.

References

1. Fauci, A. S., Haynes, B. F., and Katz, P. (1978). The spectrum of vasculitis. Clinical, pathologic, immunologic, and therapeutic considerations. *Ann. Intern. Med.* **89**:660-676.
2. De Remee, R. A., Weiland, L. H., and McDonald, T. J. (1980). Respiratory vasculitis. *Mayo Clin. Proc.* **55**:492-498.
4. Dreisin, R. B. (1982). Pulmonary vasculitis. *Clin. Chest Med.* **3**:607-618.
5. Fulmer, J. D., and Kaltreider, H. B. (1982). The pulmonary vasculitides. *Chest* **82**:615-624.
6. Daniele, R. P., Henson, P. M., and Fantane, J. C. (1981). Immune complex injury of the lung. *Am. Rev. Respir. Dis.* **124**:738-755.
7. Leavitt, R. Y., and Fauci, A. S. (1986). Pulmonary vasculitis. *Am. Rev. Respir. Dis.* **134**:149-166.
8. Fauci, A. S., and Wolff, S. M. (1973). Wegener's granulomatosis: Studies in 18 patients and a review of the literature. *Medicine (Baltimore)* **52**:535-561.
9. Klinger, H. (1931). Grenzformen der Periarteritis Nodosa. *Frankfurt. Z. Path.* **42**:455-488.
10. Wegener, F. (1936). Uber Generalisierte, Septische Gefasserkrankungen *Verh. Dtsch. Pathol. Ges.* **29**:202-209.
11. Wolff, S. M., Fauci, A. S., Horn, R. G., and Dale, D. C. (1974). Wegener's granulomatosis. *Ann. Intern. Med.* **81**:513-525.
12. Haynes, B. F., Fishman, M. C., Fauci, A. S., Wolff, S. M. (1977). The ocular manifestations of Wegener's granulomatosis. Fifteen years experience and review of the literature. *Am. J. Med.* **63**:131-140.
13. Bohlman, M. E., Ensor, R. E., and Goldman, S. M. (1984). Primary Wegener's granulomatosis of the trachea: Radiologic manifestations. *South. Med. J.* **77**:1318-1319.
14. Noritake, D. T., Weiner, S. R., Bassett, L. W., Paulus, H. E., and Weiobart, R. (1987). Rheumatic manifestations of Wegener's granulomatosis. *J. Rheum.* **14**:949-951.
15. Reed, W. B., Jensen, A. K., Konwaler, B. E., and Hunter, D. (1963). The cutaneous manifestations in Wegener's granulomatosis. *Acta Derm. Venerol.* **43**:250-264.

16. Fauci, A. S., Haynes, B. F., and Katz, P. (1983). Wegener's granulomatosis: Prospective clinical and therapeutic experience with 85 patients for 21 years. *Ann. Intern. Med.* **98**:76-85.
17. Goodman, G. C., and Churg, J. (1954). Wegener's granulomatosis. Pathology and review of the literature. *Arch. Pathol.* **58**:533-553.
18. Walton, E. W. (1958). Giant cell granuloma of the respiratory tract (Wegener's granulomatosis). *Br. Med. J.* **2**:265-270.
19. Drachman, D. A. (1963). Neurologic complications of Wegener's granulomatosis. *Arch. Neurol.* **8**:145-155.
20. Cupps, T. R., and Fauci, A. S. (1981). *The Vasculitiedes.* W. B. Saunders, Philadelphia, pp. 1-211.
21. Conn, D. L., McDuffie, F. C., and Holley, K. E. (1976). Immunologic mechanisms in systematic vasculitis. *Mayo Clin. Proc.* **51**:511-518.
22. Savage, C. O., Jones, S., Winearls, C. G., Marshall, P. D., and Lockwood, C. M. (1987). Prospective study of radioimmunoassay for antibodies against neutrophil cytoplasm in diagnosis of systematic vasculitis. *Lancet* **1**:1389-1393.
22a. Nolle, B., Pecks, U., Ludermann, J., Rohrbach, M. S., DeRemee, R. A., and Gross, W. L. (1989). Anticytoplasmic autoantibodies: their immunodiagnostic value in Wegener's granulomatosis. *Ann. Intern. Med.* **111**:28-40.
22b. Goldshmdeing, R., van der Schoot, C. E., ten Bokkel-Huinink, D., Hack, C. E., and van den Ende, A. E. G. Kr. (1989). Wegener's granulomatosis autoantibodies identify a novel diisopropylfluorophosphate-binding protein in the lysosomes of normal human neutrophils. *J. Clin. Invest.* **84**:1577-1587.
23. McGregor, M. B., and Sandler, G. (1964). Wegener's granulomatosis: A clinical and radiological survey. *Br. J. Radiol.* **37**:430-439.
24. Kornblum, D., and Fienberg, R. (1955). Roentgen manifestations of necrotizing granulomatosis and angiitis of the lungs. *Am. J. Roentgenol. Radium. Ther. Nucl. Med.* **74**:587-592.
25. Felson, B. (1959). Less familiar Roentgen patterns of pulmonary granulomas. *Am. J. Roentgenol. Radium Ther. Nucl. Med.* **81**:211-223.
26. Rosenberg, D. M., Weinberger, S. E., Fulmer, J. D., Flye, M. W., Fauci, A. S., and Crystal, R. G. (1980). Functional correlates of lung function tests in staging and follow-up. *Am. J. Med.* **69**:387-395.
27. Weiss, R. B., and Muggia, F. M. (1980). Cytotoxic drug-induced pulmonary disease: Update *Am. J. Med.* **68**:259-266.
28. Beidleman, B. (1963). Wegener's granulomatosis: Prolonged therapy with large doses of steroids. *J.A.M.A.* **186**:827-830.
29. Fahey, J., Leonard, E., Churg, J., and Goldman, G. (1954). Wegener's granulomatosis. *Am. J. Med.* **17**:168-179.

30. Reza, M. J., Dornfeld, L., Goldberg, L. S., Bluestone, R., and Pearson, C. M. (1975). Wegener's granulomatosis. Longterm follow-up of patients treated with cyclophosphamide. *Arthritis. Rheum.* **18**:501-506.
31. Brandywein, S., Esdaile, J., Danoff, D., and Tannenbaum, H. (1983). Wegener's granulomatosis. Clinical features and outcome in 13 patients. *Arch. Intern. Med.* **143**:476-479.
32. Weiner, S. R., and Paulus, H. E. (1983). Treatment of Wegener's granulomatosis with cyclophosphamide. Outcome analysis. *Arthritis Rheum.* **26**:565.
33. De Remee, R. A., McDonald, T. J., and Weiland, L. H. (1985). Wegener's granulomatosis: Observations on treatment with antimicrobial agents. *Mayo Clin. Proc.* **60**:27-32.
34. Carrington, C. B., and Liebow, A. A. (1966). Limited forms of angiitis and granulomatosis of Wegener's type. *Am. J. Med.* **41**:497-527.
35. Churg, J., and Strauss, L. (1951). Allergic granulomatosis, allergic angiitis and periarteritis nodosa. *Am. J. Pathol.* **27**:277-301.
36. Lanham, J. G., Elkon, K. B., Pusey, C. D., and Hughes, G. R. (1984). Systematic vasculitis with asthma and eosinophilia: A clinical approach to the Churg-Strauss syndrome. *Medicine (Baltimore)* **63**:65-81.
37. Chumbley, L. C., Harrison, E. G., and De Remee, R. A. (1977). Allergic granulomatosis and angiitis (Churg-Strauss syndrome). *Mayo Clin. Proc.* **52**:477-484.
38. Horn, R. G., Fauci, A. S., Rosenthal, A. S., and Wolff, S. M. (1979). Renal biopsy pathology in Wegener's granulomatosis. *Am. J. Pathol.* **74**:423-434.
39. Harkavy, J. (1943). Vascular allergy. *J. Allergy* **14**:507-537.
40. Abell, M. R., Limond, R. V., Blamey, W. E., and Martel, W. (1970). Allergic granulomatosis with massive gastric involvement. *N. Engl. J. Med.* **282**:665-668.
41. Rose, G. A. (1957). The natural history of polyarteritis. *Br. Med. J.* 1148-1152.
42. Crotty, C. P., De Remee, R. A., and Winkelmann, R. K. (1981). Cutaneous clinicopathologic correlation of allergic granulomatosis. *J. Am. Acad. Dermatol.* **5**:571-581.
43. Churg, J. (1963). Allergic granulomatosis and granulomatous-vascular syndromes. *Ann. Allergy* **21**:619-628.
44. Pagel, W. (1951). Polyarteritis nodosa and the "rheumatic" diseases. *J. Clin. Pathol.* **4**:137-157.
45. Churg, J., and Strauss, L. (1981). Interstitial eosinophilic pneumonitis, pleuritis and angiitis. (Letter.) *N. Engl. J. Med.* **304**:611.
46. Rose, G. A., and Spencer, H. (1957b). Polyarteritis nodosa. *Q. J. Med.* **26**:43-81.

47. Fauci, A. S., Katz, P., Haynes, B. F., and Wolff, S. M. (1979). Cyclo-phosphamide therapy of severe systemic necrotizing vasculitis. *N. Engl. J. Med.* **301**:235-238.
48. Liebow, A. A., Carrington, C. B., and Friedman, P. J. (1972). Lym-phamatoid granulomatosis. *Hum. Pathol.* **3**:457-558.
49. Hammar, S. P., Gortner, D., Sumida, S., and Bockus, D. (1977). Lym-phamatoid granulomatosis: Association with retroperitoneal fibrosis and evidence of impaired cell-mediated immunity. *Am. Rev. Respir. Dis.* **115**:1045-1050.
50. Katzenstein, A. A., Carrington, C. B., and Liebow, A. A. (1979). Lym-phomatoid granulomatosis. A clinicopathologic study of 152 cases. *Cancer* **43**:360-373.
51. Sackett, J. F., ZuRheum, G. M., and Bhimani, S. M. (1979). Lympha-matoid granulomatosis involving the central nervous system: Radiologic-pathologic correlation. *A.J.R.* **132**:823-826.
52. Patton, W. F., and Lynch, J. P. (1982). Lymphomatoid granulomato-sis. Clinicopathologic study of four cases and literature review. *Medi-cine (Baltimore)* **61**:1-12.
53. Saldana, M. J., Patchefsky, A. S., Israel, H. I., and Atkinson, G. W. (1977). Pulmonary angiitis and granulomatosis. The relationship between histological features, organ involvement, and response to treatment. *Hum. Pathol.* **8**:391-409.
54. Chen, K. T. (1977). Abdominal forms of lymphatoid granulomatosis. *Hum. Pathol.* **8**:99-103.
55. Fauci, A. S., Haynes, B. F., Costa, J., Katz, P., and Wolff, S. M. (1982). Lymphamatoid granulomatosis. Prospective clinical and therapeutic experience for 10 years. *N. Engl. J. Med.* **306**:68-74.
56. Fraga, A., Mintz, G., Valle, L., and Flores-Izquierdo, G. (1972). Taka-yasu's arteritis: Frequency of systematic manifestations (study of 22 pa-tients) and favorable response to maintenance steroid therapy with adreno-corticosteroids (12 patients). *Arthritis Rheum.* **15**:617-624.
57. Ishikawa, K. (1978). Natural history and classification of occlusive thromboaortopathy (Takayasu's disease). *Circulation* **57**:27-35.
58. Lupi-Herrera, E., Sanchez Torres, G., Marcushamar, J., Mispireta, J., Horowitz, S., and Vela, J. E. (1977). Takayasu's arteritis: Clinical study of 107 cases. *Am. Heart* **93**:94-103.
59. Nakao, K., Ikeda, M., Kimata, S., Niitani, H., Miyahara, M., and Ish-imi, Z. (1967). Takayasu's arteritis. Clinical report of 84 cases and im-munological studies of 7 cases. *Circulation* **35**:1141-1155.
60. Lupi, E. II, Sanchez, G., Horowitz, S., and Guiterrez, E. Pulmonary artery involvement in Takayasu's arteritis. *Chest* **67**:69-74.
61. Shimizu, K., and Sano, K. (1951). Pulseless disease. *J. Neuropathol. Clin. Neurol.* **1**:37-47.

62. Asherson, R. A., Asherson, G. L., and Schrire, V. (1968). Immunological studies in arteritis of the aorta and great vessels. *Br. Med. J.* 3:589-590.
63. Ueda, H., Saito, Y., Marooka, S., Itoh, I., Yamaguchi, H., and Sugiura, M. (1968). Experimental arteritis produced immunologically in rabbits. *Jpn. Heart J.* 9:573.
64. Numano, F., Isohisa, I., Kishi, U., Arita, M., and Maezawa, H. (1978). Takayasu's disease in twin sisters. Possible genetic factors. *Circulation* 58:173-177.
65. Numano, F., Isshisa, I., Maezawa, J., and Jaji, T. (1979). HLA antigens in Takayasu's disease. *Am. Heart. J.* 98:153-159.
66. Shelhamer, J. H., Volkman, D. J., Parillo, J. E., Lawley, T. J., Johnston, M. R., and Fauci, A. S. (1985). Takayasu's arteritis and its therapy. *Ann. Intern. Med.* 103:121-126.
67. Falicore, R. E., and Cooney, D. F. (1964). Takayasu's arteritis and rheumatoid arthritis. *Arch. Intern. Med.* 114:594-600.
68. Vinijchaikul, K. (1967). Primary arteritis of the aorta and its main branches (Takayasu's arteriopathy). A clinicopathologic autopsy study of 8 cases. *Am. J. Med.* 93:15-27.
69. Bonventure, M. V. (1970). Takayasu's disease revisited. *N. Y. State J. Med.* 74:1960-1967.
70. Strachan, R. W., Wigzell, F. W., and Anderson, J. R. (1966). Locomotor manifestations and serum studies in Takayasu's arteriopathy. *Am. J. Med.* 40:560-568.
71. Ask-upmark, E. (1961). On the pathogenesis of hypertension in Takayasu's syndrome. *Acta Med. Scand.* 169:467-477.
72. Inada, K., Katsumara, T., Hirai, J., and Sunada, T. (1970). Surgical treatment in the aortitis syndrome. *Arch. Surg.* 100:220-224.
73. Takayasu, M. (1908). A case with peculiar changes of the central retinal vessels. *Acta Soc. Ophthalmol. Jpn.* 12:554.
74. Sano, K., and Aiba, T. (1966). Pulseless disease, summary of our 62 cases. *Jpn. Circ. J.* 30:63.
75. Lupi, H. E., and Sanchez Torres, G. (1972). Arteritis inespecifica y paraplejia intermitente. *Arch. Inst. Cardiol. Mex.* 42:131-137.
76. Yomato, M., Lecky, J., Hiramatsu, K., and Kohda, E. (1986). Takayasu's arteritis. Radiographic and angiographic findings in 59 patients. *Radiology* 161:329-334.
77. Suzuki, Y., Konishi, K., and Hisada, K. (1973). Radioisotipe lung scanning in Takayasu's arteritis. *Radiology* 109:133.
78. Flye, M. W., Mundinger, G. H. Jr., and Fauci, A. S. (1979). Diagnostic and therapeutic aspects of the surgical approach to Wegener's granulomatosis. *J. Thorac. Cardiovasc. Surg.* 77:331-337.
79. Pinching, A. J., Lockwood, C. M., Pussell, B. A., et al. (1983). Wegener's granulomatosis: Observations of 18 patients with severe renal disease. *Q. J. Med.* 208:435-460.

13

Pulmonary Manifestations of Other Rheumatic Diseases

MAX S. LUNDBERG and JOHN R. WARD

University of Utah
Salt Lake City, Utah

Disease of the respiratory system is a well-described, if uncommon, complication in a number of rheumatic disorders. Earlier chapters in this text have dealt with pleuropulmonary disease in rheumatoid arthritis, systematic lupus erythematosus, progressive systematic sclerosis, inflammatory muscle disease, and systematic vasculitis. In this chapter we review the pleuropulmonary findings in other rheumatic diseases including the seronegative spondyloarthropathies, mixed connective tissue disease, juvenile rheumatoid arthritis and Still's disease, acute rheumatic fever, Behçet's syndrome, and Sjogren's syndrome. Although the changes seen are uncommon and not as well described, they may play an important role in each of these disorders. Physicians should be aware of the potential development of respiratory system disease in patients with these disorders.

I. Seronegative Spondyloarthropathies

A. Introduction

The seronegative spondyloarthropathies include ankylosing spondylitis, juvenile ankylosing spondylitis, Reiter's syndrome (or reactive arthritis), psoriatic arthritis, and the arthropathy associated with ulcerative colitis and Crohn's disease. As a group, these rheumatic disorders share a predilection for oligoarticular peripheral joint arthritis, enthesopathy, sacroiliitis and spondylitis, onset in young males, a strong association with the genetically determined class I antigen HLA-B27, and extraarticular inflammation of the eye, skin, and mucous membranes. Pulmonary involvement is uncommon and differs for each of these clinical syndromes. Thus each is discussed separately.

B. Ankylosing Spondylitis

Restrictive Lung Disease

Two types of respiratory system abnormalities have been described in ankylosing spondylitis. The first is restrictive lung disease. In ankylosing spondylitis, restrictive lung disease occurs with limited chest wall motion resulting from costovertebral joint inflammation and ankylosis. The vital capacity is minimally reduced to 70-80% of normal because normal diaphragmatic function is preserved (1,2). Residual volume is increased owing to fixation of the chest wall. Pulmonary compliance is usually normal (3). Respiratory failure is uncommon.

There is debate concerning the role of infectious pneumonitis as a complication in this setting. Hamilton suggested that restrictive changes in the chest wall made it difficult for patients to reverse focal pneumonitis and atelectasis that occurred with upper respiratory infections or bronchitis (4). The conclusions drawn from subsequent studies of respiratory illness in ankylosing spondylitis are divided. Court-Brown and Doll reported mortality in ankylosing spondylitis from 2.6 to 2.9 times the expected rate due to pneumonia, tuberculosis, and other respiratory disease (5). They acknowledged that some of their patients may have actually had apical fibrosis, which is discussed below. On the other hand, several pathology studies failed to show specific pulmonary lesions, or a higher incidence of pulmonary disease at autopsy in patients with ankylosing spondylitis than was seen in unselected autopsies (1,6).

Apical Pulmonary Fibrosis

The second type of respiratory abnormality described in ankylosing spondylitis is the uncommon development of upper lobe pulmonary fibrosis (4-10). The clinical picture in reported patients is similar. Pulmonary fibrosis occurs in patients who developed ankylosing spondylitis in early adult life. Symptoms usually begin in the fifth decade and include mild dyspnea and cough. The cough is generally dry but may become productive. With prolonged disease, significant parenchymal destruction takes place with cyst formation.

In late disease, colonization and infection with fungal pathogens have been reported, and hemoptysis is not uncommon. Early X-ray changes include pleural thickening with development of unilateral or more often bilateral upper lobe mottling. When followed over time, the mottling becomes more widespread in the upper lung fields, and eventually fibrosis and cystic changes are seen. The lesions on X-ray closely resemble those seen in pulmonary tuberculosis, so much so that a number of the early reported cases were treated in sanatoria even though repeated attempts to isolate the tubercle bacillus were unsuccessful. Autopsy studies also failed to demonstrate tuberculosis. Early histologic changes include patchy round cell infiltration and fibroblast proliferation which may later progress to extensive intraalveolar fibrosis with large areas of hyalinization (7-9). These changes appear to be a primary effect of the disease rather than changes secondary to other problems such as infection. Although fungal infection has been demonstrated in late lesions, it is not seen in early lesions and likely occurs after development of bronchiectasis and cyst formation (10).

Treatment

The management of restrictive lung disease is aimed at maintaining chest wall motion by early implementation of breathing exercises and erect posture. The spondylitic with truncal flexion will not have full diaphragmatic function. Treatment of pulmonary fibrosis in ankylosing spondylitis is difficult. Aside from prompt treatment of infections and supportive therapy with good pulmonary toilet, no specific therapy is proven. The standard treatment of ankylosing spondylitis with nonsteroidal antiinflammatory agents appears to have no effect on the development of pulmonary lesions. Immunosuppressive and corticosteroid treatments have not been adequately studied and may be contraindicated in late disease when colonization by fungal pathogens has occured.

C. Reiter's Syndrome

Significant pulmonary disease is very unusual in other seronegative spondyloarthropathies. Two case reports suggest the development of Reiter's syndrome as a complication of pulmonary infection with chlamydial organisms (11,12). Rarely, amyloid has been found in pulmonary nodules seen in Reiter's syndrome (13). Pleural disease and fleeting pulmonary infiltrates have also been reported (14).

II. Mixed Connective Tissue Disease

A. Introduction

Mixed connective tissue disease was initially described as a distinct clinical entity in 1972 (15). It is a multisystem disease characterized by clinical features which overlap other specific disorders—systematic lupus erythematosus, progressive systematic sclerosis, and polymyositis. Erosive arthritis such as that seen in rheumatoid arthritis may be seen. This disorder is also defined by a high titer of an antinuclear antibody directed against ribonucleoprotein (16).

Respiratory system disease in rheumatoid arthritis, systematic lupus erythematosus, progressive systematic sclerosis, and inflammatory muscle disease is the topic of earlier chapters in this text. One would expect similar pulmonary problems to occur in mixed connective tissue disease, as this disorder overlaps other clinical features of these disorders. Although the initial description by Sharp et al. (15) did not mention pulmonary disease as a prominent feature of mixed connective tissue disease, subsequent reviews have described a variety of pleuropulmonary abnormalities often causing significant morbidity and mortality (15,17-19). The same pulmonary complications have been seen in both childhood-onset and adult-onset mixed connective tissue disease (20).

B. Pleural Disease

Pleural thickening or pleural effusion on chest X-ray is recognized in patients with mixed connective tissue disease. In the initial description of this disorder by Sharp et al. (15), 6 of 25 patients had serositis. In 4 patients, pleuritis or pericarditis was the presenting clinical problem (15). Rarely, marked bilateral exudative pleural effusions are described as the presenting abnormality (17). In a retrospective review of 81 patients followed at the Mayo Clinic between 1973 and 1977, pleural disease was noted specifically in 7 of 20 patients who had pleuropulmonary manifestations of mixed connective tissue disease (18). In a prospective review, Sullivan carefully studied 33 patients and noted a 40% incidence of pleuritic chest pain, although pleural thickening on chest X-ray was mentioned in only 1 patient, and pleural effusions were not described (19). Characteristics of pleural fluid are not reported in most of the studies cited. In one patient, pleural fluid was reported to be exudative with 95% polymorphonuclear leukocytes, protein concentration of 4.2 mg/dl, pH of 7.6, and LDH of 411 IU/L (17).

C. Parenchymal Lung Disease

Pulmonary parenchymal disease has also been described in patients with mixed connective tissue disease. This includes parenchymal infiltrates on chest X-ray often accompanied by symptoms of respiratory difficulty and abnormal pulmonary function tests. The incidence of reported parenchymal lung disease ranges from 15% to as high as 80% (18,19,21). Pulmonary infiltrates are most commonly seen in the lower to middle lung fields, although diffuse involvement occurs (18,19,22). Abnormalities of pulmonary function are more common than chest X-ray changes. The most common abnormality of pulmonary function is a reduction in carbon monoxide diffusing capacity. Reductions may be seen in vital capacity, total lung capacity, and 1-s forced expiratory volume. Resting hypoxemia has also been demonstrated.

Wallaert et al. performed bronchoalveolar lavage in eight patients with mixed connective tissue disease who were asymptomatic for any pulmonary disease and who had normal chest X-rays (23). Three of the eight patients studied had abnormal differential cell counts of the lavage fluid suggestive of a neutrophil alveolitis. Longer-term follow-up on these patients is needed to determine the clinical significance of this finding. Pathologic changes described on the biopsy and autopsy specimens include mild to moderate interstitial fibrosis, with occasional alveolar cell hypertrophy and infiltration of the alveolar septa by plasma cells and lymphocytes (18-20,24). Immunofluorescent staining for IgM, IgA, and IgG has been unremarkable (22).

Chapman et al. examined sera from 122 patients with cryptogenic fibrosing alveolitis with or without associated connective tissue diseases for the presence of specific antinuclear antibodies. Antinuclear antibodies were found in 39 with 15 having antibody to ribonucleoprotein, although the titer in some was low (25). Clinical features noted in patients with ribonucleoprotein antibodies included arthritis, Raynaud's phenomenon, sclerodactyly, scleroderma, vasculitis, hemolytic anemia, pulmonary hypertension, pericarditis, pleuritis, Sjogren's syndrome, primary biliary cirrhosis, and ocular myasthenia gravis. Although the ribonucleoprotein antibody was not helpful in diagnosing mixed connective tissue disease in patients with cryptogenic fibrosing alveolitis, the association may indicate similar underlying mechanisms.

Pulmonary hemorrhage associated with nephritis has been reported on one occasion (26).

D. Pulmonary Hypertension

Pulmonary hypertension has emerged as one of the more serious complications of mixed connective tissue disease. Although not noted in early reports, later studies have reported this complication as an important cause of morbidity and mortality (19,22,24,27). It is often found in those patients who have features of progressive systemic sclerosis as part of their clinical presentation (19). The onset of pulmonary hypertension is generally insidious. The most common clinical symptoms are pleuritic chest pain and dyspnea on exertion (19,22,24,27). When dyspnea is noted, laboratory evaluation will often show signs of pulmonary hypertension. Chest X-rays may show hilar enlargement or parenchymal disease or may be normal. Echocardiography may show right ventricular hypertrophy, and EKG changes of right ventricular hypertrophy have been noted (18,24). Measurement of pulmonary artery pressure and pulmonary vascular resistance by righ theart catheterization can confirm pulmonary hypertension in patients with clinical symptoms (19,22,24). Gallium scanning is not helpful in diagnosing pulmonary hypertension in mixed connective tissue disease. Characteristic changes on nail fold capillary microscopy may be associated with pulmonary hypertension and parenchymal disease (19).

The pulmonary pathology in these patients is interesting. Although parenchymal changes may be seen in association with pulmonary hypertension, such changes are often minimal in the presence of significant vascular lesions (19,22,24,27). Histologic changes include prominent intimal proliferation with marked muscular hypertrophy of small pulmonary arterioles (19,22, 24). Marked luminal stenosis is occasionally described, but thromboembolic disease has not been present. Immunofluorescent studies are generally unremarkable in involved pulmonary vessels.

E. Treatment

The results of treatment of the pulmonary complications of mixed connective tissue disease are variable (17-19,22,24). Pleuritis may not require treatment (17). When treatment is required, nonsteroidal antiinflammatory agents or corticosteroids usually provide symptomatic relief. Interstitial fibrosis and pulmonary hypertension are more resistant to treatment. Some improvement in pulmonary function testing has been noted with corticosteroid treatment, although marked improvements in the clinical course are uncommon. Aside from a few reports of improvement with cyclophosphamide or chlorambucil, pulmonary hypertension has been resistant to pharmacologic intervention. The prognosis in mixed connective tissue disease is poorer in the face of significant pulmonary hypertension and parenchymal disease.

III. Juvenile Rheumatoid Arthritis and Still's Disease

A. Introduction

Juvenile rheumatoid arthritis is a disease in children characterized by inflammatory polyarthritis that may present with extraarticular manifestations (28). It appears to be a disease distinct from rheumatoid arthritis in adults and can be subdivided into three classes based on the clinical pattern of articular involvement and by the presence of systemic features. Oligoarticular arthritis with fewer than five joints involved accounts for 50% of all cases of JRA, while a polyarticular presentation is seen in 40%, and systemic features are seen in the remaining 10%. Extraarticular features are commonly seen in the patients with systemic onset disease but are less common in the polyarticular presentation and are uncommon in patients with oligoarticular arthritis. Systemic onset juvenile rheumatoid arthritis (Still's disease) is characterized by inflammatory polyarthritis and prominent systemic features which include high spiking fevers, an evanescent macular rash, leukocytosis, lymphadenopathy, and occasionally chronic uveitis, polyserositis, hepatosplenomegaly, carditis, or pulmonary parenchymal disease. Systemic onset "juvenile rheumatoid arthritis" may also present in adults. The clinical features of "adult" Still's disease are the same as those seen in childhood. Aside from pleural disease, clinical involvement of the respiratory system in juvenile rheumatoid arthritis is uncommon.

B. Juvenile Rheumatoid Arthritis

Pleural and Parenchymal Disease

Pleural and parenchymal pulmonary findings may occur individually or together in patients with juvenile rheumatoid arthritis. In many cases, pleural involvement is asymptomatic. Pleuritis is often seen with accompanying pericarditis and may occur with parenchymal disease (29). Calabro in a review of 100 patients with juvenile rheumatoid arthritis followed over 15 years reported pneumonitis and/or pleuritis in 6 of 20 patients with systemic onset disease (30,31). In the same study only 2 of 48 patients with polyarticular onset had pneumonitis or pleuritis. No respiratory system involvement was found in 32 patients with monoarticular or pauciarticular disease.

One of the more serious extraarticular manifestations of juvenile rheumatoid arthritis is pneumonitis. This has been described in a number of patients and may occur prior to the onset of articular symptoms (29,32-34). Chronic interstitial infiltrates have been described that show microscopic changes of interstitial lymphocytic pneumonitis (32,33). Other rare pulmonary disease has been seen in juvenile rheumatoid arthritis including pulmonary hemosiderosis, cor pulmonale, and cavitary pulmonary nodules (34-36). Transient parenchymal infiltrates with pleuritis and pericarditis have also been reported (34).

Laboratory Abnormalities

Chest X-ray may show pleural effusions or parenchymal infiltrates as described above. Characteristics of the pleural fluid are similar to those seen in adult rheumatoid arthritis. The fluid is exudative with white blood cell counts ranging from 2,000 to 25,000 cells/mm^3, primarily polymorphonuclear leukocytes (29,32,34). Glucose concentrations may be low or normal

(29,32,34). Protein and LDH concentrations are elevated. Pulmonary function tests have shown abnormalities in asymptomatic patients with normal radiographs. Abnormalities of pulmonary function have been reported in as many as two thirds of patients with polyarticular juvenile arthritis, and single-breath carbon monoxide diffusing capacity was abnormal in 7 of 15 patients studied (35). The incidence of respiratory complaints in patients with juvenile rheumatoid arthritis, however, is much lower than this, and the clinical significance of these numbers is uncertain. Resting oxygen saturation is normal in patients with juvenile rheumatoid arthritis, and although desaturation may occur with exercise in some patients, this has not been well studied (35).

Treatment

Treatment is directed at the underlying problem. Pleuritis with or without effusion usually responds to aspirin or nonsteroidal antiinflammatory medications. Parenchymal lung disease may require additional therapy. In both instances of chronic interstitial pneumonitis cited above, improvement was noted with systemic corticosteroid treatment but not with aspirin (32,33). Caution must be exercised when treating patients with corticosteroids or other immunosuppressive drugs in the presence of symptomatic respiratory disease unrelated to the arthritis. One patient was reported to develop a septic ankle following the injection of steroid into a different joint at a time when she was symptomatic with an upper respiratory tract infection (38).

C. Adult Still's Disease

Respiratory system involvement is reportedly more common in adult Still's disease than it is in childhood. The incidence reported in the literature is usually about 30%, but some estimates report an incidence as high as 60% (39-42). The most common symptom is pleuritic chest pain with or without effusions. Pleural fluid findings are similar to those reported in juvenile rheumatoid arthritis (41). Transient parenchymal infiltrates have been reported less commonly, and, very rarely, more serious pulmonary complications are described (40). One patient with adult Still's disease developed adult respiratory distress syndrome with a complicating opportunistic infection (43). Another patient developed a severe restrictive disease with mild chronic interstitial inflammation and patchy interstitial fibrosis on transbronchial biopsy (44).

Patients with pleural disease generally respond to nonsteroidal antiinflammatory medications but may require corticosteroids. Cytotoxic therapy was given to one patient reported with adult respiratory distress syndrome with initial improvement, although the patient later developed profound leukopenia and died from sepsis (44).

IV. Acute Rheumatic Fever

A. Introduction

Rheumatic fever is a multisystem disorder characterized by inflammation that occurs subsequent to pharyngeal infections with group A streptococci. In past decades rheumatic fever was more common. Although the incidence of acute rheumatic fever has been decreasing over the past several decades, one recent report shows a regional increase in this disease (45). Thus it remains a clinical problem that requires continued attention. The diagnosis of acute rheumatic fever is made with the aid of a number of major and minor findings from a list of manifestations known as the Jones criteria (46). The major criteria include carditis, polyarthritis, chorea, erythema marginatum, and subcutaneous nodules. The minor criteria include fever, arthralgias, elevated erythrocyte sedimentation rate or positive C-reactive protein, prolonged P-R interval, and previous rheumatic fever or rheumatic heart disease. When two major or one major and two minor criteria are found with evidence of a preceding streptococcal infection such as a culture of the throat growing group A *Streptococcus*, increased ASO or other streptococcal antibody titer, or recent scarlet fever, a diagnosis of acute rheumatic fever is likely, provided other causes of inflammatory joint disease are ruled out.

Although respiratory system disease has been described in acute rheumatic fever, it is not one of the major or minor criteria and thus has received scant attention in most recent reviews of this disorder. Only one short paragraph on pulmonary disease in acute rheumatic fever with a single reference is found in a recent comprehensive textbook of rheumatology (47).

B. Rheumatic Pneumonitis

Prior to 1940 there were reports of respiratory system disease seen in association with initial and recurrent episodes of acute rheumatic fever. From the mid 1940s to the mid 1960s, a number of large reviews appeared in the literature describing patients with pneumonitis seen in severe acute rheumatic fever along with descriptions of clinical features and the pathologic findings in those patients (48-55).

Pneumonitis generally presents with symptoms of dyspnea, cough, chest pain, hemoptysis, fever, and arthralgias (48,51,53). Although most cases are associated with carditis, many have occurred in the absence of significant congestive failure (50,51,56). In most of the early reviews specimens for study were selected based on the finding of pathologic evidence for carditis, making it difficult to separate these two manifestations in those studies. The pulmonary involvement is usually seen prior to or after the onset of the initial episode of acute rheumatic fever but has also been described as a complication of recurrent attacks (48,49,53,54). Although it is more commonly described in children ages 5-15, it may be seen in older patients (48,49,52,54). The estimated incidence of rheumatic pneumonitis ranges from 11% to 65% in early autopsy and clinical reviews (49,57-61). In a review of 1,046 cases of rheumatic fever seen at the U.S. Naval Hospital prior to 1946, the incidence of pneumonitis was 11.3% (49). In this review the author did not list specific criteria for a diagnosis of pneumonitis, nor was the incidence of mortality in affected patients given. The most common findings on physical examination were tachypnea and tachycardia with abnormalities on auscultation and percussion of the lung fields consistent with pulmonary infiltrates.

C. Laboratory Studies

X-ray findings have included cardiomegaly with pulmonary infiltrates that were typically patchy, multifocal, and sometimes fleeting (48-51,53-56,62, 63). Pleural effusions were seen in a minority of cases. In some patients, pathologic changes were noted in the lungs with normal chest X-rays (50,54). In most cases the X-rays were initially interpreted as consistent with congestive failure or pneumonia, although these findings were often disproved at autopsy.

The microscopic changes seen in autopsy and biopsy specimens are characteristic but not specific for this disorder. Described changes include alveolar hemorrhage and alveolar wall necrosis, presence of hyaline membranes, interstitial mononuclear cell infiltrate and fibroblast proliferation, and vessel wall involvement with intimal and internal elastic lamina necrosis and cellular infiltrates (48-55,64). A granulomatous lesion termed a "Masson body" has been described (50). This lesion shows hyaline and cellular collections within terminal alveolar ducts. However, it is not specific for rheumatic fever, being seen in a number of other conditions (55,64).

D. Diagnosis and Treatment

The diagnosis of this entity has classically been based on the exclusion of other causes of pneumonitis with confirmation at autopsy. Often the diagnosis of rheumatic pneumonitis is not suspected until autopsy. In one series suspected diagnoses included pneumonia, congestive heart failure with or without pneumonia, subacute bacterial endocarditis alone or with congestive heart failure or pneumonia, pulmonary embolus, myocarditis, salicylate intoxication, and uncomplicated acute rheumatic fever (48).

In the early series, treatment was supportive with oxygen, sulfonamides, salicylates, and later penicillin. The outcome has been uniformly dismal, with high reported mortality (48-55,62,64). In one report, 12 of 23 patients treated with ACTH in 1958 also showed disappointing results (54). Even recently, with the incidence of acute rheumatic fever much less than in the past, cases of fatal fulminant acute rheumatic fever with rheumatic pneumonitis are reported (63,65). The most recent cases reported in 1985 showed improvement with high-dose corticosteroids in one and improvement on salicylates in the other (56,63). Although treatment with cytotoxic agents has been suggested for patients not responding to corticosteroids, there are not data at present to support this recommendation.

In summary, rheumatic pneumonitis is a well-described but poorly understood manifestation of acute rheumatic fever. When present in the fulminant form it is often fatal, making it important to suspect the diagnosis early and institute supportive measures along with corticosteroid therapy (63).

V. Behcet's Syndrome

A. Introduction

In 1937, Behçet described the syndrome of oral and genital mucosal ulcerations with uveitis that now bears his name (66). Since that time, additional features of this syndrome have been recognized including synovitis, vasculitis, meningoencephalitis, large artery aneurysms, and thrombophlebitis. Vasculitis of both the arterial and venous systems accounts for the most significant pathology in this disorder (76). Although criteria have been suggested for the diagnosis of Behçet's syndrome, the diagnosis remains clinical, as there are no pathognomonic serologic or pathologic tests (68). Pulmonary involvement is an unusual complication in this rare disorder and thus is not commonly described.

B. Incidence and Clinical Presentation

The incidence of pulmonary lesions observed in an autopsy study of patients dying with Behçet's syndrome is quite high (69). Although a number of these are probably complications of debilitating illness and immunosuppressive treatment, many are likely due to the underlying disease.

Pleurisy has been described, and in one patient pseudochylothorax developed as a complication of superior vena caval occlusion (70-72). Infectious complications have been reported, usually thought to be due in part to immunosuppressive therapy of the underlying Behcet's syndrome. Serious infections include tuberculosis and mucormycosis (73-76). Recurrent pneumonitis has also been described. In some patients, pulmonary infiltrates are due to localized infarcts from vascular occlusion (77). Interstitial infiltrates with increased fibroblast activity and marked nodular mononuclear cell infiltration have also been observed, sometimes in the absence of vasculitis

(69,78-80). Upper airway disease with pharyngeal obstruction has been described (81). Large airway involvement in the lower respiratory tract also occurs, which may produce symptoms of obstructive lung disease (82-84). In some cases the obstructive symptoms reverse with bronchodilators, although such treatment is often ineffective.

C. Pulmonary Vascular Disease

The most serious pulmonary complication in Behçet's syndrome involves vascular changes in the pulmonary vessels. Over the years, a number of patients have been described with recurrent hemoptysis and pulmonary infiltrates (77,85-87). These patients present with hemoptysis usually accompanied by fever, chest pain, and dyspnea. They also show a high incidence of venous thrombosis and superficial thrombophlebitis. Radiographic changes include parenchymal infiltrates, prominent pulmonary vessels in the hilum, and occasional pleural effusions or pleural thickening. Radioisotope studies of ventilation and perfusion are much like those seen in pulmonary embolic disease. In some cases, the presence of an abnormal ventilation-perfusion study with a clinical history of chest pain and hemoptysis has led to the erroneous diagnosis of pulmonary embolus. Pulmonary arteriography may demonstrate single or multiple arterial occlusions, especially in proximal vessels.

As noted above, patients with pulmonary vascular involvement in Behçet's syndrome may present with symptoms similar to those seen in patients with pulmonary embolus. Pulmonary embolism is much more common than Behcet's syndrome with pulmonary vascular involvement. Unless the patient is known to have Behçet's syndrome or is evaluated by a very astute physician, he may be given the diagnosis of pulmonary embolus and treated with anticoagulation. Anticoagulation in these patients has led to worsening hemoptysis; in fact, a major cause of death in this group of patients is massive hemoptysis.

D. Treatment

The treatment of pulmonary disease in Behçet's syndrome depends on the manifestation (85). Infections should be diagnosed promptly and treated as indicated. Although experience is limited, the vascular involvement appears to be best treated with corticosteroids. Cyclophosphamide appears to have been of benefit in patients who did not respond to corticosteroids alone. Although other agents have been tried in Behçet's syndrome including azathioprine, chlorambucil, colchicine, levamisole, cyclosporin, thalidomide, and others, there are few data on their use with pulmonary manifestations.

In summary, there are a number of reported pleuropulmonary manifestations of Behcet's syndrome. The most serious involves vasculitis with the development of pulmonary infarction, aneurysms, and significant hemoptysis. Behcet's syndrome should be considered in the differential diagnosis of hemoptysis and venous occlusive disease, especially in large vessels.

VI. Sjögren's Syndrome

A. Introduction

Sjögren's syndrome is the result of lymphocyte-mediated destruction of exocrine glands that leads to diminished or absent glandular secretions and mucosal dryness (88). The most common clinical manifestations are the keratoconjunctivitis sicca syndrome, dryness of the mouth (xerostomia), and salivary gland enlargement (88). Sjögren's syndrome has also been associated with the development of neurologic complications, pulmonary disease, and impairment of other organ systems. It has been estimated that as many as 75% of patients with primary Sjögren's syndrome may have measurable pulmonary abnormalities though in many cases these are not clinically significant (89). In one series, significant pulmonary disease with symptoms and abnormal chest radiographs was found in 9% of 343 patients (90). Respiratory system involvement may include upper and lower airway abnormalities (89, 90-95), interstitial pneumonitis/fibrosis (89,90,92), pleural effusions (90), pseudolymphoma (90,93,96), and lymphoma (90,97). Rarely vasculitis, amyloidosis, and diaphragmatic myopathy have been reported with Sjögren's syndrome (90).

Sjögren's syndrome may be classified as primary or secondary. When Sjögren's syndrome occurs in the absence of other connective tissue disease it is categorized as primary Sjögren's syndrome. Secondary Sjögren's syndrome has all the clinical manifestations of primary Sjögren's syndrome but occurs in association with an established rheumatic disease. Pulmonary disease is reported in both primary and secondary Sjögren's syndrome; however, in secondary Sjögren's syndrome it is often difficult to determine if the lung process is the result of the Sjögren's syndrome or the associated rheumatic disease.

B. Clinical Manifestations

Although efforts have been made to classify the pulmonary manifestations of Sjögren's syndrome, many patients will not conform to a single type of pulmonary problem, often showing several components of the disease simultaneously (89,90). Interpretation and comparison of the different reports require that one recognize differences in patient populations. In more recent studies efforts have been made to limit investigations to nonsmokers with primary Sjögren's syndrome, though this has not always been the case (93, 94,98).

Efforts have been made to determine if differences exist between the pulmonary involvement in patients with primary and secondary Sjögren's syndrome (92,99). Vitali et al. suggested that pulmonary involvement may be more severe in patients with secondary Sjögren's syndrome, but the differences were generally not clinically or statistically significant (99). In this discussion we will concentrate on pulmonary abnormalities in primary Sjögren's syndrome with references to secondary Sjögren's syndrome when appropriate.

Upper Airway Disease

Dryness of the airways is reported in patients with primary Sjögren's syndrome and may precede the diagnosis (100). As many as 17% of primary Sjögren's syndrome patients may report nonproductive cough with no abnormalities identified on pulmonary function testing or chest X-ray to explain these symptoms (89,92). Constantopoulos et al. have used the term "xerotrachea" to describe this condition (89). The xerotrachea appears more commonly in patients with primary extraglandular Sjögren's syndrome (92). Xerotrachea has been incorrectly diagnosed and treated as tuberculosis, asthma, and chronic bronchitis (89).

Although infiltration of the bronchial mucosa with mononuclear cells is reported, there is no evidence to document a decrease in bronchial secretions in patients with Sjögren's syndrome (91,93,98). The mucociliary clearance rate was found to be normal, and the whole lung clearance was significantly increased in Sjögren's syndrome when compared with normal controls (94).

In addition to the tracheal abnormalities described above, a case is reported of a patient with primary Sjögren's syndrome who developed a tracheal lymphoma which caused airway obstruction (97). Tracheostomy was required to manage this complication.

Lower Airways

Obstructive and restrictive pulmonary changes have been reported in primary Sjögren's syndrome (89-95). Obstructive lung disease has been reported in 2.5-35% of patients with primary Sjögren's syndrome (91,92). In a comparison of obstructive disease in 40 patients with primary Sjögren's syndrome and 26 patients with secondary Sjögren's syndrome, Papthanasiou et al. reported prevalences of 19% and 2.4%, respectively (92). In contrast, obstructive pulmonary disease was seen in 40% of 40 age- and sex-matched rheumatoid arthritis patients without Sjögren's syndrome. Radoux et al. (101) and Begin et al. (102), on the other hand, have suggested that patients with rheumatoid arthritis and secondary Sjögren's syndrome may have a higher prevalence of obstructive pulmonary disease than patients with rheumatoid arthritis alone.

The differences in incidence of obstructive pulmonary disease in these studies may be due to a lack of uniformity in the definition of what constitutes obstructive pulmonary disease. For example, in one study, small airway obstruction was defined as a MEF_{25} (maximum expiratory flow at 25% of forced vital capacity), less than 60% of predicted. By this definition 22.5% of Sjögren's patients were abnormal; however, 30% of normal controls also tested below this level. In the same population, only 2.5% of patients had an FEV_1/FVC less than 70% of predicted (92).

No differences have been found in the protease inhibitor phenotype of Sjögren's syndrome patients with and without pulmonary disease (103). Thus, alpha-1-antitrypsin level deficiency is not a viable explanation for the obstructive disease seen in these patients (92). A combined restrictive and obstructive defect is reported in 10% of subjects in some series (91,100).

Pneumonitis/Fibrosis

The restrictive lung disease that is reported in up to 15% of patients probably represents pneumonitis and pulmonary fibrosis (91). The incidence of pneumonitis depends on the sensitivity of the test used to evaluate the problem. The pulmonary status of 29 patients with primary Sjögren's syndrome and 21 control subjects was compared by bronchoalveolar lavage (BAL) (104). All individuals were nonsmokers, reported no symptoms or signs of pulmonary disease, and had normal chest radiographs. Bronchoscopy showed no abnormality of the airways or signs of pulmonary infections. Total cell counts were similar in Sjögren's syndrome patients and controls; however, there were differences in the white cell differential counts. The patients with Sjögren's syndrome showed an increase in the percentages of lymphocytes and neutrophils. There were no differences in the percentages of eosinophils. On the basis of the BAL findings, the patients with Sjögren's syndrome (n = 29) were classified as either having no abnormalities (n = 13), neutrophilic (n = 5), or lymphocytic (n = 11) patterns of alveolitis. The patients with normal BALs were compared to those with neutrophil or lymphocyte alveolitis. There were no differences in the prevalence of clinical features (age, recurrent parotitis, Raynaud's phenomenon, nonerosive polyarthritis, vasculitis, myositis, lymphadenopathy, or renal or hepatic involvement) between the two groups. In contrast, laboratory measurements showed higher levels of gamma globulin and beta$_2$ microglobulin and higher prevalence of rheumatoid factor and antinuclear antibodies in patients with abnormal BAL results. Pulmonary function tests in these patients were normal.

These data show a high frequency of subclinical inflammatory alveolitis in primary Sjögren's syndrome. The clinical importance and prognostic significance of these findings are as yet unknown.

In other reports investigating the prevalence of interstitial lung disease in Sjögren's syndrome using chest radiographs and pulmonary function tests, 37.5% have been reported to have diffuse interstitial disease (92). These patients presented with cough, dyspnea, pleuritic chest pain, and infiltrates on chest X-ray (90,92). Patients with extraglandular disease and cryoglobulins may be at increased risk for interstitial disease.

Pseudolymphoma

Pseudolymphoma is an uncommon complication that most often presents as lymphadenopathy in a patient with known Sjögren's syndrome (90,105). However, there are also well-documented cases of pseudolymphoma presenting as pulmonary nodules. Pagani et al. reported a case with pulmonary pseudolymphoma that presented as a pulmonary nodule in a patient without symptoms of exocrine gland compromise (96). Two years after the initial diagnosis, clinical features of Sjögren's syndrome developed. Cavities in pseudolymphomas are reported (90,93).

Lymphoma

Lymphomas may develop in patients with Sjogren's syndrome but are quite rare (90). Pulmonary involvement with these lymphomas has been documented but is not often the primary presentation or complication. As described previously, there is a case report of airway obstruction secondary to a lymphoma of the trachea in a patient with Sjögren's syndrome (97).

C. Radiographic Findings

Radiographic abnormalities are described in Chapter 4. The findings include diffuse interstitial parenchymal infiltrates that may progress to honeycombing, pleural effusions, pulmonary nodules, and hilar adenopathy (90,91).

D. Pathology

Pathology of Sjogren's syndrome is described in Chapter 6. Airway abnormalities include atrophy of the submucosal glands of the trachea, peribronchial and peribronchiolar infiltrates with or without fibrosis, and/or lymphoid hyperplasia and bronchiolitis obliterans (89,98). Interstitial pathologic abnormalities include bronchiolitis obliterans, infiltrations of the interstitium with lymphocytes and histiocytes which may aggregate into granulomas with giant cell formation, and interstitial fibrosis (90,95,105). Two patients with secondary Sjogren's syndrome and interstitial pneumonitis have also been reported to have amyloidosis (90). The pseudolymphoma of Sjogren's syndrome is characterized by lymphocytes, reticulum cells, and large mononuclear cells that have large nucleoli and little cytoplasm (105).

E. Management

There is little information to suggest that any therapeutic intervention is successful in altering the status of pulmonary involvement in Sjogren's syndrome. Fortunately, many of the pulmonary manifestations of Sjogren's syndrome are subclinical or not of sufficient significance to warrant treatment. There are case reports of improvement after treatment with corticosteroids, but there are also reports of corticosteroid failures (90,97,106). In most cases, observation coupled with the avoidance of potential exacerbating factors, such as smoking and allergens, and a program of immunization against pulmonary infections would seem to be the most expedient course (107).

F. Summary

Although pulmonary involvement is frequent in Sjogren's syndrome, it is rarely clinically significant. The manifestations are cough, which can be related to xerotrachea; obstructive and restrictive airway disease; and pulmonary infiltrates or nodules that may represent pneumonitis/fibrosis, pseudolymphoma, or lymphoma. Management involves symptomatic control and, in severe cases, corticosteroid drugs, though there are few data to establish their efficacy.

References

1. Zorab, P. (1962). The lungs in ankylosing spondylitis. *Q. J. Med.* **31**: 267-280.
2. Miller, J. M., and Sproule, B. J. (1964). Pulmonary function in ankylosing spondylitis. *Am. Rev. Respir. Dis.* **90**:376.
3. Sharp, J. T., Sweany, K., Henry, J. P., Pietras, R. J., Meadows, W. R., Amarel, E., and Rubenstein, H. M. (1964). Lung and thoracic compliance in ankylosing spondylitis. *J. Lab. Clin. Med.* **63**:254.
4. Hamilton, K. A. (1949). Pulmonary manifestations of ankylosing spondylitis. *Ann. Intern. Med.* **31**:216-227.
5. Court-Brown, W. M., and Doll, R. (1965). Mortality from cancer and other causes after radiotherapy for ankylosing spondylitis. *Br. Med. J.* **2**:1327-1332.

6. Cruikshank, B. (1960). Pathology of ankylosing spondylitis. *Bull. Rheum. Dis.* **10**:211.
7. Campbell, A. H., and McDonald, C. B. (1965). Upper lobe fibrosis associated with ankylosing spondylitis. *Br. J. Dis. Chest* **59**:90-101.
8. Jessamine, A. G. (1968). Upper lung lobe fibrosis in ankylosing spondylitis. *Can. Med. Assoc. J.* **98**:25-33.
9. Cohen, A. A., Natelson, E. A., and Fechnar, R. E. (1971). Fibrosing interstitial pneumonitis in ankylosing spondylitis. *Chest* **59**:369-371.
10. Editorial (1971). The lungs in ankylosing spondylitis. *Br. Med. J.* **3**: 492-493.
11. Bhopal, R. S., and Thomas, G. O. (1982). Psittacosis presenting with Reiter's syndrome. *Br. Med. J.* **284**:1606.
12. Bradlow, A., and Mowat, A. G. (1983). Reiter's syndrome in a 73-year-old man with bronchiectasis. *Scand. J. Rheumatol.* **12**:207-208.
13. Mohowald, M. L., Pritzker, M., Sarosi, G. A., Valls, A. A., and Sumner, H. W. (1980). Amyloid in a patient with Reiter's syndrome—secondary or coincidental? Differentiation with potassium permanganate. *J. Rheumatol.* **7(6)**:903-906.
14. Thiers, H., and Pinet, A. (1950). Syndrome de Reiter avec uretrite a inclusions, infiltrat pulmonaire labile et keratodermie. *Lyons Med.* **184**:51.
15. Sharp, G. C., Williams, S. I., Tan, E. M., Gould, R. G., and Holman, H. R. (1972). Mixed connective tissue disease—an apparently distinct rheumatic disease syndrome associated with a specific antibody to an extractable nuclear antigen (ENA). *Am. J. Med.* **52**:148-159.
16. Sharp, G. C. (1975). Mixed connective tissue disease—overlap syndromes. *Clin. Rheum. Dis.* **1**:561-572.
17. Hoogsteden, H. C., Van Dongen, J. J. M., Van der Kwast, T. H., Hooijkaas, H., and Hilvering, C. (1985). Bilateral exudative pleuritis, an unusual pulmonary onset of mixed connective tissue disease. *Respiration* **48**:164-167.
18. Prakash, U. B. S., Luthra, H. S., and Divertie, M. B. (1985). Intrathoracic manifestations in mixed connective tissue disease. *Mayo Clin. Proc.* **60**:813-821.
19. Sullivan, W. D., Hurst, D. M., Harmon, C. E., et al. (1984). A prospective evaluation emphasizing pulmonary involvement in patients with mixed connective tissue disease. *Medicine* **63**:92-107.
20. Singsen, B. H., Bernstein, B. H., Kornreich, H. K., King, K. K., Hanson, V., and Tan, E. M. (1977). Mixed connective tissue disease in childhood. *J. Pediatr.* **90(6)**:893-900.
21. Harmon, C., Wolfe, F., Lillard, S., Held, C., Cordon, R., and Sharp, G. C. (1976). Pulmonary involvement in mixed connective tissue disease (MCTD). *Arthritis Rheum.* **19**:801 (abstract).

22. Wiener-Kronish, J. P., Solinger, A. M., Warnock, M. L., Church, A., Ordonez, N., and Golden, J. A. (1981). Severe pulmonary involvement in mixed connective tissue disease. *Am. Rev. Respir. Dis.* **124**:499-503.

23. Wallaaert, B., Hatron, P., Grosbois, J. M., Tonnel, A. B., Devulder, B., and Vaisin, C. (1986). Subclinical pulmonary involvement in collagen-vascular diseases assessed by broncho-alveolar lavage. *Am. Rev. Respir. Dis.* **133**:574-580.

24. Hosoda, Y., Suzuki, Y., Takana, M., Tojo, T., and Homma, M. (1987). Mixed connective tissue disease with pulmonary hypertension: A clinical and pathological study. *J. Rheumatol.* **14(4)**:826-830.

25. Chapman, J. R., Charles, P. J., Venables, P. J. W., et al. (1984). Definition and clinical relevance of antibodies to nuclear ribonucleoprotein and other nuclear antigens in patients with cryptogenic fibrosing alveolitis. *Am. Rev. Respir. Dis.* **130**:439-443.

26. Germain, M. J., and Davidman, M. (1984). Pulmonary hemorrhage and acute renal failure in a patient with mixed connective tissue disease. *Am. J. Kidney Dis.* **3(6)**:420-424.

27. Agia, G. A., Reddy, V. C., Maltby, J., Madigan, N. P., Sandock, K., and Hurst, D. J. (1980). Pulmonary involvement in MCTD. *Am. Rev. Respir. Dis.* **121**:105A.

28. Cassidy, J. T. (1985). *Juvenile Rheumatoid Arthritis. Textbook of Rheumatology.* W.B. Saunders, Philadelphia, pp. 1247-1277.

29. Yousefzadeh, D. K., and Fishman, P. A. (1979). The triad of pneumonitis, pleuritis, and pericarditis in juvenile rheumatoid arthritis. *Pediatr. Radiol.* **8**:147-150.

30. Calabro, J. (1977). Other extra-articular manifestations of juvenile rheumatoid arthritis. *Arthritis Rheum.* **20**(2 Suppl.):237-240.

31. Calabro, J. J., Holgerson, W. B., Sonpal, G. M., et al. (1976). Juvenile rheumatoid arthritis: A general review and report of 100 patients observed for 15 years. *Semin. Arthritis Rheum.* **5**:257-298.

32. Martel, W., Abell, M. R., Millensen, W. M., and Whitehouse, W. M. (1968). Pulmonary and pleural lesions in rheumatoid disease. *Radiology* **90**:641-653.

33. Lovell, D., Lindsley, C., and Langston, C. (1984). Lymphoid interstitial pneumonia in juvenile rheumatoid arthritis. *J. Pediatr.* **105(6)**:947-950.

34. Athreya, B. H., Doughty, R. A., Bookspan, M., Schumacher, H. R., Sewell, E. M., and Chatten, J. (1981). Pulmonary manifestations of juvenile rheumatoid arthritis. *Clin. Chest Med.* **1**:361.

35. Wagener, J. S., and Taussig, L. M. (1981). Pulmonary function in juvenile rheumatoid arthritis. *J. Pediatr.* **99**:108-110.

36. Weekly Clinico-Pathological Conference. (1968). *N. Engl. J. Med.* **279**:987-996.

37. Jordan, J. D., and Snyder, C. H. (1964). Rheumatoid disease of the lung and cor pulmonale: Observations in a child. *Am. J. Dis. Child.* **108**:174-180.
38. Shore, A., and Rush, P. J. (1987). Possible danger of intraarticular steroid injection in children with respiratory tract infections. (Letter.) *Br. J. Rheum.* **26**:73.
39. Bywaters, E. G. L. (1971). Still's disease in the adult. *Ann. Rheum. Dis.* **30**:121-133.
40. Bujak, J. S., Aptekar, R. G., Decker, J. L., and Wold, S. M. (1973). Juvenile rheumatoid arthritis presenting in the adult as fever of unknown origin. *Medicine (Baltimore)* **52**:431-444.
41. Esdaile, J. M., Tannenbaum, H., and Hawkins, D. (1980). Adult Still's disease. *Am. J. Med.* **68**:825-830.
42. Wouters, J. M. G. W., Van Rijswijk, M. H., and Van de Putte, L. B. A. (1985). Adult onset Still's disease in the elderly: A report of two cases. *J. Rheumatol.* **12**:791-793.
43. Hirohata, S., Kamoshita, H., Takentani, T., and Maeda, S. (1986). Adult Still's disease complicated with adult respiratory distress. *Arch. Intern. Med.* **146**:2409-2410.
44. Corbett, A. J., Zizic, T. M., and Stevens, M. B. (1983). Adult-onset Still's disease with an associated severe restrictive pulmonary defect: A case report. *Ann. Rheum. Dis.* **42**:452-454.
45. Veasy, L. G., Wiedmeier, S. E., Orsmond, G. S., et al. (1987). Resurgence of acute rheumatic fever in the intermountain area of the United States. *N. Engl. J. Med.* **316**:421-427.
46. Stollerman, G. H., Markowitz, M., Taranta, A., Wanamaker, L. W., and Whittemore, R. (1965). Jones criteria (revised) for guidance in the diagnosis of rheumatic fever. *Circulation* **32**:664-668.
47. Stollerman, G. H. (1985). *Rheumatic Fever. Textbook of Rheumatology.* W.B. Saunders, Philadelphia, pp. 1277-1293.
48. Lustok, M. J., and Kuzma, J. F. (1956). Rheumatic fever pneumonitis: A clinical and pathological study of 35 cases. *Ann. Intern. Med.* **44**:337-351.
49. Griffith, G. C., Phillips, A. W., and Asher, C. (1946). Pneumonitis occurring in rheumatic fever. *Am. J. Med. Sci.* **212**:22-30.
50. Neubuerger, K. T., Geever, E. F., and Rutledge, E. K. (1944). Rheumatic pneumonia. *Arch. Pathol. Lab. Med.* **37**:1-15.
51. Levy, H. B., Coffey, J. D., and Anderson, C. E. (1948). Rheumatic pneumonitis in childhood. *Pediatrics* **2**:688-693.
52. Scott, R. F., Thomas, W. A., and Kissane, J. M. (1959). Rheumatic pneumonitis: Pathologic features. *J. Pediatr.* **54**:60-67.
53. Brown, G., Goldring, D., and Behrer, M. R. (1958). Rheumatic pneumonia. *J. Pediatr.* **52**:598-619.

54. Goldring, D., Behrer, M. R., Brown, G., and Elliott, G. (1958). Rheumatic pneumonitis. *J. Pediatr.* **53**:547-565.
55. Massumi, R. A., and Legier, J. F. (1966). Rheumatic pneumonitis. *Circulation* **33**:417-427.
56. Raz, I., Fisher, J., Israeli, A., Gottehrer, N., Chisin, R., and Kleinman, Y. (1985). An unusual case of rheumatic pneumonia. *Arch. Intern. Med.* **145**:1130-1131.
57. Thayer, W. S. (1925). Notes on acute rheumatic disease of the heart. *Bull. Johns Hopkins Hosp.* **36**:99.
58. Paul, J. R. (1928). Pleural and pulmonary lesions in rheumatic fever. *Medicine* **7**:383.
59. McClenahan, M. V., and Paul, J. R. (1929). A review of the pleural and pulmonary lesions in 28 fatal cases of active rheumatic fever. *Arch. Pathol.* **8**:595.
60. Colburn, A. F. (1933). Relationship of the rheumatic process to the development of alterations in tissues. *Am. J. Dis. Child.* **45**:933.
61. Epstein, E. Z., and Greenspan, E. B. (1941). Rheumatic pneumonia. *Arch. Intern. Med.* **68**:174.
62. Serlin, S. P., Rimsza, M. E., and Gay, J. H. (1975). Rheumatic pneumonia: The need for a new approach. *Pediatrics* **56**:1075-1078.
63. Yamamoto, L. G., Seto, D. S. Y., and Reddy, D. V. (1987). Pneumonia associated with acute rheumatic fever. *Clin. Pediatr.* **26**:198-200.
64. Grunow, W. A., and Esterly, J. R. (1972). Rheumatic pneumonitis. *Chest* **61(3)**:298-301.
65. Escudero, J., Stanislawsky, E., and Escudero, X. (1983). Fulminant acute rheumatic fever with multisystem involvement. *Am. Heart J.* **105**:161-162.
66. Behcet, H. (1937). Uber rezidivierende aphthose, durch ein virus verursachte geschwure am mund, am auge und an den genitalien. *Derm. Wschr.* **105**:1152.
67. O'Duffy, J. D. (1985). *Behcet's Disease. Textbook of Rheumatology.* W.B. Saunders, Philadelphia, pp. 1174-1178.
68. O'Duffy, J. D., and Goldstein, N. P. (1976). Neurologic involvement in seven patients with Behcet's disease. *Am. J. Med.* **61**:170.
69. Lakhanpal, S., Tani, K., Lie, J. T., Katoh, K., Ishigatsubo, Y., and Ohokubo, T. (1985). Pathologic features of Behcet's syndrome: A review of Japanese autopsy registry data. *Hum. Pathol.* **16**:790-795.
70. Dilsen, N., Konice, M., Gazioglu, K., Cavdar, T., Ulagay, T., and Ovul, O. (1979). Pleuropulmonary manifestations in Behcet's disease. *Excerpta Med. Int. Cong. Ser.* **467**:163-167.
71. France, R., Buchanan, R. N., Wilson, M. W., and Sheldon, M. B. (1951). Relapsing iritis with recurrent ulcers of the mouth and genitalia (Behcet's syndrome). *Medicine (Baltimore)* **30**:335-355.

72. Hannun, Y., and Frayha, R. (1985). Behçet's disease with pseudochylothorax. *J. Rheumatol.* **12(4)**:817-818.

73. Berlin, C. (1944). Behcet's syndrome with involvement of the central nervous system. *Arch. Dermatol. Syph.* **49**:227-230.

74. Nazarro, P. (1966). Cutaneous manifestations of Behcet's disease: Clinical and histopathological findings. In *International Symposium on Behçet's Disease.* Edited by Monacelli, M., and P. Nazarro. Karger, New York, pp. 15-16.

75. Ohta, G., Nishino, T., Onchi, K., et al. (1974). An autopsy case of Behcet's syndrome associated with pulmonary arteritis and tuberculosis. *Jpn. Circ. J.* **38**:35-45.

76. Santo, M., Levy, A., Levy, M. J., et al. (1986). Pneumonectomy in pulmonary mucormycosis complicating Behcet's disease. *Postgrad. Med. J.* **62**:485-486.

77. Balduin, R., Murer, L., Drigo, R., and Glorioso, S. (1986). Behcet's syndrome: A rare case of pulmonary involvement. *Eur. J. Respir. Dis.* **69**:288-290.

78. Akoglu, T., Paydas, S., Sarpel, S., Tunali, N., and Tuncer, I. (1987). Incomplete Behcet's syndrome with unusual manifestations. *Ann. Rheum. Dis.* **46**:632-633.

79. Boe, J., Dalgaard, J. B., and Anderson, S. R. (1959). Behcet's syndrome. Report of case with complete autopsy performed. *Acta Pathol. Microbiol. Scand.* **45**:145-158.

80. Petty, T. L., Scoggin, C. H., and Good, J. T. (1977). Recurrent pneumonia in Behcet's syndrome. *J.A.M.A.* **238**:2529-2530.

81. Brookes, G. B. (1983). Pharyngeal stenosis in Behçet's syndrome. The first reported case. *Arch. Otolaryngol.* **109**:338-340.

82. Gibson, J. M., O'Hara, J. M. B., and Stanford, C. F. (1982). Bronchial obstruction in a patient with Behcet's disease. *Eur. J. Respir. Dis.* **63**: 356-360.

83. Ahonen, A. V., Steinus-Aarniala, B. S. M., Viljanen, B. C., Halttunen, P. E. A., Oksa, P., and Mattson, K. V. (1978). Obstructive lung disease in Behcet's syndrome. *Scand. J. Respir. Dis.* **59**:44-50.

84. Rosenthal, T., Band, H., Aladjem, M., David, R., and Gafni, J. (1975). Systematic amyloidosis in Behçet's disease. *Ann. Intern. Med.* **83**:220-223.

85. Efthimiou, J., Johnston, C., Spiro, S. G., and Turner-Warwick, M. (1986). Pulmonary disease in Behçet's syndrome. *Q. J. Med.* **58**:259-280.

86. Gibson, R. N., Morgan, S. H., Krausz, T., and Hughes, G. R. V. (1985). Pulmonary artery aneurysms in Behcet's disease. *Br. J. Radiol.* **58**:79-82.

87. Grenier, P., Bletry, O., Cornud, F., Godeau, P., and Nahum, H. (1981). Pulmonary involvement in Behcet's disease. *A. J. R.* **137(3)**:565-569.

88. Haralampos, M., Moutsopoulos, M. D., et al. (1980). Sjogren's syndrome (sicca syndrome): Current issues. *Ann. Intern. Med.* **92(1)**:212-226.
89. Constantopoulos, M. D., Papadimitrious, M. D., and Moutsopoulos, M. D. (1985). Respiratory manifestations in primary Sjogren's syndrome. A clinical, functional and histologic study. *Chest* **88(2)**:226-229.
90. Strimlan, C. V., Rosenow, E. C., Divertie, M. B., and Harrison, E. G. (1976). Pulmonary manifestations of Sjogren's syndrome. *Chest* **70(3)**:354-361.
91. Segal, I., Fink, G., Machtey, I., Gura, V., and Spitzer, S. A. (1981). Pulmonary function abnormalities in Sjogren's syndrome and the sicca complex. *Thorax* **36**:286-289.
92. Papathanasiou, M. P., Constantopoulos, S. H., Tsampoulas, C., Drosos, A. A., and Moutsopoulos, H. M. (1986). Reappraisal of respiratory abnormalities in primary and secondary Sjogren's syndrome. *Chest* **90(3)**: 370-374.
93. Newball, H. H., and Brahim, S. A. (1977). Chronic obstructive airway disease in patients with Sjogren's syndrome. *Am. Rev. Respir. Dis.* **115**:295-304.
94. Fairfax, A. J., Haslam, P. L., Pavia, D., et al. (1981). Pulmonary disorders associated with Sjogren's syndrome. *Q. J. Med.* **50**:279-295.
95. Forman, M. B., Zwi, S., Gear, A. J., Kallenbach, J., and Wing, J. (1982). Severe airway obstruction associated with rheumatoid arthritis and Sjogren's syndrome. A case report. *S. Afr. Med. J.* **61(18)**:674-676.
96. Pagani, J. J., Collins, J. D., and Reza, M. J. (1979). Sjogren syndrome presenting as pulmonary pseudolymphoma: Report of a case. *J. Natl. Med. Assoc.* **71(7)**:677-678.
97. Kamholz, S., Sher, A., Barland, P., Rosen, N., Rakoff, S., and Becker, N. (1987). Sjogren's syndrome: Severe upper airways obstruction due to primary malignant tracheal lymphoma developing during successful treatment of lymphotic interstitial pneumonitis. *J. Rheumatol.* **14(3)**:588-594.
98. Bariffi, F., Pesci, A., Bertorelli, G., Mangenelli, P., and Ambanelli, U. (1984). Pulmonary involvement in Sjogren's syndrome. *Respiration* **46**:82-87.
99. Vitali, C., Tavoni, A., Viegi, G., Begliomini, E., Agnesi, A., and Bombardieri, S. (1985). *Ann. Rheum. Dis.* **44**:455-461.
100. De Cremoux, H., Georges, R., Battesti, J. P., et al. (1980). Pneumopathies interstitielles diffuses au cours du syndrome de Sjogren limite (sans connectivite associee). *Nouv. Presse Med.* **9**:3445-3447.
101. Radoux, V., Menard, H. A., Begin, R., Decary, F., and Koopman, W. J. (1987). Airways disease in rheumatoid arthritis patients. One element of a general exocrine dysfunction. *Arthritis Rheum.* **30(3)**:249-256.

102. Begin, R., Masse, S., Cantin, A., Menard, H. A., and Bureau, M. A. (1982). Airway disease in a subset of nonsmoking rheumatoid arthritis patients. *Am. J. Med.* **72**:743-750.

103. Karsh, J., Moutsopoulos, H. M., Vergalla, J., and Jones, E. A. (1981). Protease inhibitor phenotypes and pulmonary disease in patients with Sjogren's syndrome. *Respiration* **41**:60-65.

104. Hatron, P., Wallaert, B., Gosset, D., et al. (1987). Subclinical lung inflammation in primary Sjogren's syndrome. *Arthritis Rheum.* **30(11)**:1226-1231.

105. Talal, N., Sokoloff, L., and Barth, W. F. (1967). Extrasalivary lymphoid abnormalities in Sjogren's syndrome (reticulum cell sarcoma, "pseudolymphoma," macroglobulinemia). *Am. J. Med.* **43**:50-65.

106. Ferreiro, J. E., Robalino, B. D., and Saldana, M. J. (1987). Primary Sjogren's syndrome with diffuse cerebral vasculitis and lymphocytic interstitial pneumonitis. *Am. J. Med.* **82**:1227-1232.

107. Editor. (1981). Pneumococcal vaccination for patients with Sjogren's syndrome. *J.A.M.A.* **245**:2288.

14

Pulmonary Reactions Induced by Antirheumatic Drugs

GRANT W. CANNON

University of Utah and VA Medical Center
Salt Lake City, Utah

I. Introduction

When pulmonary problems develop in a patient with a rheumatic disease, the possibility of an adverse drug reaction must always be considered. Prompt recognition and proper management of this problem can often lead to a complete reversal of the pulmonary process. The systematic approach to drug-induced pulmonary disease requires the knowledge of the clinical presentations of this problem, an awareness of the agents that can produce pulmonary disease, and the proper attention to exclude other causes of lung complaints.

II. Classification of Drug-Induced Pulmonary Disease

The spectrum of drug-induced pulmonary disease can range from a mild dyspnea to progressive fatal pulmonary failure (1-5). The most common pulmonary syndromes caused by medications includes pneumonitis (6-59), fibrosis (6,12,26,44,60-65), bronchospasm (67-76), bronchiolitis obliterans (77-83), noncardiogenic pulmonary edema (84-92), and pulmonary/renal syndromes (93-96) (Table 1). With such a wide variety of presentations, the

Table 1 Clinical Manifestations of Drug-Induced Pulmonary Disease

Pneumonitis
  Methotrexate (6-30)
  Gold (31-36)
  D-penicillamine (37,38)
  Cyclophosphamide (39-42)
  Chlorambucil (43,44)
  Azathioprine (45-47)
  Sulfasalazine (48-51)
  Nonsteroidal antiinflammatory drugs (52-59)

Fibrosis
  Methotrexate (6,26,60,61)
  Cyclophosphamide (62-64)
  Chlorambucil (44,65)
  Azathioprine (45)
  Sulfasalazine (66)

Bronchospasm
  Salicylate (67-72)
  Nonsteroidal antiinflammatory drugs (73-76)

Bronchiolitis obliterans
  Gold (77,78)
  D-penicillamine (79-82)
  Sulfasalazine (83)

Noncardiogenic pulmonary edema
  Methotrexate (84,85)
  Cyclophosphamide (86)
  Salicylate (87-89)
  NSAIDs (90,91)
  Colchicine (92)

Pulmonary/renal syndromes
  D-penicillamine (93-96)

recognition that the clinical manifestations may vary significantly between patients is more important than focusing on a limited number of signs and symptoms which are presently recognized. It is not uncommon for a patient to have features of more than one pathologic process during a drug-induced injury (1,6,45,83). This could not only represent multiple manifestations of a drug-induced reaction, but an adverse drug reaction superimposed on an underlying pulmonary disease.

A. Pneumonitis

Clinical Manifestations

Pneumonitis is the most common manifestation of drug-induced pulmonary disease (2). The severity can range from a mild disease (6) with insidious onset to an acute fulminant hypersensitivity reaction which may be fatal (7-9). Shortness of breath, nonproductive cough, and general malaise are the most common symptoms reported (6,10). Chest pain may be present or absent (6). A case of severe chest pain with pneumothorax is reported (31). In acute hypersensitivity pneumonitis, systematic features including fever and chills may also be a prominent component (9). Physical examination is usually unremarkable except for crackles on chest auscultation. These inspiratory rales are most common at the bases and in a symmetric distribution (6).

Laboratory Findings

Laboratory findings are helpful in evaluating the severity of the pulmonary injury but are not useful in establishing the diagnosis. In the hypersensitivity reactions, eosinophilia may be present (7,11,12). Arterial blood gases often show hypoxemia, which may be severe (6). Negative cultures and stains for microorganisms are helpful in excluding infectious agents and suggesting a drug-induced reaction.

Radiographs

Although there are rare instances of patients with normal chest X-rays during drug-induced lung disease (32,46), chest roentgenograms are almost always abnormal. Several patterns of pulmonary infiltrates occur (13). These patterns include increased interstitial markings, reticulonodular patterns, and interstitial/alveolar infiltrates. Pulmonary infiltrates are often bilateral and located in the lower lung fields, although there are situations where unilateral disease has occurred (6,9). Pleural effusions may be present (97). These effusions are most common during the acute hypersensitivity reactions. Pleural effusions may be found at autopsy (33) and surgery (31) that are not detected on chest X-ray.

Pulmonary Function Tests

Pulmonary function tests have been reported to show a restrictive or an obstructive ventilatory defect (7,14) and a reduced carbon monoxide diffusing capacity (DLCO); however, few studies have included baseline pulmonary tests for comparison.

Pathology

Lung biopsy can demonstrate characteristic changes and exclude infectious agents. Interstitial and often alveolar inflammation is characterized by mononuclear cell infiltrations (3,98) (see pathology illustration, Chap. 6, Fig. 5), although polymorphonuclear leukocytes can occasionally be seen. Epithelial abnormalities include proliferation of both type I and type II (3) pneumocytes with some dysplastic changes. In the patients with an acute hypersensitivity reaction, bronchiolitis, giant cells, granuloma formation (9,10,15), and infiltration with eosinophils (9,11) may develop. Diffuse alveolar damage, although infrequent, is seen in the more severe cases (6,9). Fibrosis may be seen on some biopsies. Chapter 1 reviews the present understanding of pathogenesis of pulmonary fibrosis and its relationship to pneumonitis. The possibility that fibrosis seen on lung biopsies is the result of the patient's underlying rheumatic diseases must always be considered. The role of bronchoalveolar lavage (BAL) in evaluation of pneumonitis is reviewed in Chapter 5. BAL may become helpful in the future evaluation of pneumonitis and hypersensitivity reactions (99,100); however, at present, lung biopsy remains the gold standard.

B. Pulmonary Fibrosis

It is postulated that pulmonary fibrosis results from chronic pneumonitis (3) (see Chap. 1). Proving that pulmonary fibrosis is the result of an adverse drug effect in patients with rheumatic diseases is diffucult because pulmonary fibrosis may be the result of the underlying disease. However, patients with malignancies or psoriasis, conditions that are not associated with the development of pulmonary fibrosis, have developed pulmonary fibrosis after receiving methotrexate (60,61) or cyclophosphamide (62,63). These data would suggest that pulmonary fibrosis can develop after treatment with antirheumatic drugs, although it is impossible in many cases to determine the exact etiology of the process.

The most frequent clinical manifestation of pulmonary fibrosis is the insidious onset of shortness of breath with or without a nonproductive cough. There are usually no other associated symptoms. Physical examination may reveal diffuse bibasilar "dry" inspiratory rales. Laboratory data are usually only abnormal for hypoxemia and a decrease in DLCO. Pulmonary function tests show a restrictive lung pattern. The clinical course after the diagnosis of drug-induced pulmonary fibrosis is poorly defined in the literature. It would appear prudent to stop the suspected agent, but there are no data at present to state whether this will alter the course of the disease.

C. Bronchospasm

Acute bronchospasm has developed in patients treated with salicylates (62-72) and nonsteroidal inflammatory drugs (NSAIDs) (73-76). These episodes usually occur early in the course of treatment and can be seen even after a single dose of medication (74). After withdrawal of the offending medication, the symptoms will usually resolve, although it is often necessary to employ supportive therapy including supplemental oxygen, beta-agonists, and corticosteroids in severe cases (74). Unfortunately, deaths have been reported with NSAID-induced bronchospasm (75).

The mechanism by which bronchospasm is produced is not clearly defined. It appears that multiple mechanisms including inhibition of prostaglandin synthesis, allergic idiosyncratic hypersensitivity reactions, and reactions to formulation components of the medications may all be possible (68). Successful attempts to "desensitize" patients with aspirin-sensitive asthma have been reported (72), although this is not always effective (101,102).

D. Bronchiolitis Obliterans

Most reports of bronchiolitis obliterans occurred in patients with rheumatoid arthritis who were receiving gold (77,78), D-penicillamine (79-82), or sulfasalazine (83). A close temporal relationship between the development of this pulmonary disease and the drug therapy is often reported. Thus, there is a strong implication that many episodes of bronchiolitis obliterans are drug induced.

These patients usually present with progressive dyspnea (83) and nonproductive cough (83). Systemic symptoms such as fever (83) are reported but are uncommon. Physical examination may show dullness to percussion over the lung fields (83), reduced breath sounds (75), and wheezing (75). Pulmonary function tests have shown a reduced diffusing capacity with evidence of airflow obstruction at low lung volumes (83).

Lung biopsy will show signs of interstitial pneumonia and marked bronchiolitis obliterans characterized by distended bronchioles obstructed by polypoid plugs made up of epithelioid cells and fibroblasts set in a loose stroma (75,83). The surrounding lung parenchyma may have alveolar septa which are thickened and a mild eosinophilic infiltrate. The alveoli may be filled with edema fluid and macrophages with rare granuloma (83) (see also Chap.6).

The prognosis of bronchiolitis obliterans is poor, with little evidence that intervention with corticosteroids is helpful (75), although there is a case report of reversal of gold-induced bronchiolitis obliterans with cyclophosphamide and methylprednisolone (78).

E. Noncardiogenic Pulmonary Edema

Although noncardiogenic pulmonary edema has been reported with methotrexate (84-85), cyclophosphamide (86), salicylates (87-89), NSAIDs (90-91) and colchicine (92), these episodes did not occur in rheumatic disease patients. Most cases are reported in individuals who received an overdose (88) of these agents or who received the drug for the first time (3,86,90-92).

Symptoms usually develops within minutes to hours after drug administration and present as acute dyspnea, diffuse pulmonary infiltrates, and other manifestations of respiratory compromise. Although deaths are reported (75), the majority of patients will recover after withdrawal of the offending agent and appropriate supportive measures (74).

F. Pulmonary/Renal Syndromes

Although only rarely reported, D-penicillamine treatment has been associated with the development of acute pulmonary/renal syndromes similar to Goodpasture's syndrome (93-96). The patients with acute pulmonary/renal syndromes usually present with prominent pulmonary symptoms including dyspnea, chest pain, and hemoptysis (93). Renal abnormalities are present on urinalysis with hematuria, proteinuria, and red cell casts (93). Antiglomerular basement membrane antibodies may be present (93), though these antibodies are not always detected (94). Although complete remissions are reported after discontinuing D-penicillamine and instituting corticosteroids and cyclophosphamide (93), some patients have died (95) or progressed to end-stage renal disease (96). The mechanism by which D-penicillamine induced this reaction is unknown, but it could to be through the induction of an autoimmune reaction (93).

III. Potential Mechanisms for Induction of Drug-Induced Pulmonary Disease

Investigations of potential mechanisms of drug-induced pulmonary disease have included work in animal models (103-105) and observations in patients with these diseases. These studies often emphasize the acute direct toxicity of these drugs rather than the long-term and indirect effects of these agents. Often the histology in humans suggests a chronic inflammatory change during drug-induced lung disease, while the injury in animal models is more acute. With the use of BAL, longitudinal data during drug treatment are being collected (106).

Direct toxicity has been noted with cyclophosphamide, which can produce direct tissue-damaging oxidants such as superoxide anions, hydrogen peroxide, and hydroxyl radicals (3). Indirectly, antirheumatic drugs may encourage pulmonary injury by disrupting the lung's natural protective and reparative mechanisms, thus leaving the lung vulnerable to injury from other sources (3). Glutathione is a molecule that is important in oxidant defense in the lung and serves as a cofactor in several enzyme reactions. Cyclophosphamide may interfere with the production of this compound and thus reduce the protection rendered by glutathione (3). Methotrexate may decrease pulmonary macrophages (103-105). The proinflammatory and antiinflammatory compounds produced during arachidonic acid metabolism may also be altered by antirheumatic drugs and influence the development of pulmonary reactions.

Although there are no proven mechanisms by which these agents produce pulmonary disease, increasing evidence is accumulating in this area. The effects of these agents may be indirect, and the development of pulmonary reactions to antirheumatic drugs may represent a disturbance of the natural lung defense mechanisms.

IV. Potential Risk Factors

Several reports have suggested risk factors that may predispose patients to develop drug-induced pulmonary disease. Although this area is controversial, efforts to prospectively identify patients at risk for the development of pulmonary reactions to antirheumatic drugs have been unsuccessful (107). An understanding of these possible risk factors may assist in selecting an antirheumatic drug therapy and alert the physician to patients who should be closely monitored during treatment. For scientific endeavors, the identification of risk factors may assist in understanding the pathophysiology of drug-induced pulmonary disease.

A. Drug Dosing

Because an idiosyncratic reaction may occur early in the course of therapy (84,85), patients should be closely monitored for the development of pulmonary disease during the intial treatment. Drug-induced pulmonary disease can, however, occur at any point during treatment (6). Fibrosis may be the result of long-standing interstitial inflammation. In this condition, it appears that the duration of therapy and cumulative dose may correlate with the risk for the development of pulmonary fibrosis (3). Overall, however, there are no data to clearly show that a modification of dosing schedules can reduce the potential for drug-induced pulmonary injury in patients receiving these agents.

B. Concurrent Pulmonary Disease

It has been suggested that chronic underlying pulmonary disease may predispose rheumatoid arthritis patients to develop methotrexate-induced pulmonary reactions (26,27), though this is not confirmed by all authors (6). Patients with limited pulmonary reserves may be more likely to manifest severe symptoms when a drug-induced pulmonary event occurs. Despite the lack of firm evidence to show that pulmonary reactions are more common in patients with chronic pulmonary disease, it would be prudent to withhold agents that can cause serious pulmonary complications in patients with significant lung disorders. The primary rationale for this recommendation is the lack of pulmonary reserve in these patients if pulmonary difficulties were to develop.

C. Concurrent Illness

The role of concurrent medical illness in the development of drug-induced lung disorders is unknown in the development of pulmonary reactions. The role that diseases that alter antirheumatic drug metabolism may play in the development of pulmonary disease with these agents is also unknown. Renal insufficiency has been associated with an increase in pulmonary (6) and non-pulmonary adverse reactions in patients receiving methotrexate (108). Previous radiation therapy may increase the likelihood of developing pulmonary fibrosis with cyclophosphamide (64). Elderly patients may have an increase in adverse drug reactions for multiple reasons. However, there are no data specifically evaluating adverse pulmonary drug reactions in elderly patients (6).

V. Screening for Pulmonary Disease During Treatment with Antirheumatic Drugs

The pulmonary status of a rheumatic patient should be appraised before the initiation of a new agent. The recommendations on the extent of this evaluation have been debated and are based primarily on clinical observations and not prospective data. It would appear prudent to review the pulmonary disease history and perform a chest examination. A baseline chest roentgenogram should be obtained on any patient with significant abnormalities. If significant pulmonary abnormalities are detected, further investigations should be undertaken as clinically indicated. There are no data to suggest that pulmonary function testing is of any value in detecting patients at risk for the development of significant drug-induced pulmonary disease. However, after the problem develops, serial pulmonary function testing may be helpful in monitoring the patient's progress (see Chap. 3).

After the pulmonary status is known, the antirheumatic agent to be employed may be selected. Instructions reviewing adverse drug effects at the initiation of new treatments should include a description of potential pulmonary reactions. Patients should be instructed to inform their physician of new pulmonary complaints. Although attention to pulmonary symptoms throughout treatment is required, vigilance during the first few weeks is particularly important.

VI. Diagnosis of Drug-Induced Pulmonary Disease

Since there are no clinical, laboratory, or pathologic findings that are pathognomonic for drug-induced pulmonary disease, the diagnosis of this condition is based on clinical features consistent with a drug-induced reaction and the exclusion of other diseases that could produced similar findings. Most important, infection must be excluded. Lung biopsy is often required to evaluate for infection and to determine the histopathology of the lesion. We have developed the following criteria for the diagnosis of drug-induced pulmonary disease (6): (a) clinical course consistent with a drug-induced reaction; (b) infiltrates on chest roentgenogram; (c) exclusion of infection and other pulmonary diseases; and (d) pathology consistent with drug-induced injury. For a diagnosis of probable drug-induced pulmonary disease, a patient must meet at least three of the above criteria. For a diagnosis of possible drug-induced pulmonary disease, a patient should meet two of the above criteria. The term "definite" is not used with these criteria because the diagnosis of drug-induced pulmonary disease is always presumptive and, although well accepted, should be subject to reassessment and review during the evaluation of each patient.

The need for open lung biopsy to establish a diagnosis of drug-induced lung disease must be evaluated in each patient. In some cases, transbronchial biopsy has been reported to be adequate to establish a diagnosis (9), while other patients have been managed without any pathologic examination of lung tissue (6). In some patients, open lung biopsy was required to make the diagnosis after transbronchial biopsy was inconclusive (6,15). The exclusion of infections is a major concern in evaluating pulmonary diseases in patients receiving antirheumatic drugs. Although rare, opportunistic pulmonary infections with *Pneumocystis carinii* (16,109) and *Candida albicans* (124) have been documented in patients receiving methotrexate. Most evidence would suggest that open lung biopsy has some advantages over transbronchial biopsy (110) and needle biopsy (111) in detecting pulmonary infections. The evaluation and management of infections in patients with rheumatic diseases is fully described in Chapter 7. While mild respiratory complaints can be observed in some patients without lung biopsy, it would seem prudent to perform lung biopsy in all patients with significant respiratory compromise. The methods needed to firmly exclude infectious agents and obtain adequate tissue samples for pathologic evidence of a drug-induced reaction should be employed. Lung biopsies should be considered early in the patient's evaluation before the institution of empiric antibiotic therapy if possible. BAL may become more helpful in the future evaluation of hypersensitivity reactions (34,96) and to exclude infection; however, at present, lung biopsy must remain the gold standard (see Chap. 5).

VII. Management of Drug-Induced Pulmonary Disease

Most drug-induced pulmonary disease will resolve after the withdrawal of the offending agent. Supportive care is important in patients with severe respiratory compromise and may include supplemental oxygen, respiratory therapy, and, in severe cases, assisted ventilation. Although there are no controlled studies to confirm their benefit, corticosteroids are reported effective in accelerating the resolution of severe acute pneumonitis (6,9,10,15, 18). The possibility of residual disease is difficult to determine, as many patients may have pulmonary compromise at baseline. The potential for developing pulmonary fibrosis appears to correlate with the duration of pneumonitis. Thus, more residual disease may occur in patients who have prolonged pneumonitis than in patients with acute pneumonitis, provided the offending agent is discontinued.

There is no evidence to firmly establish that corticosteroids are beneficial to treat pulmonary fibrosis and bronchiolitis obliterans. The most appropriate therapy for these diseases would appear to be discontinuation of the offending agent and supportive care as indicated.

VIII. Specific Agents Inducing Pulmonary Disease

A.   Methotrexate

Methotrexate is associated with acute pneumonitis (6-28), pulmonary fibrosis (6,26,60,61), noncardiogenic pulmonary edema (84,85), and pleural effusions (97). With the increasing use of methotrexate in multiple rheumatic disease, there must be an increase in the awareness of this potential problem. In rheumatoid arthritis patients receiving methotrexate, the prevalence of pulmonary disease has been estimated by Carson et al. at 5.5% and an incidence of 3.9 cases per 100 patient-years of treatment (6). St. Clair et al.

reported a 3.1% prevalence (9). However, some large series have not reported any significant drug-induced disease during treatment with methotrexate (112-115). In nonrheumatic disease, the prevalence rates have varied from 40% (16) to 2.4% (25). The former calculation is certainly an overestimate, as infections were not vigorously excluded with one case of *Pneumocystis carinii* documented (16).

There are no clear predisposing factors, although it has been suggested that methotrexate-induced pulmonary disease may be more likely in patients with underlying lung disease (26,27) and renal insufficiency (6).

The clinical features in these patients are typical of that seen in an acute pneumonitis as described earlier in this chapter. The pathology is characterized by mononuclear cell infiltration. Granulomas with giant cell formation and bronchiolitis are also often seen (6,9,10,15,18).

The general management of acute pneumonitis is described above. Although there are reports of pulmonary disease resolving despite the continuation of methotrexate (11,16), this management is not recommended. The most prudent practice would appear to be permanent discontinuation of the medication. Although there are instances when methotrexate has been reinstituted without recurrent pulmonary disease (6,7), there are well-documented cases of recurrent methotrexate-induced pulmonary disease after rechallenging with the drug (6,14). In addition to discontinuing the drug and instituting the needed supportive therapy, corticosteroids appear to benefit the patient with severe disease (6,9,10,60), although there are reports of spontaneous improvement without these agents (6,8). Case reports have suggested that daunorubicin may be effective in treatment of this disorder (116). There is no indication that leucovorin rescue is of any value in treatment of this problem (4,103).

In Sostman's review, it was suggested that methotrexate-induced pneumonitis was "not likely to develop" in patients receiving doses less than 20 mg per week (7). It was initially hoped that methotrexate-induced pulmonary complications would not be seen in patients receiving 7.5-15 mg doses used in the treatment of rheumatoid arthritis. There have now been multiple reports of methotrexate-induced lung disease occurring with doses as low as 7.5 mg per week (6,10,18,31,32) with a severe reaction reported after a cumulative dose of 12.5 mg over 2 weeks (31). In rheumatoid arthritis patients, studies have shown no differences in cumulative dose or weekly dose of methotrexate in patients who developed methotrexate-induced pulmonary disease when compared to patients who did not develop this condition (6). Also the clinical features of the disease are very similar despite the differences in dose. Thus it would appear that the drug-induced reactions are similar at all doses. One exception to these observations is noncardiogenic pulmonary edema, which has only been reported in patients receiving "high" dose methotrexate

(84,85), although it must be recognized that this rare condition may yet occur at low dose.

Long-term follow-up suggests that most patients with methotrexate-induced lung disease return to their baseline pulmonary status after resolution of their acute pulmonary process (6,10,27). Although the prognosis of acute methotrexate-induced pulmonary disease is favorable, there are reports of deaths during the treatment of malignancies (7,8) and rheumatoid arthritis (8,9). Pulmonary superinfection may have played a significant role in these patients. Methotrexate-induced pulmonary fibrosis has also been fatal in patients receiving this agent for psoriasis and malignances (60).

B. Gold

Gold therapy has been associated with the development of hypersensitivity pneumonitis (31-36) and bronchiolitis obliterans (75). Although the majority of cases of gold-induced pulmonary disease have been seen in rheumatoid arthritis patients, acute pneumonitis has been seen in patients treated with gold who do not have rheumatoid arthritis (36). The prevalence of gold-induced pneumonitis is not known, but it is certainly infrequent. A recent review of 1,019 patients treated with gold between 1933 and 1979 did not identify any cases of pulmonary toxicity (117). A study combining 14 prospectively and 96 retrospectively evaluated patients could not demonstrate any change in pulmonary function studies in rheumatoid arthritis patients receiving gold (107). The clinical spectrum can vary, with significant morbidity and fatalities reported (33). The duration of gold therapy before the onset of pulmonary diseases varies significantly. In a review of 90 reported cases, the length of gold treatment ranged from 4 to 78 weeks with a mean of 15 (34). The mean cumulative dosage was 582 mg (range 120-1,660 mg) (34).

The acute pneumonitis generally presents with cough and shortness of breath. Leukocytosis and eosinophilia are reported in 63% and 43% of the patients, respectively (34). Chest roentgenograms are usually abnormal, but normal chest X-rays have been seen with biopsy-proven pneumonitis (32). BAL has shown an increase in lymphocytes consistent with drug-induced hypersensitivity pneumonitis in several cases (34). Analysis of these cells has shown a predominance of T-cells with an inversion of the helper/suppressor ratio (34). In vitro tests of lymphocytes from BAL and peripheral blood have produced variable results. Generally the BAL lymphocytes have been reactive with gold while the peripheral blood lymphocytes have been nonreactive (36). This may be the result of recruitment of cells to the site of sensitization. Also it is known that the addition of gold to lymphocyte cultures can suppress T-cell activation (118,119). It may well be that a critical balance between the in vitro stimulatory and inhibitory effects of gold makes it difficult to completely define the immunologic effect of gold in this system (34). Exacerbations after rechallenging with gold are reported (33,36).

Bronchiolitis obliterans has also been seen with gold treatment (77,78). Although fibrosis has been seen in association with acute pneumonitis in patients receiving gold (36), this may not be a gold-induced pulmonary reaction.

C. D-Penicillamine

Hypersensitivity pneumonitis (37,38), bronchiolitis obliterans (79-82), and pulmonary/renal syndromes (93-96) have been seen in patients receiving D-penicillamine. The incidence of D-penicillamine-induced pulmonary disease is quite rare, with a prevalence of probably less than 1%. Patients with bronchiolitis obliterans present with progressive dyspnea and cough, usually without systemic symptoms. Chest roentgenograms in bronchiolitis obliterans may vary from normal to bilateral reticular infiltrates or localized infiltrates. Patients with bronchiolitis obliterans have generally had a very poor prognosis, with a 50% mortality from the pulmonary disease. Acute pulmonary hemorrhage without signs of drug-induced systemic lupus erythematosus or Goodpasture's syndrome has also been reported (120). D-penicillamine has also been associated with the development of several autoimmune phenomena including myasthenia gravis, polymyositis, pemphigus, lupuslike disease, and Sjogren's syndrome, which may affect pulmonary function (121).

D. Cyclophosphamide and Chlorambucil

The incidence of cyclophosphamide-induced pulmonary disease has been estimated at less than 1% (5). There appears to be no relationship to cumulative dose. There are reports of cyclophosphamide-induced pulmonary toxicity in patients with rheumatic diseases, although the majority of information on this reaction is in the oncology literature. The most common manifestations of alkylating agent-induced pulmonary toxicity are acute pneumonitis (39-42) and pulmonary fibrosis (6,26,62-65), although there is one case of noncardiogenic pulmonary edema (86). Pulmonary fibrosis may be progressive despite discontinuing cyclophosphamide (62) and may be fatal in some cases (41,63). Radiation therapy may increase the risk of pulmonary fibrosis during cyclophosphamide therapy (64).

E. Azathioprine

Pulmonary reactions with azathioprine are rare. Acute hypersensitivity pneumonitis (45-47) and pulmonary fibrosis (44) are the only reported presentations. Clinical features and biopsy findings are typical of interstitial pneumonitis (45) and diffuse alveolar damage (45). Fibrosis has been reported in one case with current interstitial pneumonitis (45). The reports of this condition are so uncommon that it is difficult to make specific recommendations other than those made for other types of hypersensitivity pneumonitis.

F. Sulfasalazine

Adverse drug reactions with sulfasalazine can be classified in two groups. One group of symptoms includes the common generalized side effects such as nausea, vomiting, headache, and malaise, and a second group includes idiopathic hypersensitivity reactions such as skin rash, aplastic anemia, hepatic abnormalities, and pulmonary reactions (122). The first group appears to be dose related and more common in patients with slow acetylator phenotypes, while the second type of reactions, including pulmonary disease, is not related with acetylator phenotype (122). Pulmonary disease with sulfasalazine is rare. A review of 774 rheumatoid arthritis patients treated with sulfasalazine over 11 years did not identify any cases of pulmonary disease (123).

Hypersensitivity pneumonitis (48-51), fibrosing alveolitis (66), and bronchiolitis obliterans (83) have been associated with sulfasalazine therapy. The majority of patients present with characteristic features of a drug-induced pulmonary event with cough, dyspnea, chest tightness, fever, and peripheral eosinophils (49). BAL may show an increase in eosinophils and a decrease in lymphocytes (51). One patient is reported to have reinstituted sulfasalazine without recurrent pulmonary disease (3).

G. Salicylates

Bronchospasm (67-72), noncardiogenic pulmonary edema (87-89), and adult respiratory distress syndrome (124,125) have all been reported with salicylates. The triad of asthma, nasal polyps, and aspirin sensitivity has long been recognized. The prevalence of aspirin sensitivity has ranged from 1% in the normal population (126) to 78% patients with asthma and nasal polyps (69). It was initially assumed that an immunologic reaction was responsible for the development of aspirin-induced bronchospasm. However, later work has suggested that the alteration of arachidonic acid metabolism is responsible for the bronchospasm (70). In one case, it was suggested that coronary artery spasm could be part of the aspirin-induced asthma (71). Some aspirin-sensitive patients may be desensitized to aspirin without recurrent bronchospasm (72); however, this is not always successful (97,102).

Noncardiogenic pulmonary edema is associated with high serum salicylate levels, generally over 30 mg/dl (3). In a review of 111 cases of salicylate toxicity (admission salicylate level >30 mg/dl), Walters et al. reported six (5%) cases of noncardiogenic pulmonary edema (87), while Heffner and

Sahn reported eight cases of pulmonary edema in a review of 36 instances of salicylate toxicity (88). Risk factors for the development of noncardiogenic pulmonary edema are cigarette smoking, chronic salicylate ingestion, a component of metabolic acidosis, and the presence of neurological symptoms on presentation (87,88). The mechanism for the development of noncardiogenic pulmonary edema is unknown. There appears to be an increase in permeability of the pulmonary vasculature with an increase in protein concentration in pulmonary secretions (89). BAL shows an increase in leukocytes that are predominantly polymorphonuclear leukocytes (124). Generally with prompt recognition and supportive care, the prognosis of noncardiogenic pulmonary edema is good. Only one death was reported in a review of 111 consecutive cases of salicylate intoxication (87). Recurrent episodes are reported on rechallenging with salicylates (124).

H. Nonsteroidal Antiinflammatory Drugs

Nonsteroidal antiinflammatory drugs (NSAIDs) have been associated with the development of acute pneumonitis (52-59), bronchospasm (73-76), and noncardiogenic pulmonary edema (90,91). Most frequently these symptoms develop early in the course of treatment (53,57) and can return with rechallenge (53,57). BAL has shown an increase in eosinophils (55).

I. Colchicine

One case of noncardiogenic pulmonary edema was seen in a patient who consumed 150 mg of colchicine (92). There are no reported pulmonary abnormalities during treatment with recommended colchicine doses.

IX. Summary

Drug-induced lung disease during treatment with antirheumatic drugs should be considered in all patients receiving these agents who develop new pulmonary symptoms. When a potential drug-related reaction is identified, the possible offending agents should be discontinued, needed respiratory support initiated, and a thorough investigation for other causes of respiratory disease launched to exclude infection or other pulmonary processes. Lung biopsy may be needed to completely define the disorder. In patients with acute pneumonitis, the use of corticosteroids should be considered. Although significant morbidity and even mortality may occur with drug-induced pulmonary events, proper and prompt evaluation and treatment of this disorder can often result in a complete resolution of the pulmonary disease.

Acknowledgments

Supported in part by the Veterans Administration Medical Research Program and the Nora Eccles Harrison Foundation. We thank Jean Armour for her excellent secretarial support of this project.

References

1. Allen, J., Cooper, D. Jr., White, D. A., and Matthay, R. A. (1986). Drug-induced pulmonary disease. 2. Noncytotoxic drugs. *Am. Rev. Respir. Dis.* **133**:488-505.
2. Gockerman, J. P. (1982). Drug-induced interstitial lung diseases. *Clin. Chest* **3**:521-536.
3. Cooper, J. A. D., and Matthay, R. A. (1987). Drug-induced pulmonary disease. *Disease-a-Month* **33**:61-120.
4. Batist, G., and Andrews, J. L. Jr. (1981). Pulmonary toxicity of anti-neoplastic drugs. *J.A.M.A.* **246**:1449-1453.
5. Allen, J., Cooper, D. Jr., White, D. A., and Matthay, R. A. (1986). Drug-induced pulmonary disease. 1. Cytotoxic drugs. *Am. Rev. Respir. Dis.* **133**:321-340.
6. Carson, C. W., Cannon, G. W., Egger, M. J., Ward, J. R., and Clegg, D. O. (1987). Pulmonary disease during the treatment of rheumatoid arthritis with low dose pulse methotrexate. *Semin. Arthritis Rheum.* **16**:186-195.
7. Sostman, H. D., Matthay, R. A., Putman, C. E., and Smith, G. J. W. (1976). Methotrexate-induced pneumonitis. *Medicine* **55**:371-388.
8. Gispen, J. G., Alarcon, G. S., Johnson, J. J., Acton, R. T., Barger, B. O., and Koopman, W. J. (1987). Toxicity to methotrexate in rheumatoid arthritis. *J. Rheumatol.* **14**:74-79.
9. St. Clair, E. W., Rice, J. R., and Snyderman, R. (1985). Pneumonitis complicating low-dose methotrexate therapy in rheumatoid arthritis. *Arch. Intern. Med.* **145**:2035-2038.
10. Cannon, G. W., Ward, J. R., Clegg, D. O., Samuelson, C. O. Jr., and Abbott, T. M. (1983). Acute lung disease associated with low-dose pulse methotrexate therapy in patients with rheumatoid arthritis. *Arthritis Rheum.* **26**:1269-1274.
11. Clarysse, A. M., Cathey, W. J., Cartwright, G. E., and Wintrobe, M. M. (1969). Pulmonary disease complicating intermittent therapy with methotrexate. *J.A.M.A.* **209**:1861-1864.
12. Whitcomb, M. E., Schwarz, M. I., and Tormey, D. C. (1972). Methotrexate pneumonitis: Case report and review of the literature. *Thorax* **27**:636-639.

13. Everts, C. S., Westcott, J. L., and Bragg, D. G. (1973). Methotrexate therapy and pulmonary disease. *Radiology* **107**:539-543.
14. Goldman, G. C., and Moschella, S. L. (1971). Severe pneumonitis occurring during methotrexate therapy. *Arch. Dermatol.* **103**:194-197.
15. Engelbrecht, J. A., Calhoon, S. L., and Scherrer, J. J. (1983). Methotrexate pneumonitis after low-dose therapy for rheumatoid arthritis. *Arthritis Rheum.* **26**:1275-1278.
16. Acute Leukemia Group B (1969). Acute lymphocytic leukemia in children. *J.A.M.A.* **207**:923-928.
17. Dickey, B. F., and Myers, A. R. (1984). Pulmonary disease in polymyositis/dermatomyositis. *Semin. Arthritis Rheum.* **14**:60-76.
18. Kremer, J. M., and Lee, J. K. (1986). The safety and efficacy of the use of methotrexate in long-term therapy for rheumatoid arthritis. *Arthritis Rheum.* **29**:822-831.
19. Searles, G., and McKendry, R. J. R. (1987). Methotrexate pneumonitis in rheumatoid arthritis: Potential risk factors. Four case reports and a review of the literature. *J. Rheumatol.* **14**:1164-1171.
20. Filip, D. J., Logue, G. L., Harle, T. S., and Farrar, W. H. (1971). Pulmonary and hepatic complications of methotrexate therapy of psoriasis. *J.A.M.A.* **216**:881-882.
21. Gutin, P. H., Green, M. R., Bleyer, W. A., Bauer, V. L., Wiernik, P. H., and Walker, M. D. (1976). Methotrexate pneumonitis induced by intrathecal methotrexate therapy. *Cancer* **38**:1529-1534.
22. Nesbit, M., Krivit, W., Heyn, R., and Sharp, H. (1976). Acute and chronic effects of methotrexate on hepatic, pulmonary, and skeletal systems. *Cancer* **37**:1048-1054.
23. White, D. A., Orenstein, M., Godwin, R. A., and Stover, D. E. (1984). Chemotherapy-associated pulmonary toxic reactions during treatment for breast cancer. *Arch. Intern. Med.* **144**:953-956.
24. Arnett, F. C., Whelton, J. C., Zizic, T. M., and Stevens, M. B. (1973). Methotrexate therapy in polymyositis. *Ann. Rheum. Dis.* **32**:536-546.
25. Green, D. M., Brecher, M. L., Blumenson, L. E., Gorssi, M., and Freeman, A. I. (1982). The use of intermediate dose methotrexate in increased risk childhood acute lymphoblastic leukemia. A comparison of three versus six courses. *Cancer* **50**:2722-2727.
26. Bell, M. H., Geddie, W. R., Gordon, D. A., and Reynolds, W. J. (1986). Preexisting lung disease in patients with rheumatoid arthritis may predispose to methotrexate lung. *Arthritis Rheum.* **29**:S75.
27. Boh, L. E., Schuna, A. A., Pitterle, M. E., Adams, E. M., and Sundstrom, W. R. (1986). Low-dose weekly oral methotrexate therapy for inflammatory arthritis. *Clin. Pharm.* **5**:503-508.

28. Williams, H. J., Cannon, G. W., and Ward, J. R. (1986). Methotrexate-induced pulmonary toxicity in patients with rheumatoid arthritis. *Rheumatology* **9**:244-251.

29. Ridley, M. G., Wolfe, C. S., and Mathews, J. A. (1988). Life threatening acute pneumonitis during low dose methotrexate treatment for rheumatoid arthritis: A case report and review of the literature. *Ann. Rheum. Dis.* **47**:784-788.

30. Green, L., Schattner, A., and Berkenstadt, H. (1988). Severe reversible interstitial pneumonitis induced by low dose methotrexate: Report of a case and review of the literature. *J. Rheumatol.* **15**:110-112.

31. Nickels, J., Van Assendelft, A. H., and Tukiainen, P. (1983). Diffuse pulmonary injury associated with gold treatment. *Acta Pathol. Microbiol. Immunol. Scand.* **91**:265-267.

32. Franzen, P., and Pettersson, T. (1983). Alveolitis during chrysotherapy for rheumatoid arthritis. *Acta Med. Scand.* **214**:249-251.

33. Gould, P. W., McCormack, P. L., and Palmer, D. G. (1977). Pulmonary damage associated with sodium aurothiomalate therapy. *J. Rheumatol.* **4**:252-260.

34. Evans, R. B., Ettensohn, D. B., Fawaz-Estrup, F., Lally, E. V., and Kaplan, S. R. (1987). Gold lung: Recent developments in pathogenesis, diagnosis, and therapy. *Semin. Arthritis Rheum.* **16**:196-205.

35. Levinson, M. L., Lynch, J. P. III, and Bower, J. S. (1981). Reversal of progressive life-threatening gold hypersensitivity pneumonitis by corticosteroids. *Am. J. Med.* **71**:908-912.

36. Winterbauer, R. H., Wilske, K. R., and Wheelis, R. F. (1976). Diffuse pulmonary injury associated with gold treatment. *N. Engl. J. Med.* **294**: 919-921.

37. Camus, P., Degat, R., Justrabo, E., and Jeannin, L. (1982). D-penicillamine-induced severe pneumonitis. *Chest* **81**:376-378.

38. Eastmond, C. J. (1976). Letter to the Editor. Diffuse alveolitis as a complication of penicillamine treatment for rheumatoid arthritis. *Br. Med. J.* **1**:1506.

39. Mark, G. J., Lehimgar-Zadeh, A., and Ragsdale, B. D. (1978). Cyclophosphamide pneumonitis. *Thorax* **33**:89-93.

40. Spector, J. I., Zimbler, H., and Ross, J. S. (1979). Early-onset cyclophosphamide-induced interstitial pneumonitis. *J.A.M.A.* **242**:2852-2854.

41. Tsukamoto, N., Matsukuma, K., Matsuyama, T., et al. (1984). Cyclophosphamide-induced interstitial pneumonitis in a patient with ovarian carcinoma. *Gynecol. Oncol.* **17**:41-51.

42. Topilow, A. A., Rothenberg, S. P., and Cottrell, T. S. (1973). Interstitial pneumonia after prolonged treatment with cyclophosphamide. *Am. Rev. Respir. Dis.* **108**:114-117.

43. Godard, P., Marty, J. P., and Michel, F. B. (1979). Interstitial pneumonia and chlorambucil. *Chest* **76**:471-473.

44. Cole, S. R., Myers, T. J., and Klatsky, A. U. (1978). Pulmonary disease with chlorambucil therapy. *Cancer* **41**:455-459.

45. Bedrossian, C. W. M., Sussman, J., Conklin, R. H., and Kahan, B. (1984). Azathioprine-associated interstitial pneumonitis. *Am. J. Clin. Pathol.* **82**:148-154.

46. Krowka, M. J., Breuer, R. I., and Kehoe, T. J. (1983). Azathioprine-associated pulmonary dysfunction. *Chest* **83**:696-698.

47. Carmichael, D. J. S., Hamilton, D. V., Evans, D. B., Stovin, P. G. I., and Calne, R. Y. (1983). Interstitial pneumonitis secondary to azathioprine in a renal transplant patient. *Thorax* **38**:951-952.

48. Jones, G. R., and Malone, D. N. S. (1972). Sulphasalazine induced lung disease. *Thorax* **27**:713-717.

49. Moseley, R. H., Barwick, K. W., Dobuler, K., and DeLuca, V. A. Jr. (1985). Sulfasalazine-induced pulmonary disease. *Dig. Dis. Sci.* **30**:901-904.

50. Wang, K. K., Bowyer, B. A., Fleming, C. R., and Schroeder, K. W. (1984). Pulmonary infiltrates and eosinophilia associated with sulfasalazine. *Mayo Clin. Proc.* **59**:343-346.

51. Valcke, Y., Pauwels, R., and Van der Straeten, M. (1987). Bronchoalveolar lavage in acute hypersensitivity pneumonitis caused by sulfasalazine. *Chest* **92**:572-573.

52. Albazzaz, M. K., Harvey, J. E., Hoffman, J. N., and Siddorn, J. A. (1986). Alveolitis and haemolytic anaemia induced by azapropazone. *Br. Med. J.* **293**:1537-1538.

53. Nader, D. A., and Schillaci, R. F. (1983). Pulmonary infiltrates with eosinophilia due to naproxen. *Chest* **83**:280-282.

54. Fein, M. (1981). Letter to the Editor. Sulindac and pneumonitis. *Ann. Intern. Med.* **95**:245.

55. Flint, K. C., and Johnson, N. (1987). Pulmonary eosinophilia associated with naproxen therapy. *J. R. Soc. Med.* **80**:120-121.

56. Buscaglia, A. J., Cowden, F. E., and Brill, H. (1984). Pulmonary infiltrates associated with naproxen. *J.A.M.A.* **251**:65-66.

57. Gheysens, B., and Van Mieghem, W. (1984). Pulmonary infiltrates with eosinophilia due to glafenine. *Eur. J. Repir. Dis.* **65**:456-459.

58. Reeve, P. A., Moshiri, M., and Bell, G. D. (1987). Letter to the Editor. Pulmonary oedema, jaundice and renal impairment with naproxen. *Br. J. Rheumatol.* **26**:70-71.

59. Sheehan, N. J. (1985). Letter to the Editor. Pulmonary infiltrates and eosinophilia associated with naproxen. *Br. J. Rheum.* **24**:302-303.

60. Bedrossian, C. W. M., Miller, W. C., and Luna, M. A. (1979). Methotrexate-induced diffuse interstitial pulmonary fibrosis. *South. Med. J.* **72**:313-318.
61. Kaplan, R. L., and Waite, D. H. (1978). Progressive interstitial lung disease from prolonged methotrexate therapy. *Arch. Dermatol.* **114**: 1800-1802.
62. Stentoft, J. (1987). Progressive pulmonary fibrosis complicating cyclophosphamide therapy. *Acta Med. Scand.* **221**:403-407.
63. Burke, D. A., Stoddart, J. C., Ward, M. K., and Simpson, C. G. B. (1982). Fatal pulmonary fibrosis occurring during treatment with cyclophosphamide. *Br. Med. J.* **285**:696.
64. Trask, C. W. L., Joannides, T., Harper, P. G., et al. (1985). Radiation-induced lung fibrosis after treatment of small cell carcinoma of the lung with very high-dose cyclophosphamide. *Cancer* **55**:57-;60.
65. Lane, S. D., Besa, E. C., Justh, G., and Joseph, R. R. (1979). Abstract. Fatal interstitial lung disease following high dose chlorambucil therapy. *Proc. Am. Soc. Clin. Oncol.* **20**:313.
66. Davies, D., and MacFarlane, A. (1974). Fibrosing alveolitis and treatment with sulphasalazine. *Gut* **15**:185-188.
67. McDonald, J. R., Mathison, D. A., and Stevenson, D. D. (1972). Aspirin intolerance in asthma. Detection by oral challenge. *J. Allergy Clin. Immunol.* **50**:198-207.
68. Szczeklik, A., Gryglewski, R. J., and Czerniawska-Mysik, G. (1977). Clinical patterns of hypersensitivity to nonsteroidal anti-inflammatory drugs and their pathogenesis. *J. Allergy Clin. Immunol.* **60**:276-284.
69. Falliers, C. J. (1973). Aspirin and subtypes of asthma: Risk factor analysis. *J. Allergy Clin. Immunol.* **52**:141-147.
70. Slepian, I. K., Mathews, K. P., and McLean, J. A. (1985). Aspirin-sensitive asthma. *Chest* **87**:386-391.
71. Habbab, M. A., Szwed, S. A., and Haft, J. I. (1986). Is coronary arterial spasm part of the aspirin-induced asthma syndrome? *Chest* **90**:141-143.
72. Pleskow, W. W., Stevenson, D. D., Mathison, D. A., Simon, R. A., Schatz, M., and Zeiger, R. S. (1982). Aspirin desensitization in aspirin-sensitive asthmatic patients: Clinical manifestations and characterization of the refractory period. *J. Allerg. Clin. Immunol.* **69**:11-19.
73. Bretza, J. A., and Novey, H. S. (1985). Anaphylactoid reactions to tolmetin after interrupted dosage. *West. J. Med.* **143**:55-59.
74. Lewis, R. V. (1987). Letter to the Editor. Severe asthma after naproxen. *Lancet* **1**:1270.
75. Ayers, J. G., Fleming, D. M., and Whittington, R. M. (1987). Letter to the Editor. Asthma death due to ibuprofen. *Lancet* **1**:1082.

76. Botha, J. J., and Weich, D. J. V. (1984). Hypersensitivity to non-steroidal anti-inflammatory drugs—asthma precipitated by zomepirac. *S. Afr. Med. J.* **65**:180-182.
77. Holness, L., Tenenbaum, J., Cooter, N. B. E., and Grossman, R. F. (1983). fatal bronchiolitis obliterans associated with chrysotherapy. *Ann. Rheum. Dis.* **42**:593-596.
78. Fort, J. G., Scovern, H., and Abruzzo, J. L. (1988). Intravenous cyclophosphamide and methylprednisolone for the treatment of bronchiolitis obliterans and interstitial fibrosis associated with crysotherapy. *J. Rheumatol.* **15**:850-854.
79. Stein, H. B., Patterson, A. C., Offer, R. C., Atkins, C. J., Teufel, A., and Robinson, H. S. (1980). Adverse effects of D-penicillamine in rheumatoid arthritis. *Ann. Intern. Med.* **92**:24-29.
80. Epler, G. R., Snider, G. L., Gaensler, E. A., et al. (1979). Bronchiolitis and bronchitis in connective tissue disease. A possible relationship to the use of penicillamine. *J.A.M.A.* **242**:528-532.
81. Murphy, K. C., Atkins, C. J., Offer, R. C., Hogg, H. C., and Stein, H. B. (1981). Obliterative bronchiolitis in two rheumatoid arthritis patients treated with penicillamine. *Arthritis Rheum.* **24**:557-560.
82. Lyle, W. H. (1977). D-penicillamine and fatal obliterative bronchiolitis. *Br. Med. J.* **1**:105.
83. Williams, T., Eidus, L., and Thomas, P. (1982). Fibrosing alveolitis, bronchiolitis obliterans, and sulfasalazine therapy. *Chest* **81**:766-768.
84. Lascari, A. D., Strano, A. J., Johnson, W. W., and Collins, J. G. P. (1977). Methotrexate-induced sudden fatal pulmonary reaction. *Cancer* **40**:1393-1397.
85. Bernstein, M. L., Sobel, D. B., and Wimmer, R. S. (1982). Noncardiogenic pulmonary edema following injection of methotrexate into the cerebrospinal fluid. *Cancer* **50**:866-868.
86. Maxwell, I. (1974). Letter to the Editor. Reversible pulmonary edema following cyclophosphamide treatment. *J.A.M.A.* **229**:137-138.
87. Walters, J. S., Woodring, J. H., Stelling, C. B., and Rosenbaum, H. D. (1983). Salicylate-induced pulmonary edema. *Radiology* **146**:289-293.
88. Heffner, J. E., and Sahn, S. A. (1981). Salicylate-induced pulmonary edema. *Ann. Intern. Med.* **95**:405-409.
89. Hormaechea, E., Carlson, R. W., Rogove, H., Uphold, J., Henning, R. J., and Weil, M. H. (1979). Hypovolemia, pulmonary edema and protein changes in severe salicylate poisoning. *Am. J. Med.* **66**:1046-1050.
90. Van den Ouweland, F. A., and Gribnau, F. W. J. (1987). Letter to the Editor. Nonsteroidal anti-inflammatory drugs as a prognostic factor in the acute pulmonary edema. *Arch. Intern. Med.* **147**:176-177.

91. Smally, A. J. (1983). Letter to the Editor. Acute pulmonary edema precipitated by NSAIDs. *J. Family Prac.* **17**:777-778.
92. Hill, R. N., Spragg, R. G., Wedel, M. K., and Moser, K. M. (1975). Letter to the Editor. Adult respiratory distress syndrome associated with colchicine intoxication. *Ann. Intern. Med.* **83**:523-524.
93. Peces, R., Riera, J. R., Arboleya, L. R., Lopez-Larrea, C., and Alvarez, J. (1987). Goodpasture's syndrome in a patient receiving penicillamine and carbimazole. *Nephron* **45**:316-320.
94. Natloff, D. S., and Kaplan, M. M. (1980). D-penicillamine-induced Goodpasture's like syndrome in primary biliary cirrhosis—successful treatment with plasmapheresis and immunosuppressives. *Gastroenterology* **78**:1046-1049.
95. Sternlieb, I., Bennett, B., and Scheinberg, I. H. (1975). D-penicillamine induced Goodpasture's syndrome in Wilson's disease. *Ann. Intern. Med.* **82**:673-676.
96. Gibson, R., Burry, H. C., and Ogg, C. (1976). Letter to the Editor. Goodpasture syndrome and D-penicillamine. *Ann. Intern. Med.* **84**:100.
97. Walden, P. A. M., Mitchell-Heggs, P. F., Copping, C., Dent, J., and Bagshawe, K. D. (1977). Pleurisy and methotrexate treatment. *Br. Med. J.* **2**:867.
98. Katzenstein, A. A., and Askin, F. B. (1982). Immunologic lung disease. In *Surgical Pathology of Non-Neoplastic Lung Disease.* W.B. Saunders, Philadelphia, pp. 108-138.
99. Costabel, U., Bross, K. J., Marxen, J., and Hatthys, H. (1984). T-lymphocytosis in bronchoalveolar lavage fluid of hypersensitivity pneumonitis. *Chest* **85**:514-518.
100. Delaval, M., Genetet, P. M., Merdriganc, G., and Coetmeur, D. (1985). Communications to the Editor. T-lymphocytosis in bronchoalveolar lavage fluid of hypersensitivity pneumonitis. *Chest* **87**:133.
101. Dankner, R. E., and Wedner, H. J. (1983). Aspirin desensitization in aspirin-sensitive asthma: Failure to maintain a desensitized state during prolonged therapy. *Am. Rev. Respir. Dis.* **128**:953-955.
102. Stevenson, D. D., Simon, R. A., and Mathison, D. A. (1984). Letter to the Editor. Aspirin desensitization in aspirin-sensitive asthma: Failure to maintain a desensitized state during prolonged therapy. *Am. Rev. Respir. Dis.* **129**:1031-1032.
103. Pesce, C., Mansi, C., Bogliolo, G., Tobia, F., and Pannacciulli, I. (1985). Pulmonary toxicity in mice after high-dose methotrexate administration with and without leucovorin rescue. *Eur. J. Cancer Clin. Oncol.* **21**:875-880.

104. Zeller, J. M., Buys, C. M., and Gudewicz, P. W. (1984). Effects of high-dose methotrexate on rat alveolar and inflammatory macrophage populations. *Inflammation* **8**:231-239.

105. Springmeyer, S. C., Kopecky, K. J., Deeg, H. J., Whitehead, J., Altman, L. C., and Storb, R. (1984). Pulmonary bronchoalveolar cell and protein kinetics in dogs given total-body irradiation, autologous marrow grafts and methotrexate. *Transplantation* **37**:335-339.

106. Furst, D. E., Zavala, D., Monick, M., Hauser, M., and Hunninghake, G. (1986). Pulmonary function testing and bronchoalveolar lavage in rheumatoid arthritis patients on low dose methotrexate. *Arthritis Rheum.* **39**:S17.

107. Cooke, N. T., and Bamji, A. N. (1983). Gold and pulmonary function in rheumatoid arthritis. *Br. J. Rheum.* **22**:18-21.

108. Mackinnon, S. K., Starkebaum, G., and Willkens, R. F. (1985). Pancytopenia associated with low dose pulse methotrexate in the treatment of rheumatoid arthritis. *Semin. Arthritis Rheum.* **15**:119-126.

109. Perruquet, J. L., Harrington, T. M., and Davis, D. E. (1983). *Pneumocystis carinii* pneumonia following methotrexate therapy for rheumatoid arthritis. *Arthritis Rheum.* **26**:1291.

110. Katzenstein, A. A., and Askin, F. B. (1982). Handling and interpretation of lung biopsies. In *Surgical Pathology of Non-Neoplastic Lung Disease.* W.B. Saunders, Philadelphia, pp. 1-8.

111. Greenman, R. L., Goodall, P. T., and King, D. (1975). Lung biopsy in immunocompromised hosts. *Am. J. Med.* **59**:488-496.

112. Groff, G. D., Shenberger, K. N., Wilke, W. S., and Taylor, T. H. (1983). Low dose oral methotrexate in rheumatoid arthritis: An uncontrolled trial and review of the literature. *Semin. Arthritis Rheum.* **12**:333-347.

113. Hoffmeister, R. T. (1983). Methotrexate therapy in rheumatoid arthritis: 15 years experience. *Am. J. Med.* **12**:S69-S73.

114. Weinstein, A., Marlow, S., Korn, J., and Farouhar, F. (1985). Low-dose methotrexate treatment of rheumatoid arthritis, long-term observations. *Am. J. Med.* **79**:331-337.

115. Wilke, W. S., Calabrese, L. H., and Segal, A. M. (1983). Incidence of untoward reactions in patients with rheumatoid arthritis treated with methotrexate. *Arthritis Rheum.* **26**:S56.

116. Pasquinucci, E., Ferrara, P., and Casterllari, R. (1971). Daunorubicin treatment in methotrexate pneumonia. *J.A.M.A.* **216**:2017.

117. Lockie, L. M., and Smith, D. M. (1985). Forty-seven years experience with gold therapy in 1,019 rheumatoid arthritis patients. *Semin. Arthritis Rheum.* **14**:238-246.

118. Lipsky, P. E., and Ziff, M. (1977). Inhibition of antigen- and mitogen-induced human lymphocyte proliferation by gold compounds. *J. Clin. Invest.* **59**:455-466.

119. Cannon, G. W., Cole, B. C., and Ward, J. R. (1986). Differential effects of in vitro gold sodium thiomalate on the stimulation of human peripheral blood mononuclear cells by *Mycoplasma arthritidis* mitogen, concanavalin A, and phytophenagglutinin. *J. Rheumatol.* **13**:52-57.

120. Louie, S., Gamble, C. N., and Cross, C. E. (1986). Penicillamine associated pulmonary hemorrhage. *J. Rheum.* **13**:963-966.

121. Jaffe, I. A. (1985). D-penicillamine. In *Textbook of Rheumatology*, Vol. 1. Edited by W. N. Kelley. W.B. Saunders, Philadelphia, pp. 809-815.

122. Taffet, S. L., and Das, K. M. (1983). Sulfasalazine. Adverse effects and desensitization. *Dig. Dis. Sci.* **28**:833-842.

123. Amos, R. S., Pullar, T., Bax, D. E., Stiunayake, D., Capell, H. A., and McConkey, B. (1986). Sulphasalazine for rheumatoid arthritis: Toxicity in 774 patients monitored for one to 11 years. *Br. Med. J.* **293**:420-423.

124. Suarez, M., and Krieger, B. P. (1986). Bronchoalveolar lavage in recurrent aspirin-induced adult respiratory distress syndrome. *Chest* **90**:452-453.

125. Leatherman, J. W., and Drage, C. W. (1982). Adult respiratory distress syndrome due to salicylate intoxication. *Minn. Med.* **65**:677-678.

126. Settipane, G. A., Chafee, F. H., and Klein, D. E. (1974). Aspirin intolerance. *J. Allergy Clin. Immunol.* **53**:200-204.

Part IV

**MULTISYSTEM DISORDERS INVOLVING
THE LUNGS AND JOINTS**

15

Cystic Fibrosis

PERRY J. RUSH

Mount Sinai Hospital
and University of Toronto
Toronto, Ontario, Canada

ABRAHAM SHORE

Hospital for Sick Children
and University of Toronto
Toronto, Ontario, Canada

I. Introduction

Cystic fibrosis (CF) is a genetic disease characterized by abnormal secretions from exocrine glands. The main clinical features include obstructive pulmonary disease and pancreatic insufficiency (1). The median age of survival has dramatically improved from 7 years in 1968 to 24 years in 1985 (2). Thus CF and its complications have become a problem seen by both pediatricians and adult internists.

A review of the world literature as of 1988 reveals 48 reported cases of arthritis occurring in patients with CF not attributable to any other known cause (3-15). The arthritis of CF is likely a distinct entity based on its epidemiology as well as its clinical and laboratory features. In the main, the arthritis of CF has been described as benign, episodic, and nondestructive. However, recent evidence suggests that CF arthritis may progress to a persistent erosive synovitis with progressive joint changes requiring long-term therapy with antiinflammatory or second-line, slow-acting antirheumatic drugs (13).

Table 1 Clinical Characteristics of CF Arthritis (48 cases)

Sex		Course of arthritis	
Male	21	Episodic	35
Female	22	Persistent	7
Not stated	5	Not stated	6
Age at onset		Pattern of arthritis	
Range	2-29	Poly	20
Mean	12	Mono	10
Age at presentation		Pauci	18
Range	2-33	Treatment	
Mean	16	ASA	6
Presenting Features		Other NSAID	9
Arthritis	48	Gold	2
Episodic	39	Chloroquine	2
Persistent	3	Prednisone	2
Not stated	6		
Rash	16		
Raynaud's	2		

Abbreviations: ASA, aspirin; NSAID, nonsteroidal antiinflammatory drug.
Source: Modified from Rush et al. (13).

II. Epidemiology

The prevalence of arthritis in CF patients under the age of 16 years is about 2% (13). This is much higher than the prevalence of juvenile rheumatoid arthritis (JRA) in the general population, which is estimated at 0.02-0.1% (16). Over the age of 16 the prevalence of CF arthritis is 2.6% (13), which is also much higher than the prevalence of adult rheumatoid arthritis (RA) from the ages of 15 to 34 (estimated at 0.4%) (17).

The 48 patients reported consist of almost equal numbers of males and females (Table 1). This is in contrast with the sex ratio found in CF patients in general. Although at birth there are equal numbers of males and females with CF, twice as many males as females survive until adulthood (18). Thus considering the usual 2:1 male:female ratio in older CF patients, there is actually a relative female preponderance in CF arthritis. The average age at the time of presentation of CF arthritis to physicians is 16. The average age of onset of joint syndrome is 12 years with a range from age 2 to 29. Females are younger at the onset of articular manifestations (mean 11 years vs. 13 years for males). Eighteen of the 32 patients who first had joint involvement under the age of 16 were females. There were slightly more males than females with symptoms beginning after the age of 16.

III. Clinical Features of Arthritis

Most patients present with recurrent, short-lived, episodic attacks of a debilitating, asymmetric, nonnodular, effusive but nonerosive synovitis. Involvement includes both large and small joints above and below the waist in a classic palindromic temporal pattern. The attacks usually last from hours to 2 weeks but may last up to several months. The frequency of attacks varies between one every several years to three each week, but they usually occur every few months. Involvement during each palindrome may be polyarticular, pauciarticular, or monoarticular.

Most patients continue to have episodic attacks with varying severity and frequency. Some patients with an episodic onset, however, eventually progress to a persistent synovitis requiring therapy with nonsteroidal antiinflammatory drugs as well as gold, hydroxychloroquine, and prednisone. Patients requiring slow-acting antirheumatic drugs have radiographic and clinical signs of permanent joint damage (e.g., juxtaarticular erosions, laxity of knee ligaments, and subluxation of metacarpophalangeal joints).

Three patients have been described who presented with no previous history of episodic attacks and instead at onset had a persistent, rheumatoid

Table 2 Clinically Involved Joints in CF Arthritis (44 patients)

Knee	30
Ankle	16
Wrist	12
Elbow	10
MTP	9
PIP	8
Shoulder	8
Hip	4
MCP	4
Sternoclav	1
MTP	1

Source: Modified from Rush et al. (13).

factor (RF)-positive polyarthritis (8,13). In two, the arthritis occurred in an asymmetric distribution, and in one the arthritis was in symmetrical pattern.

In the group as a whole, large joints (82 joints) are involved more commonly than small joints (23 joints) with some sparing of metacarpophalangeals and to a lesser extent, sparing of proximal interphalangeal joints (Table 2). There has never been a relationship found between joint symptoms and any medication, a worsening in pulmonary disease, or a change in sputum culture results.

IV. Associated Features

The most common associated feature is a rash, which has been reported in 15 patients. This has included erythema nodusum (6,7), vasculitic nodules (11), rheumatoid nodules (8), purpura (6,11), nonpainful nodules (6), and psoriasis with nail pitting (15). Other cutaneous associations noted are photosensitivity, hyperpigmentation, and Raynaud's phenomenon (13). A fever may also occur during the attacks of arthritis (14).

A. Neck and Back Pain

Both thoracic scoliosis and kyphosis are found relatively frequently in the CF population (19-22). Thoracic kyphosis has been found in up to 26% of CF patients, and thoracic scoliosis in 10% (21). It has been suggested that these deformities may relate to lung disease, but a recent study suggests that kyphosis arises from a high incidence of vertebral wedging found in patients with CF (22). Vertebral wedging may be due to osteopenia secondary to malabsorption and vitamin D deficiency (22). It is uncertain whether the spinal deformities contribute to the development of back or neck pain. However, CF patients commonly also complain of mechanical neck and back pain independently of the CF arthritis symptom complex (13). This pain may be so severe as to interfere with the performance of activities of daily living (22).

B. Laboratory Findings

A positive RF has been measured in 8 out of 38 reported patients (Table 3). No patient has had a positive antinuclear antibody (ANA). All patients reported have also had normal complement and uric acid levels and a normal urinalysis. Immunoglobulins may be normal or elevated. As with all patients

Table 3 Laboratory Features in CF Arthritis

RF (+)	8/38
ANA (+)	0/33
LE cell (+)	0/5
C3 (N)	26/27
C4 (N)	25/25
Uric acid (N)	22/22

Abbreviations: RF, rheumatoid factor; ANA, antinuclear antibody; N, normal.
Source: Modified from Rush et al. (13).

with CF, patients with CF arthritis have positive sputum cultures. Most have either *Pseudomonas aeroginosa* or *Pseudomonas cepacia* cultured from their sputum. Occasionally *Staphylococcus, Klebsiella,* or *Hemophilus* is also found. CF patients with arthritis do not have different sputum cultures from other CF patients (13).

Synovial fluid has been obtained infrequently in CF arthritis. On three occasions, fluid from the knee of one patient showed a cell count from 4,100 to 56,000 cells per cubic millimeter with 5-32% polymorphs and 66-95% mononuclear cells (13). No bacteria or crystals were found.

In contrast to CF patients with overt hypertrophic pulmonary osteoarthropathy (HPO) (see Chap. 16), CF patients with arthritis have similar pulmonary function when compared to CF patients without arthritis (13).

Most patients have completely normal radiographs (Table 4). Ten patients have had soft tissue swelling or joint effusions, and five have demonstrated periarticular osteopenia. Five patients have had evidence of cartilage destruction with joint space narrowing and/or bony erosions (13). These changes involved both large and small joints and always were in an asymmetric pattern.

A synovial biopsy has been performed in one patient and revealed a dark red synovial membrane (15). On microscopic examination, there was increased vascularity in the synovial membrane and granulomas consisting of mononuclear and giant cells surrounded by lymphocytes.

C. Differential Diagnosis

Patients with CF arthritis must be differentiated from those with JRA and adult RA. Five patients with CF arthritis have demonstrated destructive changes with cartilage loss or bony erosions indicating irreversible damage

Table 4 Radiographic Changes in CF-
Associated Arthritis

Normal	27
Effusion	10
Periarticular osteopenia	5
Joint space narrowing	4
Erosions	2
Subluxation	1
Enthesopathy	1
Not stated	4

Source: Modified from Rush et al. (13).

(13). However, these patients did not have symmetrical small joint involvement typical of RA or the growth changes of typical JRA (23). Furthermore, the arthritis of CF is unlike that of JRA in that there are no reported cases of uveitis or a positive ANA despite 23 patients with monoarticular or pauciarticular involvement. Also, unlike adult RA, in CF arthritis large joints are usually involved with sparing of metacarpophalangeal joints. Thus CF arthritis is likely a distinct clinical entity.

Patients with CF arthritis do have a 20% incidence of a positive RF. However, RF is present in increased numbers of CF patients for other reasons, such as chronic infection (24). One study found that 6% of all CF patients have a positive RF (25). Thus the incidence of RF in CF arthritis is threefold higher than in CF patients without arthritis.

The arthritis of CF must also be differentiated from the arthritis associated with HPO (see Chap. 16). Patients with HPO may present with clinical features suggesting an inflammatory arthritis (26) with pain and swelling of the knees, ankles, hands, and wrists. Radiographs may confuse the issue by demonstrating effusions and periarticular osteopenia. However, joint space narrowing and erosions do not occur in HPO. Patients with CF arthritis do not have clinical evidence of bone tenderness or radiographic evidence of periosteal elevation typical of HPO. A bone scan is the best imaging method for the detection of early HPO. Two patients with CF arthritis have demonstrated periositis, but this was not typical of HPO since it involved the small bones of the hands and feet adjacent to diseased joints, and radiographs of the long bones were normal (13).

V. Pathophysiology

The etiology of CF arthritis is unclear. Possible explanations are (a) a common hereditary defect causes both CF and arthritis, or (b) a complication of

CF or its treatment causes arthritis (Table 5). Each of these possibilities will be discussed below.

A. CF and Arthritis Are Clinical Manifestations of a Common Defect

The possibility of a genetic defect should be considered as many rheumatic diseases have associations with HLA antigens. HLA typing in CF has been reported by six different groups from 1973 to 1980. Five of these reported no differences in the frequency of HLA A, B, or C antigens in CF patients compared with normal populations (27-31). Only Kaiser et al. reported an increase in HLA B-18; however, a relatively small sample was used (32). No study has ever been a study of the incidence of HLA A, B, and C antigens in CF arthritis patients.

B. CF Arthritis Is a Complication of CF or Its Treatment

The intestinal bypass arthritis-dermatitis syndrome, following jejunal bypass for obesity, is characterized by polyarthritis, tendinitis, rash, and fever (33). The pathogenesis of this syndrome may relate to bacterial overgrowth associated with elevated immune complexes yielding the clinical manifestations (34). Could CF arthritis result from circulating immune complexes resulting from chronic lung infection or impaired bowel function? The evidence for this hypothesis is inconclusive. A vasculitis characterized by a cutaneous necrotizing venulitis, hypergammaglobulinemia, and elevated immune complexes has been described in four patients with CF (35,36). These patients did not, however, have arthritis. One case of CF arthritis reported in the literature did have vasculitic nodules (11). Patients with CF all suffer from chronic pulmonary infection (37). All reported patients with CF arthritis as expected, had positive sputum cultures. Elevated immune complexes containing *Pseudomonas* antigen have been described in CF (38). The chronic

Table 5 Possible Pathogenic Mechanisms of CF Arthritis

Genetic
Complication of CF or its treatment
Chronic Infection: Respiratory or gastrointestinal systems
Vasculitis
Pancreatitis
Diabetes Mellitus
Amyloidosis
Polycythemia
Pancreatic Enzymes
Antibiotics

Source: Modified from Rush et al. (13).

exposure to exogenous bacterial antigen and immune complexes might conceivably result in arthritis, but CF patients with arthritis have similar sputum cultures compared to those without arthritis (13).

Patients with CF may have recurrent acute pancreatitis even with normal pancreatic enzymes (39). Arthritis associated with pancreatitis usually occurs with subcutaneous fat necrosis and lytic bone lesions (40,41). Persisting chronic arthritis has been described with alcoholic pancreatitis (42). There are no cases of pancreatitis in patients with CF arthritis, and their radiographs are not characteristic of this condition (40).

Up to 40% of CF patients demonstrate glucose intolerance (43), which becomes frank diabetes mellitus (DM) in 1-2% of cases (44,45). The rheumatic manifestations of DM include diabetic osteolysis, septic arthritis, osteomyelitis, neuropathic joints, diffuse idiopathic skeletal hyperostosis, and juvenile diabetic cheiroarthropathy (46,47). It is unlikely that any of these conditions are responsible for the arthritis in CF. There is one case of DM in a patient with arthritis, but this patient's arthritis was clinically indistinguishable from that of the arthritis patients without DM (13).

Amyloidosis can cause an arthropathy mimicking RA (48,49). Twenty-five cases of CF complicated by amyloidosis have been described. None had arthritis (50). None of the cases of CF arthritis have had amyloidosis.

Hypoxia due to pulmonary disease is common in patients with CF. One study found 33% of patients with a pO_2 of less than 70 mm Hg (51). Polycythemia secondary to the chronic hypoxia could be a cause of hyperuricemia and gout (52). No reported patients had elevated hemoglobins or uric acid levels.

Another source of uric acid is the pancreatic enzymes that CF patients consume. The pancreas is rich in purines, and therapy with pancreatic extracts may cause hyperuricosuria and hyperuricemia (53-56). None of the reported patients have had hyperuricemia.

CF patients receive chronic and intensive antibiotic therapy, usually penicillins and aminoglycosides, for pulmonary infections (57). Ampicillin has been associated with an arthritis-colitis syndrome (58). Antibiotics, especially penicillin, can also be associated with a hypersensitivity vasculitis (59). A high proportion of CF patients may be asymptomatic carriers of *Clostridium difficile,* which can be associated with an arthritis (60). However, the patients reported were not on any single antibiotic, nor was there any report of a relationship between a change in antibiotic therapy and arthritis.

Perhaps the most intriguing hypothesis for the etiology of CF arthritis is that this may represent a reactive arthritis due to a combination of both the complications of CF and its treatment. Thus, the respiratory and gastrointestinal tracts in CF patients are altered by both the disease and continuous antibiotic therapy. changes in the endogenous microflora or enhanced systematic penetrance of these organisms due to this combination of factors could cause a reactive arthritis in susceptible hosts. HLA B27-normal individuals are susceptible to reactive arthritis following infection of the gastrointestinal or genitourinary tracts (61). Although there is no firm evidence for such a hypothesis in CF arthritis, two patients with CF arthritis have been reported to be HLA B27-positive (15). Two further CF arthritis patients who were not HLA typed had periostitis and enthesopathy (13) and radiographic findings similar to those found in Reiter's syndrome (62). However, there has been no family history of iritis, psoriasis, colitis, inflammatory back pain (i.e., HLA B27-related diseases), or arthritis in any reported patient.

VI. Treatment

Patients with CF arthritis often do not require any treatment, as episodic attacks may resolve in hours. More persistent disease usually responds to an nonsteroidal antiinflammatory drug. Persistent arthritis unresponsive to these drugs should be treated with the usual second-line agents such as gold and chloroquine. Particular joints may also benefit from an intraarticular injection of a long-acting corticosteroid preparation. In general, oral prednisone should be avoided because of side effects. However, we have successfully managed one patient with prednisone (0.3-0.5 mgm/kg/day) for 18 months who initially was felt to have a limited prognosis for survival because of advanced pulmonary disease. Patient education and the use of physical therapies such as exercise and orthotics should not be neglected. Appropriate referrals should also be made to a physiotherapist, occupational therapist, and social worker.

Acknowledgments

The author's investigations were supported by grants from the Canadian Arthritis Society and the Medical Research Council of Canada. Dr. Shore is an associate of the Canadian Arthritis Association.

References

1. Gurwitz, D., Corey, M., Francis, P. W. J., Crozier, D., and Levison, H. (1979). Perspectives in cystic fibrosis. *Pediatr. Clin. North. Am.* **26**:603-615.
2. Arehart-Treichel, J. (1984). Lengthened survival raises problems in cystic fibrosis. *J.A.M.A.* **252**:2526-2527.

3. Euler, A. R., and Ament, M. E. (1976). Crohn's disease—a cause of arthritis, oxalate stones and fistulae in cystic fibrosis. *West. J. Med.* **125**:315-317.

4. Schwachman, H., Kowalski, M., and Khaw, K. T. (1977). Cystic fibrosis: A new outlook. *Medicine* **56**:129-148.

5. Mathieu, J. P., Stack, B. H. R., Dick, W. C., and Buchanan, W. W. (1978). Pulmonary infection and rheumatoid arthritis. *Br. J. Dis. Chest* **72**:57-61.

6. Newmann, A. J., and Ansell, B. M. (1979). Episodic arthritis in children with cystic fibrosis. *J. Pediatr.* **94**:594-596.

7. Vaze, E. (1980). Episodic arthritis in cystic fibrosis. *J. Pediatr.* **93**:346.

8. Sagransky, D. M., Greenwald, R. A., and Gorvoy, J. D. (1980). Seropositive rheumatoid arthritis in a patient with cystic fibrosis. *Am. J. Dis. Child.* **1134**:319-320.

9. McGuire, S., Monaghan, H., and Tempany, E. (1982). Arthritis in childhood cystic fibrosis. *Ir. J. Med. Sci.* **1151**:133-234.

10. De Lumley, L., Umdenstock, R., Boulesteix, J., et al. (1983). Polyarthrite chronique au cours d'une mucoviscidose. *Arch. Fr. Pediatr.* **40**: 723-725.

11. Schidlow, D. V., Goldsmith, D. P., Palmer, J., and Huang, N. N. (1984). Arthritis in cystic fibrosis. *Arch. Dis. Child.* **59**:377-379.

12. Blau, H., Yahav, J., and Katznelson, D. (1984). Episodic arthritis in cystic fibrosis. *Prog. Rheum.* **2**:357-360.

13. Rush, P. J., Shore, A., Coblentz, C., Wilmont, D., Curey, M., and Levison, H. (1986). The musculoskeletal manifestations of cystic fibrosis. *Semin. Arthritis Rheum.* **15**:213-225.

14. Summers, G. D., and Webley, M. (1986). Episodic arthritis in cystic fibrosis: A case report. *Br. J. Rheumatol.* **25**:393-395.

15. Phillips, B. M., and David, T. J. (1986). Pathogenesis and management of arthropathy in cystic fibrosis. *J. R. Soc. Med.* **79**(Suppl. 12):44-50.

16. Gewanter, H. L., Roghmann, K. J., and Baum, J. (1983). The prevalence of juvenile arthritis. *Arthritis Rheum.* **26**:599-603, 1983.

17. Roberts, J. (1984). Information on arthritis and other musculoskeletal disorders from the interview and examination survey programs of the national center for health statistics. In *Epidemiology of the Rheumatic Diseases.* Edited by Lawrence, R. V., and L. E. Shulman. Gower Medical Publishing, New York, pp. 341-348.

18. Logvinoff, M. M., Fon, G. T., Taussig, L. M., and Pitt, M. J. (1984). Kyphosis and pulmonary function in cystic fibrosis. *Clin. Pediatr.* **23**:389-392.

19. Erkkila, J. C., Warwick, W. J., and Bradford, D. S., (1978). Spine derformities and cystic fibrosis. *Clin. Orthop.* **131**:146-150.

20. Denton, J. R., Tietjen, R., and Gaerlan, P. F. (1981). Thoracic kyphosis in cystic fibrosis. *Clin. Orthop.* **155**:71-74.
21. Paling, M. R., and Spasovsky-Chernick, M. (1982). Scoliosis in cystic fibrosis—an appraisal. *Skeletal. Radiol.* **8**:63-66.
22. Rose, J., Gamble, J., Schultz, A., and Lewiston, M. (1987). Back pain and spinal deformity in cystic fibrosis. *Am. J. Dis. Child.* **141**:1313-1316.
23. Ansell, B. M., and Kent, P. A. (1977). Radiological changes in juvenile chronic polyarthritis. *Skeletal. Radiol.* **1**:129-144.
24. Bartfield, H. (1969). The distribution of rheumatoid factor activity in non-rheumatoid states. *Ann. N.Y. Acad. Sci.* **168**:30-38.
25. Hoiby, N., and Wiik, A. (1975). Antibacterial precipitins and autoantibodies in serum of patients with cystic fibrosis. *Scand. J. Respir. Dis.* **56**: 38-46.
26. Frank, H. A., (1952). Hypertrophic pulmonary osteoarthropathy simulating rheumatoid arthritis. *N. Engl. J. Med.* **247**:283-285.
27. Goodchild, M. C., Edwards, J. H., Glenn, K. P., Grindley, C., Harris, R., Mackintosh, P., and Wentzel, J. (1976). A search for linkage in cystic fibrosis. *J. Med. Genet.* **13**:417-419.
28. Hennecquet, A., Jehanne, M., Betuel, H., Gilly, R., Schmid, M., and Hors, J. (1978). Cystic fibrosis and HLA. *Tissue Antigens* **12**:159-162.
29. Polymenidis, Z., Ludwig, H., and Gotz, M. (1973). Cystic fibrosis and HL-A antigens. *Lancet* **2**:1452.
30. Tobin, M. J., Maguire, O., Reen, D., Tempany, E., and Fitzgerald, N. X. (1980). Autopy and bronchial reactivity in older patients with cystic fibrosis. *Thorax* **35**:807-813.
31. Safwenberg, J., Kollberg, H., and Lindblom, J. (1977). HLA frequencies in patients with cystic fibrosis. *Tissue Antigens* **10**:287-290.
32. Kaiser, G. I., Laszlo, A., and Gyurkovits, K. (1977). Cystic fibrosis: An HLA associated hereditary disease? *Acad. Sci. Hung.* **18**:27-29.
33. Stein, H. B., Schlappner, O. L. A., Boyko, W., Gourlay, R. H., and Reeve, C. E. (1981). The intestinal bypass arthritis-dermatitis syndrome. *Arthritis Rheum.* **24**:684-690.
34. Wands, J. R., LaMont, J. T., Mann, E., and Isselbacher, K. J. (1976). Arthritis associated with intestinal-bypass procedure for morbid obesity. *N. Engl. J. Med.* **294**:121-124.
35. John, E. G., Medenis, R., and Rao, S. (1980). Cutaneous necrotizing venulitis in patients with cystic fibrosis. *J. Pediatr.* **97**:505.
36. Soter, N. A., Mihm, M. C., and Colten, H. R. (1979). Cutaneous necrotizing venulitis in patients with cystic fibrosis. *J. Pediatr.* **95**:197-201.
37. Wang, E. E. L., Prober, C. G., Manson, B., Corey, M., and Levison, H. (1984). Association of respiratory viral infections with pulmonary

deterioration in patients with cystic fibrosis. *N. Engl. J. Med.* **311**: 1653-1658.

38. Moss, R. B., and Lewiston, N. J. (1980). Immune complexes and humoral response to *Pseudomonas aeroginosa* in cystic fibrosis. *Am. Rev. Respir. Dis.* **121**:23-29.

39. Shwachman, H., Lebenthal, E., and Khaw, K. T. (1975). Recurrent acute pancreatitis in patients with cystic fibrosis with normal pancreatic enzymes. *Pediatrics* **55**:86-95.

40. Boswell, S. H., and Baylin, G. J. (1973). Metastatic fat necrosis and lytic bone lesions in a patient with painless acute pancreatitis. *Radiology* **106**:85-86.

41. Lucas, P. F., and Owen, T. K. (1962). Subcutaneous fat necrosis, polyarthritis and pancreatic disease. *Gut* **3**:146-148.

42. Hammond, J., and Tesar, J. (1980). Pancreatitis-associated arthritis. *J.A.M.A.* **244**:694-696.

43. Handwerger, S., Roth, J., Gorden, P., DiSant'Agnese, P., Carpenter, D. F., and Peter, G. (1969). Glucose intolerance in cystic fibrosis. *N. Engl. J. Med.* **281**:451-460.

44. Milner, A. D. (1969). Blood glucose and serum insulin levels in children with cystic fibrosis. *Arch. Dis. Child.* **44**:351-355.

45. Rosan, R. C., Shwachman, H., and Kulczycki, L. L. (1962). Diabetes mellitus and cystic fibrosis of the pancreas. *Am. J. Dis. Child.* **104**:625-634.

46. Gray, R. G., and Gottlieb, N. L. (1976). Rheumatic disorders associated with diabetes mellitus: Literature review. *Semin. Arthritis Rheum.* **6**:19-34.

47. Holt, P. J. L. (1981). Rheumatological manifestations of diabetes mellitus. *Clin. Rheum. Dis.* **7**:723-746.

48. Gordon, D. A., Pruzanski, W., Ogryzlo, M. A., and Little, H. A. (1974). Amyloid arthritis simulating rheumatoid disease in five patients with multiple myeloma. *Am. J. Med.* **55**:142-154.

49. Wiernick, P. H. (1972). Amyloid joint disease. *Medicine* **51**:465-479.

50. McGlennen, R. C., Burke, B. A., and Dehner, L. P. (1986). Systematic amyloidosis complicating cystic fibrosis. *Arch. Pathol. Lab. Med.* **110**: 879-884.

51. Di Sant'Agnese, P. A., and Davis, P. B. (1979). Cystic fibrosis in adults. *Am. J. Med.* **66**:121-132.

52. Denman, A. M., Szur, L., and Ansell, B. M. (1964). Joint complaints in polycythemia vera. *Ann. Rheum. Dis.* **23**:139-144.

53. Davidson, G. P., Hassel, F. M., Crozier, D., Corey, M., and Forstner, G. G. (1978). Iatrogenic hyperuricemia in children with cystic fibrosis. *J. Pediatr.* **93**:976-978.

54. Nousia-Arvanitakis, S., Stapleton, F. B., Linshaw, M. A., and Kennedy, J. (1977). Therapeutic approach to pancreatic extract-induced hyperuricosuria in cystic fibrosis. *J. Pediatr.* **90**:302-305.
55. Sack, J., Blau, H., Goldfarb, D., Ben-Zaray, S., and Katznelson, D. (1980). Hyperuricosuria in cystic fibrosis patients treated with pancreatic enzyme supplements. *Isr. J. Med. Sci.* **16**:417-419.
56. Stapleton, F. B., Kennedy, J., Nousia-Arvanitakis, S., and Linshaw, M. (1976). Hyperuricosuria due to high-dose pancreatic extract therapy in cystic fibrosis. *N. Engl. J. Med.* **295**:246-248.
57. Marks, M. I. (1981). The pathogenesis and treatment of pulmonary infections in patients with cystic fibrosis. *J. Pediatr.* **98**:172-179.
58. Rothschild, B. M., Masi, A. T., and June, P. L. (1977). Arthritis associated with ampicillin colitis. *Arch. Intern. Med.* **137**:1605-1607.
59. Winkelmann, R. K., and Ditto, W. B. (1963). Cutaneous and visceral syndromes of necrotizing or allergic angiitis. *Medicine* **43**:59-89.
60. Peach, S. L., Borriello, S. P., Gaya, H., Barclay, F. E., and Welch, A. R. (1986). *Clostridium difficile* and cystic fibrosis. *J. Clin. Pathol.* **39**:1013-1018.
61. Brewerton, D. A., Caffrey, M., Nicholls, A., Walter, D., Oates, J. K., and James, D. C. O. (1973). Reiter's disease and HL-A27. *Lancet* **2**:996-998.
62. Sholkoff, S. D., Glickman, M. G., and Steinback, H. L. (1970). Roentgenology of Reiter's syndrome. *Radiology* **97**:497-503.

16

Hypertrophic Pulmonary Osteoarthropathy System Complex

PERRY J. RUSH

Mount Sinai Hospital
and University of Toronto
Toronto, Ontario, Canada

ABRAHAM SHORE

Hospital for Sick Children
and University of Toronto
Toronto, Ontario, Canada

These symptoms attend chronic empyemata . . . the nails of the hands are bent, the fingers are hot especially their extremities.

—Hippocrates

I. Introduction

The peculiar and unique fingernail deformity called clubbing has intrigued physicians since the time of Hippocrates. Clubbing is typically associated with periostitis and arthritis giving rise to the hypertrophic pulmonary osteoarthropathy (HPO) symptom complex. Some authors have dropped the term "pulmonary" because HPO has also been described in association with many extrathoracic conditions. However, since the most commonly suggested pathophysiology of HPO relates to the lung, "pulmonary" should probably remain. Primary forms of HPO and clubbing have been described in several families without any underlying condition. The primary HPO syndromes will not be discussed. Readers are referred to other reviews (1).

Some authors separate simple clubbing from full-blown HPO (2). We feel that clubbing is the earliest feature of HPO and is a definite part of the

415

symptom complex. In our experience all patients with clubbing will develop HPO if followed long enough and if the underlying condition is not removed. Both arthritis and periostitis may be mild or asymptomatic and may be easily missed. In keeping with this concept, pathological studies of synovium, periosteum, and soft tissues of distal phalanges show similar changes.

II. Epidemiology

HPO may be found in association with a wide variety of conditions (Table 1). Historically, HPO was found most commonly in association with chronic lung infections (3-6). Today, with the availability of antibiotic treatment, most cases are found in association with pulmonary malignancy. The type of lung cancer may be primary or secondary (7,8). If primary, the histology

Table 1 HPO-Associated Conditions

Thoracic
  Lung
    carcinoma
      primary
        squamous-cell carcinoma (8)
        adenocarcinoma (8)
        undifferentiated carcinoma (8)
      Hodgkin's disease (66)
      secondary metastases (7)
    pulmonary fibrosis (74)
    bronchiectasis (3)
    tuberculosis (4)
    blastomycosis (5)
    aspergillosis (6)
    abscess (3)
    cyst (3)
    cystic fibrosis (30)
  Pleura
    mesothelioma (3)
    empyema (6)
  Heart/great vessels
    endocarditis (75)
    cyanotic congenital heart disease
    tetralogy of Fallot (9)

transposition of great vessels (9)
patent ductus arteriosus (9)
other (9)
  Mediastinum
    reticulosus (10)
    nasopharyngeal carcinoma (11)
Extrathoracic
  Gastrointestinal
    inflammatory bowel disease
      ulcerative colitis (17)
      Crohn's disease (17)
    esophagitis (18)
    esophageal adenocarcinoma (18)
  Hepatobiliary
    primary biliary cirrhosis (19)
    alcohol cirrhosis (20)
    other causes of cirrhosis (19)
    biliary atresia (21)
    bile duct stricture (20)
    chronic active hepatitis (19)
    liver transplant rejection (22)
    liver carcinoma (23)
    bile duct carcinoma (20)

Table 1 continues

Table 1 Continued

Vascular	Miscellaneous
abdominal aortic prosthesis (13)	laxative abuse (24)
arterial aneurysm (14)	lupus erythematosus (25)
arterial bypass graft (15)	polyarteritis (26)
arteriovenous fistula (16)	pregnancy (27)
Other cancers	Zollinger-Ellison syndrome (28)
adenocarcinoma of uterus (45)	Idiopathic/hereditary (1)
breast cancer (32)	

may be squamous cell carcinoma, adenocarcinoma, or undifferentiated. Oat cell carcinoma is conspicuously absent (8). Other intrathoracic pathologies associated with HPO include diseases of the heart, great vessels, pleura, and mediastinum (3,6,9-11). Congenital cyanotic heart diseases are also now seen less commonly perhaps because of refined surgical techniques (9). In children, HPO is today most commonly caused by osteogenic sarcoma with pulmonary metastases (12). Chronic obstructive pulmonary disease is not associated with HPO. Gastrointestinal, hepatobiliary, or vascular diseases may also be associated with the HPO complex (13-23). There are other rare associations and also cases of HPO without any obvious underlying disorder (1,24-28). However, these single and, in many instances, quite old case reports must be interpreted with caution. These causes are recorded in Table 1 only for the sake of completeness and to facilitate further study.

There are few recent studies looking at HPO in detail. One can only assume that better and earlier treatment of infection, malignancy, and heart disease has lessened the incidence of HPO. The highest incidence of HPO has been said to be in association with pleural mesothelioma with 57% (3). In contrast, only 4-10% of patients with primary lung cancer develop HPO (3,8).

The sex and age of patients presenting with HPO are determined by the underlying diagnosis. For example, in a study of HPO and lung cancer, there were 70% males with a mean age of 56 years (29). In a study of HPO associated with cystic fibrosis (CF), there were 80% males with a mean age of 23 (30). This is in keeping with the longer survival of males with CF, who would thus form the bulk of the older CF patients in any clinic (31).

III. Clinical Features

The early recognition of HPO is of great clinical importance. HPO can be the first sign of an underlying malignancy which may more likely respond to treatment if discovered early. The classical triad of arthritis, clubbing, and periostitis may not be initially present. Both clubbing and periostitis may occur singly in isolation early on in the disease (32). In CF and other diseases, clubbing and periostitis may occur together but without arthritis (30,33). HPO may be confined to the lower or upper extremities, as seen with a patent ductus arteriosus (34) or abdominal aortic prosthesis (13). It may even only involve one extremity (15). Signs and symptoms of HPO are similar irrespective of the underlying diagnosis.

Patients with CF and musculoskeletal symptoms may have either CF arthritis (see previous chapter) or HPO. Differentiation between these two conditions is usually not difficult. CF patients with HPO never have persistent synovitis or any radiographic evidence of joint damage. The development of HPO in CF patients is associated with a worsening of pulmonary function. The FEV_1 of CF patients with HPO has been found to be significantly lower than in patients with CF arthritis alone or CF patients without joint symptoms (30). The development of HPO in these patients tends to precede episodes of pulmonary deterioration and may dramatically improve or resolve following treatment with intravenous antibiotics and intensified pulmonary toilet. Indeed, CF patients with HPO have a poor prognosis, and 6 of the 11 patients we originally described are now dead 2 years later from end-stage pulmonary disease (30).

A. Arthritis

Typically, the arthritis of HPO involves large, distal joints such as the knees and ankles. Less commonly, the small joints of the hands, wrists, and the elbows are affected. The distribution is usually bilateral and symmetrical. The articular symptoms are usually expressed in acute attacks, which can be quite severe. With progression of disease, these attacks become persistent, leading to chronic articular disease. Patients complain of joint pain, and there may be morning stiffness. On examination, there are the typical signs of inflammation including joint tenderness on palpation, warmth, and joint swelling, which may be due to joint fluid or synovial thickening.

B. Clubbing

Clubbing may involve the fingers and/or the toes and can be unilateral (14) or bilateral. In a patient with a systemic disease, clubbing has been said to be first seen in the thumb and index finger and then in the other digits (35). Other investigators suggest that all digits are affected simultaneously (36). In general, the abnormality starts at the base of the nail with an enlargement of the cuticle followed by a loss of the nail angle, nail bed softening, an increase in the curvature of the nail, and finally hyperextension of the distal interphalangeal joint (35). The normal base angle of the nail is about 160°. With the development of early clubbing, this angle is first obliterated (when it reaches 180°). With disease progression, the angle becomes greater than 180° and thus projects above the planar surface of the digit (35). There is also a painless increase in the volume of the distal phalanx caused by soft tissue swelling resulting in a bulbous finger end often described as a "drumstick" (35).

A useful bedside physical sign is the Schamroth sign, named for a physician who described clubbing in himself while suffering from endocarditis (36). This sign is a loss of the diamond-shaped space at the base of the nails when the affected digits are viewed opposing each other in silhouette (Fig. 1). Attempts at an objective measurement of clubbing include the use of finger casts and calculating a ratio of the width of the index finger at the base of the nail divided by the width at the distal interphalangeal joint (37-39). A shadowgraph to perform another measurement, that of the nail angle, has also been used (40,41). A brass plate has been used to measure the nail curvature (42).

C. Periostitis

Patients with periostitis may complain of diffuse bone pain, or, more typically, there may be difficulty in squatting or kneeling, especially with a twisting motion. On examination, tenderness on palpation can be found along the shafts of long bones, especially at the distal ends. Edema, which can be pitting or nonpitting, may be present. A thickening and widening of the bones may be appreciated clinically. Rotation of the knees, ankles, or wrists by the examiner may be particularly painful.

D. Associated Features

Associated features found with HPO include evidence of autonomic neuropathy with postural hypotension, impotence, bowel dysfunction (43), sweating—especially of the palms and soles (12,44)—and flushing. Dermatological manifestations include cutaneous vasculitis (11), alopecia (12), skin induration, hyperpigmentation (45), and thick skin with deep creases (44). Cyanosis is commonly seen in association with congenital heart disease. Endocrine abnormalities are suggested by the findings of spider naevi (45), gynecomastia (46), and mastalgia in women (46). An associated fever has also been described (12).

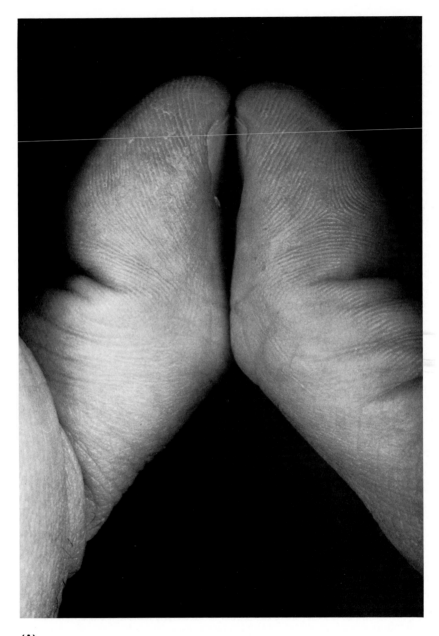

(A)

Figure 1   (A) Normal thumbs showing characteristic diamond-shaped space at the base of the nails. (B) Clubbing of the thumbs in a 16-year-old patient with cystic fibrosis showing loss of the diamond-shaped space.

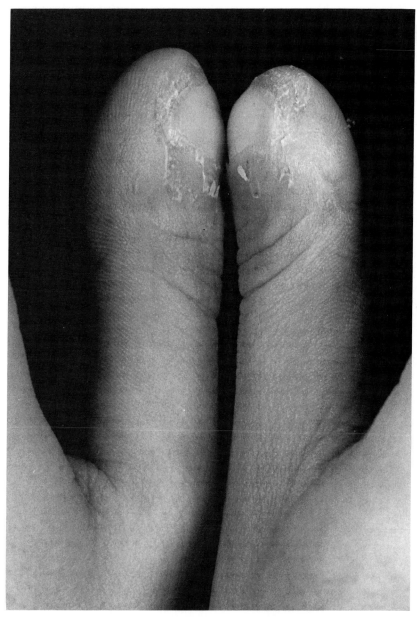

(B)

IV. Laboratory

A. Serology

The ESR is usually elevated and can reach very high levels, even over 100 mm/h Westergren (47). This probably reflects the underlying disease. Serology including rheumatoid factor and antinuclear antibodies are negative (29,47).

B. Joint Fluid Analysis

Joint aspiration in HPO arthritis reveals a noninflammatory (type 1) fluid with a clear yellow or slightly cloudy turbidity, normal viscosity, good mucin clot, few leukocytes which are mainly mononuclear, and no crystals or tumor cells (12,13,22,47-49). As both gout (50) and carcinomatous synovial metastasis (51) may occur in a patient with HPO, a search for crystals and tumor cells in the synovial fluid should not be neglected. Spontaneous clotting of the joint fluid has been reported, a finding of unknown significance (47).

C. Radiology

Plain radiographs of clubbed hands and feet have been said to be usually normal. However, recent evidence suggests that upon detailed radiographic examination, abnormalities are relatively common. In one study, up to 87% of patients with congenital heart disease and clubbing had abnormalities in their hands, and 42% had abnormal radiographs of the feet (52). These abnormalities included both new bone formation and acroosteolysis of the distal phalanges.

In areas of periostitis there may be soft tissue swelling around the affected bones. However, the main feature of periostitis is a proliferation of the periosteum along long bones, especially the femur, tibia, fibula, and phalanges (12). Less commonly, the clavicles, sternum, metatarsals, ribs, scapula, and pelvis may be involved (12,53). The periostitis appears as a line of radiodense new bone that is separated from the cortex by a translucent line (Fig. 2). Patients with long-standing HPO have thicker and more widespread periostitis. Thus patients with chronic diseases such as cystic fibrosis have worse periostitis than those with a disease of short duration such as cancer. This suggests that the degree of bony change depends more on the duration than the nature of the underlying disease (54).

In children, the periosteum is loosely attached, allowing the formation of more new bone than in adults. With resolution of the periostitis, the new bone fuses with the shaft, and the radiolucent line disappears. The cortex remains thickened, leaving a clue to the presence of previous disease. Bone scans may be positive before plain radiographs and reveal a characteristic

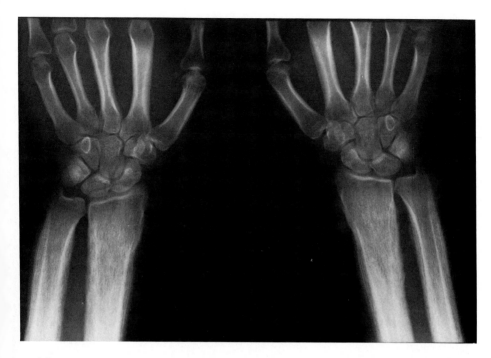

(a)

Figure 2   (a) PA radiograph of the wrists in a 21-year-old patient with cystic fibrosis, who died 1 year after this X-ray from pulmonary disease. Periosteal new bone formation is seen at the distal radius and ulna and the radial aspect of the first metacarpal. (b) AP radiograph of the same patient as in (a). There is ragged, stratified, periostitis extending from the diaphysis to the epiphysis of the tibiae and fibulae.

linear increase in activity parallel to the affected bones. The scan may also demonstrate the associated arthritis and clubbing and can be used for follow-up after treatment of the underlying disease (53).

   Radiographic evaluation of the joints reveals only soft tissue swelling. There are no reports of erosions or cartilage space loss in HPO. Juxtaarticular osteopenia may be seen (55).

D. Pathology

Pathological examination of synovium, periosteum, and phalanges is similar, suggesting a common pathophysiology for the three. The synovium shows increased capillaries with vascular congestion and minimal lympho-

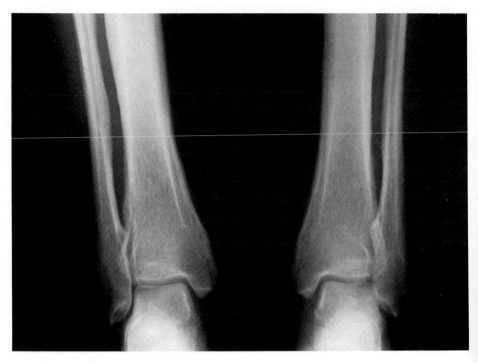

(B)

cytic infiltration. The synovial lining is an average of three cells thick, as in a normal joint (47). There is little other evidence of inflammation (44). This is as opposed to active rheumatoid arthritis, where the synovium may be hundreds of cells thick with inflammatory cell infiltrates.

Examination of clubbed digits shows only soft tissue changes. Histologically, the increased volume of the distal fingers is caused by swollen collagen bundles, widened interfascicular spaces, and mononuclear cell infiltrates composed of lymphocytes and plasma cells (56). There is also thickening of nearby arterioles with luminal narrowing.

The periosteum of involved long bones is thickened and edematous (32). New bone can be seen to be deposited along the inner surface of the periosteum separated from the cortical bone by a space. Histologically, there is again a mononuclear cell infiltrate (32).

V. Pathophysiology

The cause of HPO has never been satsifactorily explained (Table 2). Any theory would have to explain why only some patients with any of the varied

Table 2 Pathogenesis of HPO

Toxic
Genetic
Immunological
Neurogenic reflex
Endocrine

underlying conditions develop HPO. How can HPO occur only in the upper or lower limbs and even involve only one limb (14)? It is likely that, like all rheumatic diseases, the answer is multifactorial, with several pathogenic mechanisms operating, resulting in similar clinical features. There are also likely both systemic and local factors modulating clinical expression of the symptom complex.

The most commonly accepted hypothesis (57,58) theorizes the presence in the blood of a toxic substance, so far unidentified, that is normally inactivated by the lungs. Because of lung disease, or by bypassing the lungs altogether, as in congenital heart disease, this substance is able to enter the systemic circulation and exert its effects on the bones, joints, and soft tissues. In CF, HPO dramatically improves or resolves in patients treated for deterioration in their lung disease by intravenous antibiotics and intensified pulmonary toilet (30). HPO in congenital heart disease also resolves with shunt closure. Suggestions for the substance have included ferritin and prostaglandins. However, efforts to document arteriovenous differences in blood levels of these substances have been disappointing (9,59,60). However, an increase in digital capillary blood flow can be measured with radioactive isotopes (61). Other postulated mechanisms possibly contributing to HPO will be discussed below.

A. Genetic

The major histocompatibility complex has been associated with numerous diseases. However, no HLA typing has been performed in HPO. This could be important as, almost certainly, there is a hereditary component in primary HPO.

B. Neurogenic

An abnormality in a neurocirculatory reflex mechanisms of the autonomic nervous system has been postulated. Affected areas in HPO are usually supplied by the 9th and 10th (vagus) cranial nerves, suggesting that these nerves comprise the afferent portion of a reflex arc. Transection of the vagus nerve (18) or the use of anticholinergic drugs may alleviate some of the symptoms of HPO. Also, HPO has been associated with autonomic neuropathy (43). The efferent part of the arc causing the changes seen in the bones and joints, however, has never been explained.

C. Immunologic

An immunologic pathogenesis has also been considered. HPO may be found with vasculitis (11). However, immune complexes and all autoantibodies tested have been negative. Complement and immunoglobulin levels have been normal (12,47,49). Electron-dense deposits suggestive of immune complexes have been seen in pathological studies of HPO, but these deposits are negative for immunoglobulins and complement (47).

D. Hormonal

The possibility that an ectopically produced hormonal factor is the cause of HPO has been suggested. HPO patients may have an associated gynecomastia (46) and may have acromegaliclike facies. Increased levels of estrogen and growth hormone have been seen in patients with HPO and cancer (45,62). The elevated hormonal level returned to normal following tumor removal (45) and resolution of HPO symptoms. However, this likely represents an epiphenomenon.

The few case reports of clubbing associated with pregnancy and its resolution with parturition also suggest a hormonal origin (27,63). This theory has recently been revived with the description of a patient with a pancreatic tumor and the Zollinger-Ellison syndrome. The clubbing and Zollinger-Ellison syndrome resolved with tumor removal (28).

E. Crystals

The possibility that HPO is a form of gout is an old theory (64). This has not been borne out, but it should be noted that gout and HPO may coexist in the same patient (50).

VI. Course, Prognosis, and Management

Treatment or reversal of the underlying disease may result in resolution of arthritis and disappearance of clubbing and periostitis as the new bone becomes incorporated into the cortex (48). Surgical correction of congenital heart disease (65), chemotherapy for Hodgkin's disease (66), resection or radiotherapy of lung cancer (43,67), antibiotics for subacute bacterial endo-

Table 3 Treatments Used for HPO

Treat underlying disease
  medical
  surgical

Treat symptoms
  medical
    aspirin
    other NSAIDs
    steroids
      oral
      intraarticular
    anticholinergics
      atropine
      propantheline
    antiadrenergics
      propranolol
      phenoxybenzamine
  surgical
    vagotomy

carditis (33), and liver transplantation for liver cirrhosis (48) have been reported to be associated with clinical resolution of HPO. Improvement may occur in hours to days or not before months (9,65). Soft tissue changes resolve before bone changes. Patients with severe bone pain are often relieved immediately postoperatively (44). Even palliative treatment with chemotherapy, radiation or surgery of otherwise incurable lung cancer may still cause relief of intractable symptoms of HPO (67-69).

Many diverse treatment modalities have been attempted, including prednisone (13), ASA (12,47), other nonsteroidal antiinflammatory medications (47), intraarticular steroid injection, anticholinergics (propantheline bromide) (70-72), propranolol plus phenoxybenzamine (73), and subcutaneous atropine (71) (Table 3). All of these have had their proponents with varying degrees of success.

Acknowledgments

The authors' investigations were supported by grants from the Canadian Arthritis Society and the Medical Research Council of Canada. Dr. Shore is an associate of the Canadian Arthritis Association.

References

1. Diren, H. B., Kutluk, M. T., Karabent, A., Gocmen, A., Adalioglu, G., and Kenanoglu, A. (1986). Primary hypertrophic osteoarthropathy. *Pediatr. Radiol.* **16**:231-234.
2. Holling, H. E., and Brodey, R. S. (1961). Pulmonary hypertrophic osteoarthropathy. *J.A.M.A.* **178**:977.
3. Wierman, W. H., Clagett, O. T., and McDonald, J. R. (1954). Articular manifestations in pulmonary diseases. *J.A.M.A.* **155**:1459.
4. Macfarlane, J. T., Ibrahim, M., and Tor-Agbidye, S. (1979). The importance of finger clubbing in pulmonary tuberculosis. *Tubercle* **60**:45-48.
5. Yacoub, H., Simon, G., and Ohnsorge, J. (1967). Hypertrophic pulmonary osteoarthropathy in association with pulmonary metastases from extrathoracic tumours. *Thorax* **22**:226-231.
6. Magdi, H., Yacoub, H., and Simon, G. (1966). Hypertrophic pulmonary osteoarthropathy and intrathoracic inflammatory conditions. *Br. J. Dis. Chest* **60**:81-86.
7. Firooznia, N., Seliger, G., Genieser, N. B., and Barasch, E. (1975). Hypertrophic pulmonary osteoarthropathy in pulmonary metastases. *Radiology* **115**:269-274.
8. Yacoub, M. H. (1965). Relation between the histology of bronchial carcinoma and hypertrophic pulmonary osteoarthropathy. *Thorax* **20**:537.
9. Martinez-Lavin, M., Bobadilla, M., Casanova, J., Attie, F., and Martinez, M. (1982). Hypertrophic osteoarthropathy in cyanotic congenital heart disease. *Arthritis Rheum.* **25**:1186-1193.
10. Molyneux, M. E. (1973). Mediastinal reticulosis with hypertrophic pulmonary osteoarthropathy. *Br. J. Dis. Chest* **67**:66-69.
11. Miyachi, H., Akizuki, M., Yamagata, H., Minori, T., Yoshida, S., and Homme, M. (1987). Hypertrophic osteoarthropathy, cutaneous vasculitis, and mixed-typed croglobulinemia in a patient with nasopharyngeal carcinoma. *Arthritis Rheum.* **30**:825-829.
12. Petty, R. E., Cassidy, J. T., Heyn, R., Kenien, A. G., and Washburn, R. L. (1976). Secondary hypertrophic osteoarthropathy. *Arthritis Rheum.* **19**:902-906.
13. Stein, H. B., and Little, H. A. (1978). Localized hypertrophic osteoarthropathy in the presence of an abdominal aortic prosthesis. *Can. Med. Assoc. J.* **118**:947-948.
14. Gold, A. H., Bromberg, B. E., Herbstritt, J. G., and Stein, H. (1979). Digital clubbing: A unique case and a new hypothesis. *J. Hand Surg.* **4**:60-66.
15. Ho, A., Williams, D. M., and Zelenock, G. B. (1987). Unilateral hypertrophic osteoarthropathy in a patient with an infected axillary-axillary bypass graft. *Radiology* **162**:573-574.

16. Leb, D. E., and Sharma, J. K. (1978). Clubbing secondary to an arteriovenous fistula for hemodialysis. *J.A.M.A.* **240**:142.
17. McAllister, C., McNulty, J. G., and Fielding, J. F. (1986). Is hypertrophic osteoarthropathy really so rare in regional enteritis? *J. Clin. Gastroenterol.* **8**:562-568.
18. Flavell, G. (1956). Reversal of pulmonary hypertrophic osteoarthropathy by vagotomy. *Lancet* **1**:260-262.
19. Epstein, O., Dick, R., and Sherlock, S. (1981). Prospective study of periostitis and finger clubbing in primary biliary cirrhosis and other forms of chronic liver disease. *Gut* **22**:203-206.
20. Epstein, O., Ajdukiewicz, A., Dick, R., and Sherlock, S. (1979). Hypertrophic hepatic osteoarthropathy. *Am. J. Med.* **67**:88-97.
21. Rothberg, A. D., and Boal, D. K. (1983). Hypertrophic osteoarthropathy in biliary atresia. *Pediatr. Radiol.* **13**:44-66.
22. Wolfe, S. M., Aelion, J. A., and Gupta, R. C. (1987). Hypertrophic osteoarthropathy associated with a rejected liver transplant. *J. Rheumatol.* **14**:147-151.
23. Morgan, A. G., and Walker, W. C. (1972). A new syndrome associated with hepatocellular carcinoma. *Gastroenterology* **63**:340-344.
24. Pines, A., Olchovsky, D., Gregman, J., Kaplinski, N., and Frankl, O. (1983). Finger clubbing associated with laxative abuse. *South. Med. J.* **76**:1071-1072.
25. Mackie, R. M. (1973). Lupus erythematosus in association with finger-clubbing. *Br. J. Dermatol.* **89**:533.
26. Lovell, R. R. H., and Scott, G. B. D. (1956). Hypertrophic osteoarthropathy in polyarteritis. *Ann. Rheum. Dis.* **15**:46.
27. Cullen, D. R., and Maskery, P. J. K. (1966). Clubbing of the fingers and hypertrophic osteoarthropathy in pregnancy. *Lancet* **2**:473.
28. Taube, M., and Wastell, C. (1986). Finger clubbing in the Zollinger-Ellison syndrome. *Br. Med. J.* **293**:1346-1347.
29. Segal, A. M., and Mackenzie, A. H. (1982). Hypertrophic osteoarthropathy: A 10-year retrospective analysis. *Semin. Arthritis Rheum.* **12**:220-232.
30. Rush, P. J., Shore, A., Coblentz, C., Wilmot, D., Corey, M., and Levison, H. (1986). The musculoskeletal manifestations of cystic fibrosis. *Semin. Arthritis Rheum.* **15**:213-225.
31. Gurwitz, D., Corey, M., Francis, P. W. J., Crozier, D., and Levison, H. (1979). Perspectives in cystic fibrosis. *Pediatr. Clin. North Am.* **26**:603-615.
32. Shapiro, J. S. (1987). Breast cancer presenting as periostitis. *Postgrad. Med.* **82**:139-140.
33. Shapiro, L. M., and Mackinnon, J. (1980). The resolution of hypertrophic pulmonary osteoarthropathy following the treatment of subacute infective endocarditis. *Postgrad. Med. J.* **56**:513-515.

34. Williams, B., Ling, J., Leight, L., and McGaff, C. J. (1963). Patent ductus arteriosus and osteoarthropathy. *Arch. Intern. Med.* **111**:346-350.
35. Lovibond, J. L., and Camp, M. D. (1938). Diagnosis of clubbed fingers. *Lancet* **1**:363-364.
36. Schamroth, L. (1976). Personal experience. *S. Afr. Med. J.* **50**:297-300.
37. Waring, W. W., Wilkinson, R. W., Wiebe, R. A., Fawl, B. C., and Hilman, B. C. (1971). Quantification of digital clubbing in children. *Am. Rev. Respir. Dis.* **104**:166-174.
38. Sly, R. M., Buranakul, B., Gupta, S., and Waring, W. (1973). Objective assessment for digital clubbing in Caucasian, Negro and Oriental subjects. *Chest* **64**:687-689.
39. Sly, R. M., Fuqua, G., Matta, E. G., and Waring, W. (1972). Objective assessment of minimal digital clubbing in asthmatic children. *Ann. Allergy* **30**:575-578.
40. Bentley, D., Moore, A., and Shwachman, H. (1976). Finger clubbing: A quantitative survey by analysis of the shadowgraph. *Lancet* **2**:164-167.
41. Bentley, D., and Cline, J. (1970). Estimation of clubbing by analysis of shadowgraph. *Br. Med. J.* **3**:43.
42. Staven, P. (1959). Instrument for estimation of clubbing. *Lancet* **2**:7-8.
43. Vasudevan, C. P., Suppiah, P., Udoshi, M. B., and Lusins, J. (1981). Reversible autonomic neuropathy and hypertrophic osteoarthropathy in a patient with bronchogenic carcinoma. *Chest* **79**:479-481.
44. Case records of the Massachusetts General Hospital (1978). *N. Engl. J. Med.* **299**:708-714.
45. Brear, S. G., Edwards, J. D., Rademaker, M., and Doyle, L. (1985). Hypertrophic osteoarthropathy, spider naevi and estrogen hypersecretion association with adenocarcinoma. *Postgrad. Med. J.* **61**:827-828.
46. Braude, S., Kennedy, H., Hodson, M., and Batten, J. (1984). Hypertrophic osteoarthropathy in cystic fibrosis. *Br. Med. J.* **288**:822-823.
47. Schumacher, H. R. (1976). Articular manifestations of hypertrophic pulmonary osteoarthropathy in bronchogenic carcinoma. A clinical and pathologic study. *Arthritis Rheum.* **19**:629-636.
48. Huaux, J. P., Geubel, A., Maldague, B., Michielsen, P., Hemptinne, B. de, Otte, J. B., and Nagant de Deuxchaisnes, C. (1987). Hypertrophic osteoarthropathy related to end stage cholestatic cirrhosis: Reversal after liver transplantation. *Ann. Rheum. Dis.* **46**:342-345.
49. Owerbuch, M. S., and Brookss, P. M. (1981). Role of immune complexes in hypertrophic osteoarthropathy and nonmetastatic polyarthritis. *Ann. Rheum. Dis.* **40**:470-472.

50. Martinez-Lavin, M., Amigo, M. C., Castillejos, G., Padilla, L., and Vintimilla, F. (1984). Coexistence of gout and hypertrophic osteoarthropathy in patients with cyanotic heart disease. *J. Rheumatol.* **11**:832-834.
51. Fam, A. G., and Cross, E. G. (1979). Hypertrophic osteoarthropathy, phalangeal and synovial metastases associated with bronchogenic carcinoma. *J. Rheum.* **6**:680-686.
52. Pineda, C. J., Guerra, J. Jr., Weisman, M. H., Resnick, D., and Martinez-Lavin, M. (1985). The skeletal manifestations of clubbing: A study in patients with cyanotic congenital heart disease and hypertrophic osteoarthropathy. *Semin. Arthritis Rheum.* **14**:263-273.
53. Rosenthall, L., and Kirsch, J. (1976). Observations on radionuclide imaging in hypertrophic pulmonary osteoarthropathy. *Radiology* **120**: 359-362.
54. Pineda, C. J., Martinez-Lavin, M., Goobar, J. E., et al. (1987). Periostitis in hypertrophic osteoarthropathy: Relationship to disease duration. *A.J.R.* **148**:773-778.
55. Matthay, M. A., Matthay, R. A., Mills, D. M., Latshminarayan, S., and Cotton, E. (1976). Hypertrophic osteoarthropathy in adults with cystic fibrosis. *Thorax* **31**:572-575.
56. Gall, E. A., Bennett, G. A., and Bauer, W. (1951). Generalized hypertrophic osteoarthropathy. A pathologic study of seven cases. *Am. J. Pathol.* **27**:349-373.
57. Martinez-Lavin, M. (1987). Digital clubbing and hypertrophic osteoarthropathy: A unifying hypothesis. *J. Rheum.* **14**:6-8.
58. Thorburn, W., and Westmacott, F. H. (1986). The pathology of pulmonary osteo-arthropathy. *Trans. Pathol. Soc. Lond.* **47**:177-190.
59. Shneerson, J. M., and Jones, B. M. (1981). Ferritin, finger clubbing and lung disease. *Thorax* **36**:688-692.
60. Martinez-Lavin, M., and Castillejos, G. (1986). Ferritin and prostaglandins in hypertrophic osteoarthropathy. *J. Rheum.* **13**:834-836.
61. Racoceanu, S. N., Mendlowitz, M., Suck, A. F., Wolf, R. L., and Natlchi, N. E. (1971). Digital capillary blood flow in clubbing. [85]Kr studies in hereditary and acquired cases. *Ann. Intern. Med.* **75**:933-935.
62. Steiner, H., Dahlback, O., and Waldenstron, J. (1968). Ectopic growth-hormone production and osteoarthropathy in carcinoma of the bronchus. *Lancet* **1**:783-785.
63. Borden, E. C., and Holling, H. E. (1969). Hypertrophic osteoarthropathy and pregnancy. *Ann. Intern. Med.* **71**:577.
64. Thornburn, W., and Westmacott, F. H. (1896). The pathology of hypertrophic pulmonary osteo-arthropathy. *Trans. Path. Soc. Lond.* **47**: 177-190.

65. Shaffer, H. A., and Heckman, J. D. (1973). Hypertrophic osteoarthropathy associated with cyanotic congenital heart disease. *J. Can. Assoc. Radiol.* **24**:265-267.
66. Atkinson, M. K., McElwain, T. J., Peckman, M. J., and Thomas, P. R. M. (1976). Hypertrophic pulmonary osteoarthropathy in hodgkin's disease. *Cancer* **38**:1729-1734.
67. Steinfeld, A. D., and Munzenrider, J. E. (1974). The response of hypertrophic pulmonary osteoarthropathy to radiotherapy. *Radiology* **113**: 709-711.
68. Evans, W. K. (1980). Reversal of hypertrophic osteoarthropathy after chemotherapy for bronchogenic carcinoma. *J. Rheumatol.* **7**:93-97.
69. Lester, W. M., and Robertson, D. I. (1981). Hypertrophic osteoarthropathy complicating metastatic ovarian adenocarcinoma. *Can. J. Surg.* **24**:520-523.
70. Schwartz, H. A. (1981). Pro-banthine for hypertrophic osteoarthropathy. *Arthritis Rheum.* **24**:1588.
71. Lopez-Enriquez, E., Morales, A. R., and Robert, F. (1980). Effect of atropine sulfate in pulmonary hypertrophic osteoarthropathy. *Arthritis Rheum.* **23**:822-824.
72. Deal, C. J., and Canoso, J. J. (1983). Minimal response to propantheline bromide therapy in hypertrophic pulmonary osteoarthropathy: A double-blind controlled case study. *J. Rheum.* **10**:165-167.
73. Reardon, G., Collins, A. J., and Bacon, P. A. (1976). The effect of adrenergic blockade in hypertrophic pulmonary osteoarthropathy. *Postgrad. Med. J.* **52**:170-173.
74. Schechter, S., and Bole, G. (1976). Hypertrophic osteoarthropathy and rheumatoid arthritis. *Arthritis Rheum.* **19**:639-644.
75. Churchill, M. A., Garaci, J. E., and Hunder, G. G. (1977). Musculoskeletal manifestations of bacterial endocarditis. *Ann. Rheum. Dis.* **87**: 754-759.

17

Sarcoidosis

OM P. SHARMA

University of Southern California
Los Angeles, California

TAKATERU IZUMI

Chest Research Institute
Kyoto University
Kyoto, Japan

More than a century ago, Jonathan Hutchinson, a surgeon-dermatologist, described the first case of sarcoidosis at King's College Hospital in London. Although for the better part of this century the disease has remained confined to the domain of the chest physician, its multisystem nature is now being widely recognized (1,2). Clinicians of different disciplines, radiologists, pathologists, immunologists, biochemists, and geneticists face the problem of sarcoidosis. The clinical and radiologic features of the disease are relatively clear-cut, but the diagnosis is often delayed or completely missed because of its resemblance to tuberculosis, berylliosis, hypersensitivity pneumonitis, fungal infections, and collagen vascular diseases. The diagnostic difficulties are particularly common in those patients with sarcoidosis who suffer from extrapulmonary involvement. The following description combines the pathogenesis, clinical features, pulmonary and articular relationships, biochemical changes, and immunological features of the disease and provides an outline for the diagnosis and the management of the patient suffering from sarcoidosis.

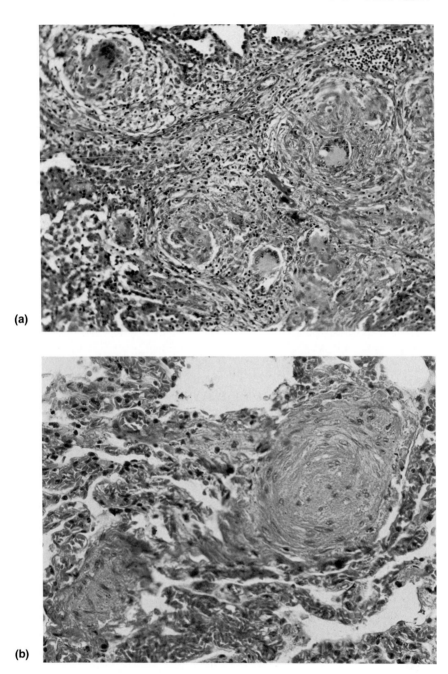

(a)

(b)

Figure 1 (a) Noncaseating granuloma of sarcoidosis (HE, ×75). (b) A hylanized sarcoid granuloma (HE, ×75).

I. Sarcoid Granuloma

The lesion of sarcoidosis is a well-defined round or oval granuloma made up of compact, radially arranged epithelioid cells with pale nuclei (Fig. 1). The typical giant cell of the sarcoid granuloma is of the Langhans' type in which the nuclei are arranged in an arc or a circular pattern around a central granular zone. Lymphocytes are usually seen at the periphery. Caseation is absent; fibrinoid necrosis may occasionally be seen in areas where several granulomas have coalesced.

Monoclonal antibody techniques and indirect immunofluorescence methods have uncovered the dynamic relationship between the various components of the granuloma and the putative causative agent (3). The center of the granuloma is composed of macrophage-derived cells and OKT4 helper lymphocytes, whereas the periphery of the granuloma has a large number of antigen-presenting interdigitating macrophages and OKT8 suppressor lymphocytes (Fig. 2). The lymphokines from the inflammatory cells recruit blood-borne monocytes, prevent macrophage migration, and keep the chronic inflammatory reaction alive and efficient. It is probable that this arrangement

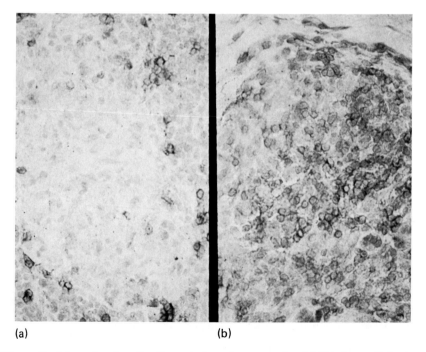

(a)   (b)

Figure 2 Monoclonal antibodies technique demonstrating (a) T-helper cells in the center of the granuloma and (b) T-suppressor cells forming a peripheral rim.

of interdigitating OKT8 cells on the periphery and the epithelioid cell-OKT4 pattern in the center provides an efficient perimeter defense to a persistent, poorly degradable "antigen" of low potency. This architectural arrangement is also found in cases of tuberculoid leprosy in which an efficient immune system keeps the bacillary load to a minimum; in lepromatous leprosy, on the other hand, the arrangement of the immune cells is disorganized and haphazard, and bacteria abound (3).

II. Natural History of a Sarcoid Granuloma

If a granuloma does not resolve spontaneously or after adequate therapy, it becomes converted into avascular, almost acellular, connective tissue. Granulomas that persist longer than a year or two show peripheral hyalinization and fibrosis resulting in tissue scarring.

The mechanisms regulating the development of fibrosis are not well understood (see Chap. 1). The alveolar macrophage, however, appears to play an important role by producing a number of active mediators, including a macrophage-derived fibroblast growth factor that activates fibroblasts, fibronectin, interleukin 1, and biologically active factor VII. The role of lymphocyte products such as interleukin 2 and gamma-interferon is unclear. Prostaglandins (PGE_2) appear to modulate fibroblast growth. Neutrophils may be involved in the pathogenesis of fibrosis. The cells are recruited from blood by a macrophage-derived factor. These lung neutrophils may participate in the development of fibrosis either by producing superoxide anion or by influencing the local concentration of immune complexes (4,5).

III. The Multisystem Nature of Sarcoidosis

Because of its diverse manifestations, sarcoidosis presents to clinicians of many different specialities. Clinical manifestations depend on the race, duration of the illness, site and extent of tissue involvement, and activity of the granulomatous process.

A. Nonspecific Constitutional Manifestations

About a third of patients with sarcoidosis complain of such nonspecific symptoms as fever, fatigue, and weight loss. Fever is generally mild, but temperature elevations to 103 or 104 °F are not unheard of. Weight loss is generally limited to 5-15 lb during the 10-12 weeks prior to presentation. Occasionally, night sweats occur. The constitutional symptoms occur more frequently in blacks and Asians from the Indian subcontinent than in Caucasians.

B. Lungs

Asymptomatic Pulmonary Sarcoidosis

At the Sarcoidosis Clinic at Los Angeles County Hospital in California, about 20% of the patients with sarcoidosis were detected by routine chest radiography. Most of these patients were asymptomatic; a few complained of vague retrosternal discomfort on careful questioning.

Respiratory Symptoms

Over a third of patients with sarcoidosis complain of dyspnea, cough, chest pain, and tightness of the chest. The cough is usually dry. Chest pain is generally confined to the retrosternal area. Occasionally it may be severe and indistinguishable from cardiac pain. In one patient the pain became intensified after drinking alcohol.

Chest Radiographic Abnormalities

We prefer the following radiographic staging system:

Stage 0   Normal chest roentgenogram

Stage I   Bilateral hilar lymphadenopathy without pulmonary infiltrates

Stage II   Bilateral hilar lymphadenopathy with pulmonary infiltrates

Stage III   Pulmonary infiltrates without hilar adenopathy

Stave IV   End-stage fibrosis, bullea, and honeycombing

Lung Function Abnormalities

Extensive physiological studies in the past emphasized functional changes characteristic of "restrictive impairment" in patients with sarcoidiosis. Vital capacity, residual volume, and total lung capacity are reduced. The loss of diffusing capacity remains perhaps the most common abnormality in sarcoidosis. The diffusing capacity is reduced even in patients with hilar adenopathy without any associated parenchymal infiltrates on chest X-ray film (stage I). Severe abnormalities of gas exchange are also more frequent than is generally realized (6). The obstruction of airways—large and small—is quite common, particularly in American black patients (7). The abnormality may result from any one, or any combination, of the following three factors: endobronchial granulomas and bronchiolitis; fibrosis and disruption of the supporting structure around the airways; and release of chemical mediators, complement products, and anaphylotoxins from activated alveolar macrophages. The presence of airways obstruction may indicate persistent and extensive disease.

C. Musculoskeletal System

The articular involvement in sarcoidosis became established through the studies of Burman and Mayer, Gendel et al., Myers et al., Sokoloff and Bunim, Spilberg et al., Grigor and Hughes, James et al., and Arnold (8-15).

The incidence of joint involvement ranges from 25% to 39% in various series. Onset of articular symptoms has occurred as early as 4 months and as late as 59 years of age. The joint disease was an initial manifestation of sarcoidosis in 74 (90%) of 83 patients in one study (16). The joint involvement may precede other manifestations of sarcoidosis by many years. In one of the 10 patients described by Patterson et al., acute arthritis preceded the established diagnosis by 16 years (17).

The joints most commonly affected by sarcoidosis are the knees, ankles, elbows, wrists, and small joints of hand. The affected joints are usually swollen, warm, tender, and painful; effusions are common, particularly in patients with chronic disease. Sarcoid arthritis may be indistinguishable from that observed in rheumatic fever, rheumatoid disease, and juvenile rheumatoid arthritis. The articular involvement in sarcoidosis may be divided into the following clinical types:

Transient, Migrating Arthralgias

There is no evidence of arthritis. The symptoms may sometimes be associated with erythema nodosum. This type of nonspecific articular reaction is also observed in other systemic diseases including primary tuberculosis and fungal or viral infections.

Migrating Polyarthritis with Fever, Erythema Nodosum, and Bilateral Hilar Adenopathy

This type of articular involvement commonly affects the small and medium-size joints including the ankles, knees, elbows, wrists, and hands (Fig. 3). Clinical manifestations include extreme pain and tenderness of the joints, especially the proximal ends of the long bones and phalanges. The joint pain is sometimes out of proportion to the degree of swelling and other objective evidence of arthritis. Uveitis is often present, particularly in children. The acute joint involvement probably reflects a circulating immune complex reaction. The erythrocyte sedimentation rate is usually elevated. Radiographic examination of the joint may reveal soft tissue swelling and periarticular osteoporosis; bones are normal. A synovial biopsy specimen may show noncaseating granulomas. It is a self-limiting lesion which resolves spontaneously within 1-2 months, leaving no sequelae; recurrence is rare. Clinical and radiological recovery is the rule.

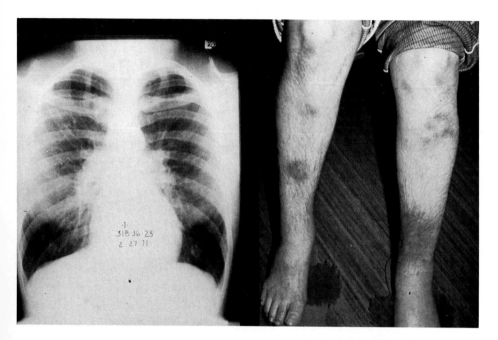

Figure 3 Acute sarcoidosis in a young woman showing bilateral hilar adenopathy, erythema nodosum, and swelling of both ankles. The disease at this stage is self-limiting and requires no specific treatment.

Acute Relapsing Mono- or Polyarticular Arthritis

The picture is similar to the one seen in type 2, but with multiple episodes. Joint deformity is likely to occur. Relapsing monoarticular arthritis of the great toe, simulating gout, has been reported. Acute monoarticular involvement of temporomandibular joint and vertebrae has been described (18).

Chronic Persistent Polyarthritis (Rarely Monoarthritis)

This type of joint involvement with recurrent acute exacerbations usually occurs in patients with advanced pulmonary fibrosis and lupus pernio. The shoulders, knees, wrists, ankles, and small joints of the hands and feet are the frequently involved articulations. Joint deformities are common; occasionally, destruction of the affected joint may occur. Eight of 28 patients studied by Spilberg et al. experienced recurrences ranging from three to seven in number, and in four patients the articular lesions became chronic (12). Synovial thickening and effusions were present in all. None of the patients with persistent arthritis had erythema nodosum, which is a feature of acute

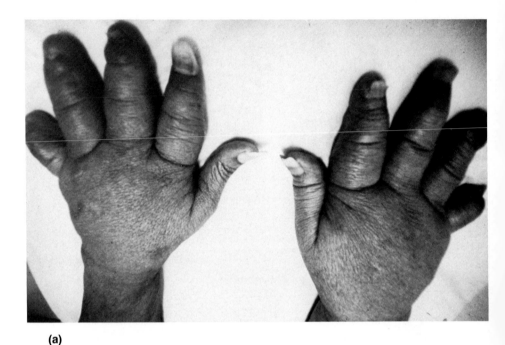

(a)

Figure 4   (a) Chronic polyarthritis of the small joints of hands in a patient with sarcoidosis of 30 years' duration. (b) Her chest X-ray showed diffuse fibrosis (stage III).

benign sarcoidosis. The process of persistent polyarthritis may result in permanent disability (Fig. 4).

Radiographic features include soft tissue swelling, periarticular osteoporosis, joint space narrowing, bone lesions, and, occasionally, articular destruction (Fig. 5). Synovial biopsy specimens may reveal noncaseating granuloma and cellular infiltrates consisting of leukocytes, plasma cells, and fibroblasts. Synovial fluid analysis often shows elevated total protein and lymphocytosis.

Miscellaneous Joint Involvements

Occasionally, osseous ankylosis of the sacroiliac joint and paravertebral ossifications may occur (1,2,9).

Sarcoid Arthritis in Children

The clinical syndrome of sarcoid arthropathy in children deserves special mention. At the time of onset the child is usually younger than 4 years. A

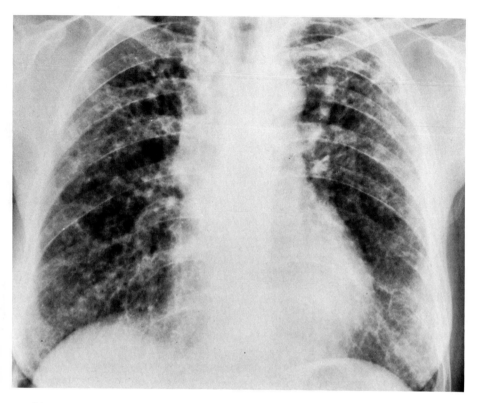

(b)

characteristic erythematous macular rash is usually present. It may be wide-spread but is more prominent on flexor surfaces. The joint involvement, in-itially pauciarticular, gradually evolves into a polyarticular pattern. Exam-ination of the joints shows edema, tenderness, and limitation of movements. The lung and mediastinum are not involved. Eye lesions occur in 80% of children with sarcoid arthropathy (19,20). Sarcoid arthritis in the older chil-dren may be associated with uveitis. The disease may mimic juvenile rheu-matoid arthritis, but the clinical features and course of uveitis may help to clinich the correct diagnosis (Table 1).

Differential Diagnosis of Sarcoid Arthritis

Sarcoidosis should be included in the differential diagnosis in a patient with arthritis. The diagnosis can be established on the basis of a typical chest roent-genographic finding and by demonstrating noncaseating granulomas in a

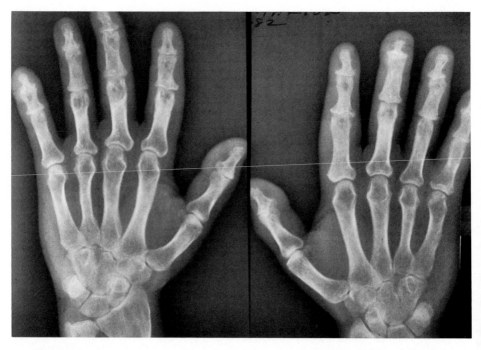

Figure 5 Mild soft tissue swelling of the small joints of hands in a 38-year-old Russian man. X-ray films of the hands show extensive bone lesions.

Table 1 Ocular Manifestations of Sarcoidosis and Juvenile Rheumatoid Arthritis: A Comparison

Lesion	Sarcoidosis	Juvenile Rheumatoid Arthritis
Conjunctiva		
Redness	May be present	May be present
Nodules	Present	Absent
Nodule biopsy	Noncaseating granuloma	Absent
Cornea		
Keratitic precipitate	Present	Present
Distribution	Near limbus	Diffuse
Band keratopathy	Rare	Rare
Iris		
Nodules	Present	Absent
Adhesions	Focal	Diffuse

synovial membrane, lymph node, skin, or lung biopsy sample. The serum angiotensin-converting enzyme (ACE) activity may be high. It is helpful to measure this variable in the diagnosis of patients with seronegative polyarthritis. At times, the distinction between "gouty" arthritis and monoarticular sarcoidosis may be difficult. This is particularly so if the patient also has elevated uric acid levels, for hyperuricemia occurs in about 20% of the sarcoidosis patients (21). In acute stages sarcoidosis may be confused with rheumatic fever or rheumatoid arthritis. However, the characteristic pulmonary lesions, normal ASO titers, negative serological tests, and demonstration of noncaseating granulomatous by organ biopsy confirm the diagnosis of sarcoidosis. Tuberculosis—typical and atypical—can produce a destructive arthritis. The isolation of appropriate organism from culture and the presence of draining skin lesions indicate myobacterioses or fungal infections rather than sarcoidosis. *Yersinia enterocolitica* infection may cause granulomatous arthritis (22).

D. Skin

Skin lesions occur in about a quarter of patients with sarcoidosis (1,2).

1. Lupus pernio, the most characteristic of all sarcoid skin lesions, is a chronic violaceious indurated skin lesion with a predilection for the nose, ears, lips, and face. It occurs commonly in women with persistent sarcoidosis with extensive pulmonary infiltration and fibrosis, chronic uveitis, and bone lesions. The nose lesion is often associated with granulomatous infiltration of the nasal mucosa. Occasionally, the bony nasal septum may be destroyed. A bulbous or sausage-shaped finger in a patient with lupus pernio indicates the presence of an underlying bone and joint lesion. Occasionally, the nails may become dystrophic and brittle (Fig. 6).

2. Skin plaques, like lupus pernio, are purplish, elevated, indurated patches commonly located on the limbs, face, back, and buttocks. The distribution is usually symmetrical. The center of the plaque is pale and atrophic; the periphery indurated, elevated, and dark.

3. Maculopapular eruptions are the most common skin manifestation of sarcoidosis in black patients. The waxy translucent lesions with a distinct flat top vary from 2 mm to 6 mm in diameter, They characteristically occur on the face, on the lids, around the orbits, in the nasolabial folds, and on the nape and upper back.

4. Subcutaneous nodules, also called Darier-Roussy sarcoidosis, are painless and arise deep in the dermis and subcutaneous tissue.

5. Scars from atrophy, trauma, surgery, or venipuncture may become purple, swollen, and tender either at the time the patient presents or during reactivation of the disease. Biopsy of these areas shows noncaseating granulomas.

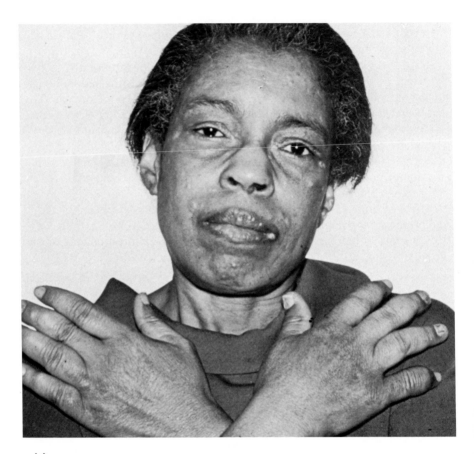

(a)

Figure 6 (a) The same patient as in Figure 5 has features of chronic sarcoidosis: chronic skin lesions and joint and bone lesions are associated with dystrophic and brittle nails. (b) A chest X-ray film shows extensive fibrosis and bullae formation (stage IV).

6. Erythema nodosum is the most common nonspecific cutaneous manifestation of sarcoidosis and is the hallmark of acute sarcoidosis. Systemic manifestations such as fever, malaise, and polyarthralgia occur in about 50% of patients with erythema nodosum.

E. Eyes

Any structure of the eye may be involved in sarcoidosis, but granulomatous uveitis is the most common eye lesion. Uveitis may be acute, subacute, or chronic (23,24).

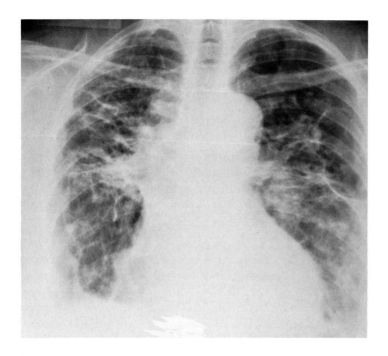

(b)

Acute uveitis presents suddenly with redness of eyes, watering, cloudy vision, and photophobia. Circumcorneal ciliary congestion is present, pupils are irregular, and "mutton fat" keratotic precipitates (KPs) may be prominent in the anterior chamber. The patient may have other manifestations of early sarcoidosis including erythema nodosum and bilateral hilar lymphadenopathy and arthralgias.

Chronic uveitis, on the other hand, develops slowly and may lead to adhesions between the iris and the lens, glaucoma, cataracts, and blindness. Ciliary congestion is absent, but KPs are present. The patient complains of pain and blurred vision. Other manifestations of chronic sarcoidosis, including lupus pernio, plaques, bone and joint lesions, and interstitial pulmonary fibrosis may be present.

Other ocular lesions include conjunctival follicles, periphlebitis retine, retinal hemorrhages, retinitis proliferans, cataracts, band keratopathy, proptosis, and exophthalmos (25).

F. Peripheral Lymph Nodes

The most frequently involved nodes are cervical, axillary, epitrochlear, and inguinal. In the neck, the posterior triangle nodes are more commonly affected than those in the anterior triangle. Enlarged nodes are discrete, shotty, mobile, painless, and free from the surrounding structures.

G. Spleen

Although the spleen is infiltrated by sarcoid granulomas in more than 50% of patients, the incidence of a clinically palpable spleen is only about 15%. Splenic enlargement is usually silent, but, as the disease progresses, pressure symptoms, anemia, leukopenia, and thrombocytopenia are likely to occur (26).

H. Gastrointestinal Tract

The esophagus is least frequently involved by sarcoidosis. Asymptomatic granulomas occur in the gastric mucosa in 10% of patients with or without hematemesis may occur (27,28).

Intestinal involvement is rare, and there are only a few documented cases. Dines et al. reported two patients with sarcoidosis and regional ileitis (29). It should be emphasized, however, that the distinction between sarcoidosis confined to the intestinal tract and Crohn's or Whipple's disease may be difficult. Joints may be involved in all three conditions.

Maher et al. found four case of pancreatic sarcoidosis in the literature and added one more with histologic evidence of noncaseating granulomas in the pancreas (30). Unexplained abdominal pain in a patient with sarcoidosis may be due to pancreatic involvement (31).

The liver is palpable in about 20% of patients with sarcoidosis, and granulomas are found in 63-87%, depending on the stage and activity of the disease. Mild elevation of alkaline phosphatase and serum bilirubin is common and may occur in as many as 80% of patients. Portal hypertension is rare (32).

I. Heart

Clinically recognizable involvement of the heart occurs in about 5% of the patients with sarcoidosis; however, at autopsy granulomas are found in as many as 27%. Myocardial involvement may present clinically in many ways including conduction disturbances, disturbances of rhythm, sudden death, congestive heart failure, valvular involvement, pericardial disease, and myocardial infarction. Endomyocardial biopsy is of limited value because of the patchy distribution of the disease (1,2).

J. Kidneys

Renal involvement in sarcoidosis may result from one or more of the following mechanisms: hypercalcemia/hypercalciuria, granulomatous infiltration of the renal parenchyma, glomerular disease, or renal arteritis secondary to granulomas. The incidence of renal granulomas in sarcoid patients varies from 4% to 40% (1).

K. Salivary Glands

Although the parotid gland is palpable in only about 6% of patients, subclinical involvement is more common and may be detected by technetium-99m scan and by measuring salivary volume and amylase. Granulomas in minor salivary glands occur in as many as 50% of patients with mediastinal sarcoidosis but seldom occur without hilar adenopathy or other evidence of multisystem involvement (2).

L. Upper Respiratory Tract

Nasal involvement is an indicator of chronic disease, and finding nasal granulomas even in the early stage of the disease constitutes an indication for corticosteroid therapy. Intralesional corticosteroid injections may be beneficial for polypoidal growths.

Laryngeal involvement occurs in about 5% of sarcoidosis patients. The granulomatous lesions most commonly affect the epiglottis, aryepiglottic folds, arytenoids, and false cords. Ulceration is rare. A large exophytic lesion may produce severe airway obstruction (1,2).

M. Endocrine Glands

The pituitary and hypothalamus are the most commonly affected endocrine glands in sarcoidosis. An elevated prolactin level may be a sensitive marker of hypothalamic sarcoidosis. Thyroid, parathyroid, and adrenal glands are rarely involved by sarcoidosis.

IV. Laboratory Investigations

The true incidence of anemia (hemoglobin of less than 11 g) in sarcoidosis is about 5%. Hemolytic anemia is rare. Although corticosteroid therapy is useful in some cases, spontaneous correction of hemolytic anemia may occur.

Leukopenia is a frequent finding. It may occur in the absence of splenomegaly and reflect bone marrow involvement. Leukemoid reactions and polycythemia are rare. The mean incidence of eosinophilia is about 24%. In many patients thrombocytopenia is associated with an enlarged spleen, but there is some evidence that it may be an expression of a generalized immune reaction. The erythrocyte sedimentation rate is high in about two thirds of patients, but this finding does not carry any diagnostic or prognostic significance.

Hypercalcemia may occur in any stage of sarcoidosis. The available evidence indicates that it is due to increased intestinal calcium absorption. In sarcoidosis, endogenous overproduction of 1,25-(OH) 2-D3 by activated pulmonary macrophages seems to be the cause of increased intestinal absorption of calcium. Corticosteroids bring down the raised calcium level to normal by inhibiting the peripheral action of 1,25-(OH) 2-D3 and by metabolizing the compound to an inactive metabolite (33).

Angiotensin converting enzyme catalyzes the conversion of angiotensin I to vasoactive angiotensin II and inactivates bradykinin. In normal individuals, ACE is primarily located in endothelial cells of the pulmonary capillaries and epithelial cells of the proximal renal tubules.

In sarcoidosis, the serum ACE level is raised to about 60% of patients. The ACE activity is higher in patients with hilar adenopathy and pulmonary infiltration (stage II) than in those with either hilar adenopathy alone (stage I) or pulmonary infiltrate/fibrosis (stage III/IV). The test is positive in patients with extrathoracic sarcoidosis. ACE reflects the granuloma load in the body because it is derived from the epithelioid cells of the granulomas.

The diagnostic value of ACE is limited because the test has a false-negative incidence of 40% and a false-positive incidence of 10%. This test is most useful in monitoring the clinical course of the disease. A raised ACE level occasionally antedates the clinical, radiographic, and physiologic alterations of sarcoidosis (34,35).

V. Immunology

A. Cutaneous Anergy

Depression of cutaneous delay-type hypersensitivity reaction has long been established as a cardinal immunologic feature of sarcoidosis. Approximately two thirds of patients with the disease do not respond to the tuberculin test in any of the conventional strengths between 1 and 250 TU. This cutaneous anergy, however, does not correlate with acitivity of the disease, and the immunologic defect persists in most patients despite clinical and radiographic recovery (36).

B. Lymphopenia and Helper/Suppressor T Lymphocyte Ratio

Cutaneous anergy in sarcoidosis seems to be due to unavailability of immune effector lymphocytes. Lymphopenia is a prominent feature of the disease. Monoclonal antibody techniques have enabled us to assess the helper-to-suppressor cell ratio of human T lymphocytes. In normal subjects this ratio in the peripheral blood is 1.8:1. The ratio is somewhat lower in low-activity sarcoidosis (1.4:1) and significantly lower in high-intensity alveolitis (0.8:1). The relatively high number of suppressor cells in the peripheral blood may partly explain the cutaneous and in vitro anergy found in sarcoidosis (37).

The helper-to-suppressor cell ratio is significantly higher (10.5:1) at the site of tissue granulomas. The cells bearing the suppressor-cytoxic antigen are located in a mantle surrounding the granuloma, while the helper-inducer cells are distributed throughout the granuloma among the aggregated epitheloid cells (3,36).

C. Humoral Response and Immune Complexes

Circulating antibody production is exaggerated in sarcoidosis. Hypergammaglobulinemia occurs in perhaps half of the patients and more frequent among blacks. Circulating immune complexes are present in about half the patients with acute sarcoidosis, particularly those with erythema nodosum. In chronic disease, immune complexes are less frequent. Direct immunofluorescence techniques have demonstrated the complexes in cutaneous granulomas. It has been suggested that they alter the distribution and function of the helper and suppressor cells and macrophages (4,37).

D. Kveim Test

Although the Kveim test is generally specific for sarcoidosis, there are many drawbacks that prevent it from being widely used: The potent validated antigen is not widely available; it requires 4-6 weeks for the Kveim nodule to mature; there is variability of interpretation of the granulomatous reaction; it is necessary to withhold corticosteroid therapy until the completion of the test (38).

VI. Bronchoalveolar Lavage

Bronchoalveolar lavage (BAL) is performed by placing a fiberoptic bronchoscope into a distal airway and instilling 100-150 m of saline in 20-ml aliquots. In normal nonsmokers, the effector population of the alveolar cells consists of 93% ± 3% alveolar macrophages, 7% ± 3% lymphocytes, and less than 1% polymorphonuclear leukocytes. In normal smokers, the number of polymorphs increases from 2% to 8%. In patients with active sarcoidosis there is a significant increase in the number of T lymphocytes. T lymphocytes in BAL fluid are also increased in such conditions as hypersensitivity pneumonitis, pulmonary lymphoma, and miliary tuberculosis (39,40).

The expansion of T lymphocytes in the BAL in active sarcoidosis consists of T helper cells. There is also an increase in other T-cell subtypes, including the T37 cell, the Ty cell, and the Tu cell. The concentration of immunoglobulin G (IgG) is also elevated in sarcoidosis. The clinical application of these observations is not yet established (4).

VII. Diagnosis

The criteria for establishing the diagnosis of sarcoidosis include (1) a compatible clinical or radiologic picture or both; (2) histologic evidence of noncaseating granulomata; and (3) negative special stains and cultures for other entities (e.g., acid-fast bacilli or fungi on sputum or tissue biopsy specimens). A diagnosis based on only one of these features is misleading, since clinical or radiographic manifestations present too wide a differential diagnosis, and histologic evidence of noncaseating granuloma may be produced by many bacterial, viral, fungal, and chemical agents (1,36).

VIII. Biopsy Procedures

A. Lung Biopsy

The transbronchial biopsy through a fiberoptic bronchoscope is the procedure of choice for obtaining tissue diagnosis in pulmonary sarcoidosis. A diagnostic yield of about 85% can be secured with four transbronchial specimens. In experienced hands, the procedure is safe, simple, and inexpensive. Mediastinoscopy and thoracotomy are only occasionally required (41).

B. Extrapulmonary Sites

Before the advent of fiberoptic bronchoscopy, lymph node biopsies (scalene, mediastinal, peripheral) were frequently performed. In the acute stage of sarcoidosis, fruitful sources of tissue biopsy include liver, skeletal muscle, and lacrimal gland. Later, in the subacute stage, biopsy of the nasal mucosa, a minor salivary gland, the conjunctiva, or spleen may provide a reliable source of epithelioid granuloma. Choice skin lesions are a good source of granuloma in some patients with advanced multisystem sarcoidosis (42).

IX. Treatment

A. Indications

In a disease like sarcoidosis, with a variable clinical course and a high spontaneous remission rate, evaluation of any therapeutic regimen is difficult.

Although corticosteroids are generally considered to be beneficial in its treatment, there is no single opinion regarding the indications for such treatment, the maximum effective dose, the duration, and the effect of therapy on the course of the granulomatous process.

Why is there such a difference of opinion? Partly because a large number of patients with sarcoidosis either undergo natural remission or follow a benign course, making controlled clinical studies impossible. Confusion has been created by the unreliability of the clinical, radiologic, and physiologic data in predicting the activity, extent, and course of the granulomatous process. Indications for the use of corticosteroids are discussed below (43-45).

B. Pulmonary Sarcoidosis

Since a major aim of the therapy is to prevent fibrosis, it is important to establish the activity and reversibility of the granulomatous process. It seems that serum ACE does not accurately reflect activity of the disease as assessed by the BAL lymphocyte count. There is a rough correlation between gallium scanning and serum ACE activity but not between gallium lung scans and BAL lymphocyte count. Much has yet to be learned about the day-to-day usefulness of these tests in assessing the activity of sarcoidosis (45).

In the meantime, some combination of these tests, along with the clinical picture, lung function changes, chest radiograph, and a dash of common sense should be used to assess the activity and extent of pulmonary involvement. Remember, not every patient needs all of the tests. Just choose one, two, or any combination appropriate to a given clinical situation. The following points should be remembered:

1. Patients with bilateral hilar adenopathy (stage I) without symptoms or extrapulmonary involvement should be left untreated, and their status should be followed radiographically.

2. Patients with bilateral hilar adenopathy and pulmonary infiltration (stage II) and symptoms (dyspnea, cough, chest pain, exercise intolerance) should be treated with corticosteroids. Serum ACE, chest radiographs, and spirometry with diffusing capacity measurement should be used to monitor the course of the disease.

3. Patients with stage II disease who are asymptomatic should be further evaluated by gallium-67 and BAL lymphocyte activity studies. If tests show very high intensity disease, the patient should be given corticosteroids. If the sarcoidosis is of low activity, then no treatment is needed, and the patient's course should be followed radiographically and clinically at reasonable intervals.

4. In stage III disease, the patients should undergo gallium-67 and BAL lymphocyte studies. The treatment is almost always needed if the disease is active.

5.   In stage IV disease (fibrosis, bullae formation, and honeycombing), the assessment of disease activity would be of great value. However, fibrosis is usually so advanced that any therapy would be ineffective. These patients have severe dyspnea. The corticosteroid therapy may provide symptomatic relief but does not influence the natural history of the disease.

C. Extrapulmonary Sarcoidosis

Indications for the treatment of ocular involvement are not controversial. In acute iridocyclitis or uveitis, the response to corticosteroid therapy is favorable. At this early stage, the treatment usually prevents further damage to the eye. Topical corticosteroids (prednisone acetate 1%) in the form of eye drops and ointments are effective for anterior uveitis. If there is no improvement within 2 weeks, or if there is evidence of posterior uveitis, papilledema, or enlarged lacrimal glands, the use of systemic corticosteroids is strongly indicated (24,47).

The arthritis associated with sarcoidosis responds to nonsteroidal anti-inflammatory drugs (NSAID), corticosteroids, colchicine, antimalarial agents, and allopurinol. Because the disease may resolve spontaneously with time, these reports are difficult to interpret. No controlled trials have been reported in this area. The goal of therapy should be to provide symptomatic relief. If the symptoms are not successfully controlled with NSAIDs, a short course of low-dose prednisone (7.5-15 mg/day) should be considered. Most patients will respond. Refractory cases with chronic arthritis may warrant trials with col-suppressive therapy.

In hypercalcemia and hypercalciuria, corticosteroids prevent urinary excretion and resultant nephrocalcinosis by blocking absorption from the gut and suppressing calcitriol production by activated sarcoid macrophages (48,49).

Heart block or cardiac arrhythmia is an indication for corticosteroid therapy. An artificial pacemaker should be considered in the management of complete heart block (50,51).

Neurologic lesions such as diabetes insipidus, epilepsy, papilledema, and peripheral neuritis respond well to corticosteroids (52,53).

Corticosteroids are effective in patients with hypersplenism. Progressive liver disease is also an indication for corticosteroid therapy; however, portacaval surgery should be considered in patients with portal hypertension and uncontrollable bleeding from esophageal varices (25,54).

Symptomatic involvement of other organs such as chest pain or cough due to enlarged hilar or mediastinal nodes, dry eye due to lacrimal gland involvement, and dry mouth due to parotid enlargement respond to corticosteroid therapy, as does sarcoidosis of the upper respiratory tract (55).

Oral or local corticosteroids may cause regression of ugly skin rash, lupus pernio, plaques, and other chronic skin lesions. Methotrexate is an effective therapy for lupus pernio. In selected cases cosmetic surgery is helpful (56-58).

D. Therapeutic Methods

Corticosteroids

Prednisone in daily single doses of 20-40 mg for a period of 8-12 weeks, gradually reducing the dosage to a maintenance level of about 5-10 mg/day, is an effective regimen for most of the indications given above. Alternate-day therapy can be effective, with considerable reduction of side effects (59).

Acute uveitis, myocardial involvement, papilledema, severe hypercalcemia, and neurologic involvement require somewhat higher dosages of prednisone—e.g., 60-80 mg. Local corticosteroids, as mentioned, are often effective for controlling low-grade uveitis and may be administered in the form of eye drops alone or reinforced by one subconjunctival injection.

Cutaneous lesions frequently respond to local corticosteroids alone. Intralesional injection of triamcinolone acetonide diluted with 1% procaine to a final concentration of 2-5 mg/m may be repeated at weekly intervals.

Chloroquine

Chloroquine or hydroxychloroquine is useful in the management of lupus pernio, pulmonary fibrosis, and chronic arthritis, starting with 200-250 mg twice daily for 6 months. Frequent eye examinations are mandatory (60).

Other Medications

Methotrexate, chlorambucil, and azathioprine have been used with satisfactory results in only a few cases. Oxyphenbutazone, colchicine, levamisole, allopurinol, and radiation have all been tried without consistent success (61-64).

X. Cause of Sarcoidosis

What causes sarcoidosis remains a mystery. Hypotheses abound; some are of only historical interest, and other merely speculative (65,66). Is it a clinical syndrome with many causes, or is it a disease produced by a lone perpetrator? There are many unanswered questions about sarcoidosis. In which organ does the disease originate? How does is disseminate? Considerations are that sarcoid spreads through either a hematogenous or a lymphatic route, or that it originates from either a hypersensitivity reaction or a vasculitis. It is probable that the initial alveolar injury that results in the formation of the immune and inflammatory reaction in sarcoidosis is caused by an inhaled antigen. The alveolitis may either resolve or remain dormant indefinitely, or it may become chronic, resulting in persistent granuloma formation and fibrosis. The exact antigen or antigens that cause the initiation of the alveolitis remain obscure, but the formation and perpetuation of the granuloma are carried out by activated T cells. The presence of hyperglobulinemia, altered suppressor T-cell function, loss of tolerance to self-antigens with the appearance of autoantibodies, uveitis, and the favorable response to immunosuppressive therapy suggest that an autoimmune mechanism plays an important role in the pathogenesis of sarcoidosis (67). The expression of the sarcoid granuloma may be influenced by hormonal or environmental stimuli. A genetic predisposition or genetic abnormality may play a role in the expression of the disease. Okabe and colleagues have shown chromosomal aneuploidy in the granuloma cells (68). It is conceivable that an environmental agent may stimulate the formation of the aneuploidy cell and the development of sarcoidosis. On the other hand, it is just as possible that chromosomal aneuploidy may be totally unrelated to granuloma formation.

During the past 15 years, conflicting reports concerning the association of HLA phenotypes and sarcoidosis have appeared. Moller et al. and Kueppers et al. found no relationship between the HLA-B7 phenotypes and sarcoidosis in a German population (69,70). Brewerton et al. reported that in sarcoidosis patients with arthritis, there was an increased incidence of B8 and the haplotype A1-B8 (71). Among black patients, there was no increase in the frequency of HLA in the A and B loci (72). Newill et al. demonstrated an association of the disease with HLA-AW30 and with a group of cell surface antigens that serologically cross-react with AW30 (73). According to Tachibana et al. there is an increase in HLA-DR-MT2 and HLA-B-W61 in Japanese sarcoidosis patients (74). Thunell et al., on the other hand, found a significant increase in HLA-B8 in patients with erythema nodosum and HLA-B27 in Swedish patients with advanced sarcoidosis (75).

The pathogenesis of sarcoidosis is still undefined, but with the facilities now at our disposal in the field of electron microscopy, virology, and immunology, we should be able to identify the etiologic agent in the not too distant future.

Acknowledgments

Supported in part by the Japan Society for Promotion of Science, Tokyo.

References

1. Sharma, O. P. (1984). *Sarcoidosis: Clinical Management*. Butterworth, London.

2. Scadding, J. G., and Mitchell, D. N. (1985). *Sarcoidosis.* Chapman and Hall, London.
3. Modlin, R. L., Hofman, F. M., Meyer, P. R., Sharma, O. P., and Rea, T. (1983). In Situ demonstration of T-lymphocyte subjects in granulomatous inflammation: Leprosy, rhinoscleroma and sarcoidosis. *Clin. Exp. Immunol.* **51**:430-438.
4. Semenzato, G. (1986). The immunology of sarcoidosis. *Semin. Respir. Med.* **8**:17-30.
5. Arnoux, A. G., and Reynolds, H. (1986). Granuloma formation and fibrosis. *Clin. Dermatol.* **4**:22-34.
6. Athos, L., Mohler, J. G., and Sharma, O. P. (1986). Exercise testing in physiologic assessment of sarcoidosis. *Ann. N.Y. Acad. Sci.* **465**:491-501.
7. Sharma, O. P., and Johnson, R. (1988). Airway obstruction in sarcoidosis: A study of 123 nonsmoker american black patients with sarcoidosis. *Chest* **94**:343-346.
8. Burman, M. S., and Mayer, L. (1936). Arthroscopic examination of the knee joint. Report of cases observed in the course of arthroscopic examination including instances of sarcoid and multiple polypoid fibromatosis. *Arch. Surg.* **32**:846-856.
9. Gendel, B. R., Young, J. M., and Greiner, D. J. (1952). Sarcoidosis: A review with 24 additional cases. *Am. J. Med.* **12**:161-175.
10. Myers, G. B., Gottlieb, A. M., Mattman, P. E., Eckley, G. M., and Chason, J. L. (1952). Joint and skeletal manifestations in sarcoidosis. *Am. J. Med.* **12**:161-169.
11. Sokoloff, L., and Bunim, J. J. (1959). Clinical and pathological studies of joint involvement in sarcoidosis. *N. Engl. J. Med.* **260**:841-845.
12. Spilberg, I., Siltzbach, L. E., and McEwen, C. (1969). The arthritis of sarcoidosis. *Arthritis Rheum.* **12**:126-130.
13. Grigor, R. R., and Hughes, G. R. (1976). Chronic sarcoid arthritis. *Br. Med. J.* **2**:1044-1046.
14. James, D. G., Neville, E., and Carstairs, I. S. (1976). Bone and joint sarcoidosis. *Semin. Arthritis Rheum.* **6**:53-81.
15. Arnold, W. J. (1985). The rheumatic manifestations of sarcoidosis. In *Textbook of Rheumatology,* 2d ed. Edited by Kelley, W. N., E. D. Harris, S. Ruddy, and C. B. Sledge. Saunders, Philadelphia, pp. 1488-1493.
16. Kaplan, H. (1963). Sarcoid arthritis: A review. *Arch. Intern. Med.* **112**:924-935.
17. Patterson, J. R., Israel, H., and Smukler, N. (1971). The musculoskeletal manifestations of sarcoidosis. In *Proceedings of the Fifth International Conferences on Sarcoidosis.* Edited by Levinsky, L., and F. Machoda. Charles University, Prague, pp. 590-595.
18. Sartoris, D., Resnick, D., and Resnick, C. (1985). Musculoskeletal manifestations of sarcoidosis. *Semin. Roentgenol.* **20**:376-386.

19. North, A. F., Fink, C. W., Gibson, W. M. et al. (1970). Sarcoid arthritis in children. *Am. J. Med.* **48**:449-455.
20. Lindsley, M. D., and Godfrey, W. A. (1985). Childhood sarcoidosis manifesting as juvenile rheumatoid arthritis. *Pediatrics* **76**:765-767.
21. Sequeira, W., and Stinar, D. (1986). Serum angiotensin converting enzyme levels in sarcoid arthritis. *Arch. Intern. Med.* **146**:125-127.
22. Agner, E., and Larsen, H. (1979). *Yersinia enterocolitica* infections and sarcoidosis: A report of 7 cases. *Scand. J. Resp. Dis.* **60**:230-234.
23. James, D. G. (1959). Ocular sarcoidosis. *Am. J. Med.* **26**:331-339.
24. Liggett, P. E. (1986). Ocular sarcoidosis. *Clin. Dermatol.* **4**:129-135.
25. Karma, A. (1979). Ophthalmic changes in sarcoidosis. *Acta Ophthalmol.* **57**:1-94. (Suppl. 14).
26. Kataria, Y., and Whitcomb, M. E. (1980). Splenomegaly in sarcoidosis. *Arch. Intern. Med.* **140**:35-39.
27. Gallagher, P., Harris, M., Turnbull, F. W. A., and Turner, L. (1984). Gastric sarcoidosis. *J. R. Soc. Med.* **77**:837-839.
28. Munker, M., and Sharma, O. P. (1987). Fatal gastrointestinal haemorrhage in sarcoidosis: A previously unreported occurrence. *Sarcoidosis* **4**:55-57.
29. Dines, D. E., DeRemee, R. A., and Green, R. A. (1971). Sarcoidosis associated with regional enteritis (Crohn's disease). *Minn. Med.* **54**:617-620.
30. Maher, L., Choi, H., and Dodds, W. J. (1981). Noncaseating granulomas of the pancreas. *Am. J. Gastroenterol.* **75**:222-228.
31. Friedman, H. Z., and Weinstein, R. A. (1983). Sarcoidosis of the pancreas. *Arch. Intern. Med.* **143**:2182-2183.
32. Tekeste, H., Latour, F., and Levitt, R. E. (1984). Portal hypertension complicating sarcoid liver disease. Report and review of the literature. *Am. J. Gastroenterol.* **79**:389-396.
33. Adams, J., Sharma, O. P., Gacad, M. A., and Singer, F. (1983). Metabolism of 25-hydroxyvitamin D3 by cultured pulmonary alveolar macrophages in sarcoidosis. *J. Clin. Invest.* **72**:1856-1860.
34. Lieberman, J. (1985). *Sarcoidosis.* Grune & Stratton, New York, pp. 145-159.
35. Sharma, O. P., and Pandya, K. (1988). Serum angiotensin converting enzyme: Role in diagnosis of sarcoidosis. *IM (Intern. Med. Specialist)* **9**:147-154.
36. James, D. G., and Williams, W. J. (1985). *Sarcoidosis and Other Granulomatous Disorders.* W. B. Saunders, Philadelphia, pp. 174-191.
37. Kataria, Y. P. (1985). Immunology of sarcoidosis. In *Sarcoidosis.* Edited by Lieberman, J. Grune & Stratton, New York, pp. 39-63.
38. Tierstein, A. (1985). The Kveim-Siltzbach test in sarcoidosis. In *Sarcoidosis.* Edited by Lieberman, J. Grune & Stratton, New York, pp. 103-116.

39. Hunninghake, G. W., and Crystal, R. G. (1981). Pulmonary sarcoidosis: A disorder mediated by excess of helper T-lymphocyte activity at sites of disease activity. *N. Engl. J. Med.* **305**:429-434.
40. Roth, C., Huchon, G., Arnoux, A., Stanislas-Lequern, G., Marsac, J. H., and Chretien, J. Bronchoalveolar cells in advanced pulmonary sarcoidosis. *Am. Rev. Respir. Dis.* **124**:9-12.
41. Tiestein, A. (1983). Fiberoptic bronchoscopy in the diagnosis of sarcoidosis. In *Sarcoidosis and other Granulomatous Disease of the Lung.* Edited by Fanburg, B. Marcel Dekker, Inc., New York, pp. 323-333.
42. James, D. G. (1983). Biopsy of tissues other than the lung in the diagnosis of sarcoidosis. In *Sarcoidosis and Other Granulomatous Diseases of the Lung.* Edited by Fanburg, B. Marcel Dekker, Inc., New York, pp. 335-345.
43. DeRemee, R. A. (1977). The present status of treatment of pulmonary sarcoidosis: A house divided. *Chest* **71**:388-394.
44. Turner-Warwick, M. (1988). Treatment of pulmonary sarcoidosis: State-of-the-art. In Sarcoidosis and Other Granulomatous Disorders. Edited by Grassi, G., G. Rizzato, and E. Pozzi. Excerpta Medica, Amsterdam, pp. 621-629.
45. Odlum, C. M., Muiris, X., and Fitzgerald. (1986). Evidence that steroids alter the natural history of previously untreated progressive pulmonary sarcoidosis. *Sarcoidosis* **3**:35-39.
46. Staton, G. W., Jr., Gilman, M. J., Pine, J. R., Fajman, W. A., and Check, I. J. (1986). Comparison of clinical parameters, bronchoalveolar lavage, gallium-67 lung uptake, and serum angiotensin converting enzyme in assessing the activity of sarcoidosis. *Sarcoidosis* **3**:10-18.
47. Angi, M. R., Cipriani, A., Chilosi, M., Ossi, E., and Semenzato, G. (1985). Asymptomatic ocular sarcoidosis. *Sarcoidosis* **2**:124-134.
48. Adams, J. S., Gacad, M. A., Anders, A., Endres, D. B., and Sharma, O. P. (1986). Biochemical indicators of disordered vitamin D and calcium homeostasis in sarcoidosis. *Sarcoidosis* **3**:1-6.
49. Sharma, O. P., and Alfaro, C. (1986). Hypercalciuria and renal stones in a sarcoidosis patient treated by extracorporeal shockwave lithotripsy. *Sarcoidosis* **3**:7-9.
50. Fleming, H. A. (1988). Death from sarcoid heart disease. United Kingdom series 1971-1986. 300 cases with 138 deaths. In *Sarcoidosis and Other Granulomatous Disorders.* Edited by Grassi, C., G. Rizzato, and E. Pozzi. Excerpta Medica, Amsterdam, pp. 19-33.
51. Sekiguchi, M. (1983). Long term prognosis of cardiac sarcoidosis patients with permanent pacemaker implantation. A Japanese study. In *Sarcoidosis and Other Granulomatous Disorders.* Edited by Chretien, J., and J. Marsac. Pergamon Press, London, pp. 650-661.

52. Sharma, O. P., and Anders, A. (1985). Neurosarcoidosis. *Sarcoidosis* **2**:96-106.
53. Oksanen, V. (1987). New cerebrospinal fluid, neurophysiological and neuroradiological examinations in the diagnosis and follow-up of neurosarcoidosis. *Sarcoidosis* **4**:105-110.
54. Maddrey, W. C., Johns, C. T., Boitnott, J. K., and Iber, F. L. (1970). Sarcoidosis and chronic heptatic disease. *Medicine (Baltimore)* **49**:75-87.
55. Hendrick, D. J., Blackwood, R. A., and Black, J. M. (1976). Chest pain in the presentation of sarcoidosis. *Br. J. Dis. Chest* **4**:75-87.
56. Veien, N. K. (1986). Cutaneous sarcoidosis: Prognosis and treatment. *Clin. Dermatol.* **4**:75-87.
57. Gibson, L. E., and Winkelmann, R. K. (1986). The diagnosis and differential diagnosis of cutaneous sarcoidosis. *Clin. Dermatol.* **4**:62-74.
58. Verdegem, T., and Sharma, O. P. (1987). Cutaneous ulcers in sarcoidosis. *Arch. Dermtol.* **123**:1531-1534.
59. Johns, C. C., Schonfeld, S. A., Scott, P. P., Zachary, J. B., and MacGregor, M. I. (1986). Longitudinal studies of chronic sarcoidosis with low dose maintenance corticosteroid therapy: Outcome and complications. *Tenth International Conference on Sarcoidosis and Other Granulomatous Disorders.* Edited by Johns, C. J. *Ann. New. Acad. Sci.* **465**:702-712.
60. Siltzbach, L. E., and Teirstein, A. S. (1964). Chloroquine therapy in 43 patients with intrathoracic and cutaneous sarcoidosis. *Acta Med. Scand.* (Suppl. 425) **176**:302-308.
61. Veien, N. K. (1977). Cutaneous sarcoidosis treated with methotrexate. *Br. J. Dermatol.* **97**:213-216.
62. Pacheco, Y., Marechal, C., Marechal, F., Biot, N., and Fayolle, M. D. (1985). Azathioprine: Treatment of chronic pulmonary sarcoidosis. *Sarcoidosis* **2**:107-113.
63. Kataria, Y. P. (1980). Chlorambucil in sarcoidosis. *Chest* **78**:36-43.
64. James, D. G., Carstairs, L. S., Trowell, J. S., and Sharma, O. P. (1967). Treatment of sarcoidosis. Report of a controlled therapeutic trial. *Lancet* **2**:526-529.
65. Van Gundy, K., and Sharma, O. P. (1987). Pathogenesis of sarcoidosis. *West. J. Med.* **147**:168-174.
66. Sharma, O. P., and Kadakia, D. (1986). Etiology of sarcoidosis. *Semin. Respir. Med.* **8**:95-102.
67. Wiesenhutter, C. W., and Sharma, O. P. (1979). Is sarcoidosis an autoimmune disease? Report of four cases and review of literature. *Semin. Arthritis Rheu.* **9**:124-144.

68. Okabe, T., Suzuki, A., and Ishikawa, H. (1986). Chromosomal aneu-ploidy in sarcoid granuloma cells. *Am. Rev. Respir. Dis.* **134**:300-304.
69. Moller, E., Hedgors, E., and Wiman, L. G. (1974). HLA genotypes and MLR in familial sarcoidosis. *Tissue Antigens* **4**:299-302.
70. Kueppers, F., Mueller-Eckhardt, G., and Heinrich, D. (1974). HLA antigens of patients with sarcoidosis. *Tissue Antigens* **4**:56-58.
71. Brewerton, D., Cockburn, G., and James, D. G. (1977). HLA antigens in sarcoidosis. *Clin. Exp. Immunol.* **27**:227-229.
72. Eisenberg, H., Terasaki, P., and Sharma, O. P. (1978). HLA associa-tion studies in black patients with sarcoidosis. *Tissue Antigens* **11**:484-486.
73. Newill, C. A., John, C. J., Cohen, H. B., Diamond, E. L., and Bias, W. B. (1981). Sarcoidosis: HLA and immunoglobulin marker in Balti-more blacks. In *Sarcoidosis and Other Granulomatous Disorders.* Per-gamon Press, Paris, pp. 253-256.
74. Tachibana, T., Shirakura, R., and Yamazaki, Y. (1985). HLA-DR antigens in sarcoidosis. *Sarcoidosis* **2**:83 (abstract).
75. Thunell, M., Sondell, K., and Stjernberg, N. (1985). HLA-antigen in pa-tients with sarcoidosis from northern Sweden. *Sarcoidosis* **2**:84.

AUTHOR INDEX

Numbers in parentheses are reference numbers and indicate that an author's work is referred to although his name is not cited in the text. Italic numbers give the page on which the complete reference is listed.

A

Abbott, T. M., 375(10), 377 (10), 384(10), 385(10), 386(10), *390*

Abbrecht, P. H., 67(90), *77*

Abdul-Kanm, F. W., 139(80), *143*

Abe, T., 185(129), *215*

Abell, M. R., 84(6), *113*, 146(23), 155(23), *176*, 231(23), 232(23), 236(23), *254*, 337(40), *348*, 357(32), 358(32), *369*

Abruzzo, J. L., 239(65), 245(65), *256*, 375(78), 376(78), 379(78), 387(78), *395*

Ackerman, G. A., 187(153), *217*

Acton, R. T., 375(8), 377(8), 384(8), 385(8), 386(8), *390*

Acute Leukemia Group B (1969), 375(16), 383(16), 384(16), 385(16), *391*

Ada, G. L., 184(102), *213*

Adalioglu, G., 415(1), 417(1), 418(1), *428*

Adams, E. M., 375(27), 382(27), 384(27), 385(27), 386(27), *391*

Adams, J., 450(33), *458*

Adams, J. S., 454(48), *459*

Adams, T. E., 67(97), *78*

Addison, I. E., 185(121), *214*

Adelberg, S., 7(47), 13(105), 14(47,113,114), *19, 23, 24*

Adelman, L. S., 305(9), *320*

Adelizzi, R. A., 6(38), *19*

Adelmann-Grill, B. C., 11(73), 16(126), *21, 25*, 125(53), 129(53), *141*, 291(80), 293(80), *300*

Adhikari, P. K., 280(16), 286(16), *296*

Adler, K. B., 10(71), 15(71,118), *21, 24*

Aerts, C., 123(44), 126(44), 128(44), 129(44), 131(64), 132(44), *140, 142*, 184(113), *214*

Aelion, J. A., 417(22), 418(22), 422(22), *430*

G

SUBJECT INDEX

A

Alanyl-tRNA synthetase, 315, 317, 318-320
Allergic angiitis (*see* Churg-Strauss disease)
Alpha-1-antiprotease, 9
  deficiency in rheumatoid lung disease, 246
Alveolar macrophage (*see* Macrophage)
Alveolar cell carcinoma, 92
  polymyositis, 93, 306-308
  systemic sclerosis, 89
Alveolar damage, 8-10
  lymphocyte alveolitis, 121
  mechanism, 118
  neutrophil alveolitis, 121
Alveolitis, 4, 6
Amyloidosis, 98
  cystic fibrosis, 408
Angiotensin converting enzyme, 450
Ankylosing spondylitis, 351-353
  apical pulmonary fibrosis, 352-353
  bronchiolitis obliterans organizing pneumonia, 170
  bullae, 106
  dead space, 67

[Ankylosing spondylitis]
  fungal infections, 106
  gas exchange, changes in, 67
  pathology, 168
  pleural disease, 38, 105
  pneumothorax, 106
  pulmonary assessment, 67-68
  radiographic findings, 105-106
  restrictive lung disease, 352
  treatment, 353
Antinuclear antibodies (*see* Auto-antibodies)
Arterial blood gas analysis (*see* Blood gas analysis)
Aspergillus, 191-192
Aspiration
  aspiration pneumonia, 93
  polymyositis, 306-308
  rheumatoid arthritis, 89
  systemic sclerosis, 166
Aspirin (*see* Salicylates)
Atelectasis, 100
  systemic lupus erythematosus, 100-104; 271-272
Autoantibodies
  antialanyl-tRNA synthetase, 315 317, 318-320
  anticytoplasmic antibodies, 314-320
  anti-DNA antibodies, 263-264